D0765475

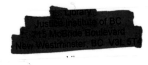

HUMANITARIAN CRISES

HUMANITARIAN CRISES

THE MEDICAL AND
PUBLIC HEALTH RESPONSE

EDITED BY

jennifer leaning

susan m. briggs

lincoln c. chen

HARVARD

UNIVERSITY

PRESS

cambridge, massachusetts

london, england

1999

Library of Congress Cataloging-in-Publication Data

Humanitarian crises : the medical and public health response / edited
by Jennifer Leaning, Susan M. Briggs, Lincoln C. Chen.

   p. cm.

  Includes bibliographical references and index.

  ISBN 0-674-15515-7 (alk. paper)

   1. Medical assistance—International cooperation.

2. International relief. 3. Humanitarian assistance. 4. Disaster
relief. 5. World health. I. Leaning, Jennifer. II. Briggs, Susan
M. III. Chen, Lincoln C.

RA394.H85   1999

362.1—dc21   98-41838

to all those who have been caught
in the wars of these times
and to the humanitarian workers
who have tried to
stem the tide

CONTENTS

CONTRIBUTORS

Jennifer Leaning, M.D., S.M.H.

Director, Human Security Program, Common Security Forum, Harvard Center for Population and Development Studies; Assistant Professor of Medicine, Harvard Medical School

Susan M. Briggs, M.D.

Attending Surgeon in General and Trauma Surgery, Massachusetts General Hospital; Assistant Professor of Surgery, Harvard Medical School

Lincoln C. Chen, M.D.

Senior Vice President for International Programs, Rockefeller Foundation

Ruth A. Barron, M.D.

Psychiatrist, Harvard Vanguard Medical Associates; Instructor, Harvard Medical School

Sissela Bok, Ph.D.

Senior Fellow, Harvard Center for Population and Development Studies

Brent T. Burkholder, M.D.

Chief, International Emergency and Refugee Health Program, U.S. Centers for Disease Control and Prevention

Frederick M. Burkle, Jr., M.D., M.P.H.

Professor of Pediatrics, Surgery and Public Health, John A. Burns School of Medicine, University of Hawaii

Thomas S. Durant, M.D.

Assistant General Director, Massachusetts General Hospital

Brian W. Flynn, Ed.D.

Director, Division of Program Development, Special Populations and Projects, Center for Mental Health Services, Substance Abuse and Mental Health Services Administration, U.S. Public Health Service

Col. Joel C. Gaydos
Director, Clinical Preventive Medicine, U.S. Army Center for Health Promotion and Preventive Medicine, Aberdeen Proving Ground

Judith B. Lee, R.N., B.S.
Manager, Logistics Response Directorate, Disaster Services, American Red Cross

Mark Leong, M.D.
Former Fellow in Disaster Medicine, Massachusetts General Hospital; attending physician in emergency medicine, Singapore

Marc Lindenberg, Ph.D.
Dean, Graduate School of Public Affairs, University of Washington; formerly Senior Vice President for Programs, CARE USA

Col. George A. Luz, M.S.
Program Manager, Environmental Noise, U.S. Army Center for Health Promotion and Preventive Medicine, Aberdeen Proving Ground

Richard F. Mollica, M.D., M.A.R.
Director, Harvard Program in Refugee Trauma

Aryeh Neier
President, Open Society Institute

Eric K. Noji, M.D., M.P.H.
Senior Medical Officer, Division of Emergency and Humanitarian Action, World Health Organization

Pierre Perrin, M.D.
Chief Medical Officer, International Committee of the Red Cross

Cdr. Trueman W. Sharp
Officer in Charge, U.S. Naval Medical Research Institute Detachment, Lima, Peru

Michael J. Toole, M.D.
Head, International Health Unit, Macfarlane Burnet Medical Research Center, Melbourne, Australia

FOREWORD by thomas s. durant

Over the many years that I have worked in humanitarian relief, I have come to realize that although each crisis has its own peculiarities, patterns have emerged. These patterns are not yet subject to scientific analysis, but are realistic and practical enough to count as valid insights gained from experience, and lessons learned. During the 1970s and 1980s, the crises to which we in the humanitarian community were prompted to respond were predominantly those of famine, flood, drought, and refugee migration. Building on what we had learned from each previous relief effort, we developed some competence in food distribution, water management, refugee education, and repatriation. We also observed and absorbed a simple powerful maxim from the people we were trying to help: anticipate, adapt, or die. This maxim is the fundamental premise that veterans in the relief community bring to current complex emergencies. The current crises, which include war in the mix of disaster and migration, are much more vast and complicated than prior events. Yet insights relating to human and technical needs, gleaned from the past, should still prove useful if they serve to anticipate new problems and to adapt previous methods for new approaches. We tend not to learn from one another across time, however, unless these insights are written down, subjected to analytic assessment, and then translated into professional education. In the field of humanitarian relief, that task is just beginning.

So instead of lessons learned we repeat mistakes. Three such repetitions are particularly painful to note in our attempts to respond to the crisis in Rwanda. First, it is well known that locating a refugee camp near a border conflict zone means that shelter can never be assumed to be permanent and that the camp can never be free of refugee-warriors. The experience of Site 2 at the Thai-Cambodia border is a case in point. For twelve years, from

1969 to 1981, the camp was continually targeted and attacked. Seven times in those years the refugees had to relocate completely, packing at a moment's notice and abandoning the site in order to avoid the fighting. We could have anticipated the security problems of the camps in the Goma region. Once they were upon us, it was much more difficult to find the international will and capacity to force an adaptation.

Second, there was a failure early in the crisis to provide potable water in these camps staked out on harsh volcanic rock. Provision of potable water is without question the paramount primary need in all humanitarian crises involving large populations torn from habitual living circumstances. Identifying water sources and planning distribution routes need to take place before 800,000 refugees surge into an area. No emergency in this century has driven that lesson home more definitively than the cholera epidemic that raged briefly through the Goma refugee camps in the summer of 1994. Although the Goma cholera experience is a failure in anticipation, the rapidity with which the epidemic was brought under control and abundant water supply mechanisms were introduced is a tribute to the power of adaptation.

Last, to maintain the quality of life in refugee camps is very difficult but it is crucial to do so. A key barometer is the effectiveness of food distribution. Making sure that food does not fall into the wrong hands, such as those of armed elements or profiteers, requires creative solutions. In Cambodia we found that the most reliable method was to distribute food to mothers and young girls no older than ten years (measured by those who came up to your elbow). Another feature is the early introduction of education, for young adults as well as for children and adolescents. A hunger for skills among the refugees in Site 2 allowed us to train many people to help us with our delivery capacities as well as prepare them for repatriation when the crisis abated. The Rwandan camps were much tougher environments, given the pervasive control of the armed Hutu extremists. Despite a general recognition of the needs for stable and equitable food distribution and productive group activities, the usual humanitarian interventions were often blocked or distorted by the tumultuous security situation. Adaptation was not possible, in part because our entire system for refugee support had been overwhelmed by numbers and organized violence.

Looking ahead, the structures and systems of international humanitarian relief need to be reorganized and strengthened. Given the refugee numbers that recent experience now forces us to anticipate, we must develop a rigorous commitment to the coordination of humanitarian aid. We must consider stockpiling extensive supplies in regionally deployed sites. We must develop consistent and sound policies relating to local labor force and economic factors, so as not to contribute to collapse in food prices, wage inflation, and trade in arms. We should select the best-trained personnel and maintain a master roster list for emergency call-up. These initiatives require at least a standing agreement among all major humanitarian relief organizations, and strong links with international agencies, with the overall goal of improving our capacities to anticipate and adapt. Steps toward greater efficiency, effectiveness, and community transparency either will come because we can collectively learn from our mistakes, or they will be forced upon us, at some point, by the people we are attempting to serve.

PREFACE

Over the course of the twentieth century, more than 150 million people have died as a result of war or genocide. The death toll from the two world wars exceeded 80 million, and nearly an equal number were exterminated during the century in genocidal campaigns. In the great wars, about as many soldiers died as civilians; the victims of genocide were all civilians. These terrible human losses have led some to label our time a "century of megadeaths."

In the closing decade of this century, a new type of conflict—called a "complex humanitarian emergency" or, more concisely, a "humanitarian crisis"—has emerged. These conflicts, as exemplified by Bosnia, Rwanda, Somalia, and Afghanistan, occur primarily within national boundaries, not between sovereign nations. While they are rife with the age-old phenomenon of war-induced death, they also bear witness to the changing nature of violence: ten civilians are killed for each combatant death, and the human suffering caused by these crises receives instantaneous public visibility because of the revolution in media and communications. These new humanitarian crises have developed in a global climate significantly different from that of the cold war: international humanitarian intervention is now politically more feasible and the international community is now much less tolerant of unnecessary deaths and violations of human rights.

For the health field, the changing nature of conflict presents unprecedented challenges and vexing dilemmas. Standards and practices for providing emergency public health and medical services have developed rapidly. The United Nations, the Red Cross, and nongovernmental organizations such as CARE, Médecins sans Frontières, and Oxfam are strengthening their organizational capacities for emergency relief.

At the height of a crisis, refugee death rates, predominantly among children, may soar, but effective relief programs can control mortality within weeks. Reality falls far short of optimal medical relief, however, because the barriers are more political, logistical, and organizational than they are technical. Confusion and uncertainty surround any crisis. But humanitarian responses to these emergencies are complicated by the internal divisiveness that spawned the violence in the first instance—usually "identity" politics based on religious or ethnic affiliation in contests for governance, territory, or resources. Complex emergencies are characterized by the breakdown of the fabric of society, the destruction of institutions and government, and often the selective targeting of civilians as a tactic of warfare.

In this fraught context, all aspects of health care, from ascertainment of need to delivery of services, must undergo marked revision and adaptation. As an example, epidemiology, the principal tool of public health, has been forced to incorporate significant changes in content and methodology in order to adapt to the conditions presented by humanitarian crises.

Epidemiology has proved to be invaluable for mapping populations at risk, for assigning priorities to health problems, and for guiding relief operations. In decades past, most disaster epidemiologic assessments have been made among refugees because they were at high risk, were geographically accessible, and were protected under international law. But in complex emergencies refugees are only the tip of an iceberg of human suffering: at least twice the number of refugees are typically either internally displaced or trapped at home. In this era of identity politics, epidemiologic assessment must also move beyond customary age and gender variables to incorporate social characteristics such as ethnicity, race, and religious affiliation. These social attributes can be predictors of health outcomes in complex emergencies many times more powerful than customary risk factors. Unlike historical studies of famine that rely on state record systems, however, epidemiologic appraisals conducted in real time during modern warfare are extremely demanding. Baseline data may be poor or absent, and time pressures are high. There are daunting logistical barriers and even threats to the safety of health workers. Successful health assessments must also be able to navigate through the "politics of information," wherein data intended for humanitarian purposes can also be used or abused for political reasons or can be sensationalized by the press and broadcast media.

Epidemiology is only one of many fronts on which complex humanitarian emergencies have challenged health professionals to modify their response to public health and to the medical needs of populations trapped in these circumstances. In addition, these recurring crises have unleashed such dehumanizing violence that a much more comprehensive health mandate must be developed. In emergencies that destroy the trust, the personal relations, and the social networks so essential for sustained human survival, the strategic approach to health must be to strengthen the coping capacity of local people and their families, communities, and institutions. Without commitment to this objective, the technical application of scientific medicine will be futile, if not impossible.

As an early step, health professionals who practice in the setting of humanitarian crises must develop an enhanced understanding of the ways in which these emergencies undermine the very structures that support human security. A realm of problems relating to psychosocial stress, sexual and reproductive health, violence and rape, and the violation of human rights is being increasingly recognized. Many, but not all, of these threats to human security are covered by international humanitarian law and human rights laws. These laws, even if not respected by combatants, nevertheless provide guidelines about legal entitlements and behavioral constraints that can operate as normative standards for planning and action.

A host of ethical quandaries highlighted by recent experiences also need to be addressed. How can health professionals, as was seen in Bosnia, work alongside military forces while maintaining the practice as well as the perception of medical neutrality among civilians and combatants? What should be the level of tolerance of "food leakages," rampant in Somalia, from intended beneficiaries to those who control access to the victims? What can be done when the witnessing and reporting of human rights abuses, as in Rwanda, are incompatible with—and can even jeopardize— the mission of those who need to maintain a presence in the field to continue serving the innocent? What should be the "health voice" when punitive economic sanctions, as in Haiti, affect not the perpetrators but the civilian populace?

The stress of working in these crises, and of interacting with many other actors and organizations in related fields, places heavy demands on health care professionals. Crisis management is characterized by high intensity and short time frames. Lower priority is usually accorded to reflection, to continuing education, and to career development. As we face the prospect of ongoing and new complex emergencies, however, the longer-term challenge to the health care profession is to improve performance and to promote dialogue and policy clarification on a range of ethical and legal dilemmas.

This volume of essays by engaged practitioners and academics signals an acceptance of that challenge and is intended to reflect and to help advance the discussion now active within the health community worldwide. The authors describe for the medical and public health practitioner the myriad health-related dimensions of these crises; they speak to what is known about the adaptations and modifications in medical relief imposed by these settings; and they explore the conceptual and practical complexities of medical humanitarian action in arenas shaped by conflict and human rights abuses.

lincoln c. chen

new york

march 1999

HUMANITARIAN CRISES

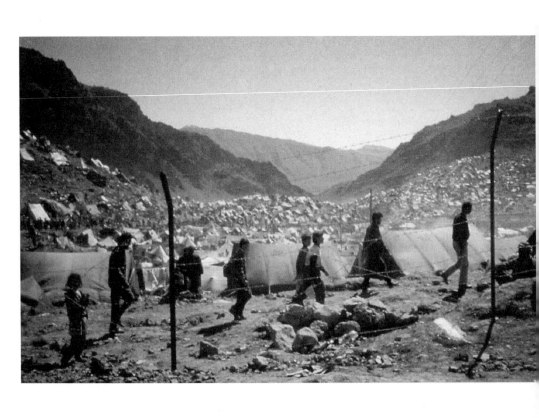

INTRODUCTION

---

jennifer leaning

The international relief community has seen its resources and coping strategies stretched to the limit by humanitarian crises, sometimes termed complex humanitarian emergencies, or CHEs. Recent events in Afghanistan, Somalia, Bosnia, Rwanda, Chechnya, and Congo/Zaire provide examples of such emergencies. Their origins are political, economic, and social, but they are in essence very bloody wars, waged within regions of collapsed or collapsing states.[1] They cause mass population dislocation and great human suffering, and they are associated with widespread human rights abuses.[2,3,4] In contrast with natural and technological disasters, the very situation that creates these emergencies also actively undermines attempts to provide an effective response.

This book is written for those in the public health and medical community worldwide who participate in creating policy and carrying out field operations with the aim of reducing morbidity and mortality in these emergencies. It seeks to present the current state of understanding regarding these actions as they are carried out within the larger framework of the overall humanitarian relief effort. The focus of the discussion thus precludes detailed treatment of several important topics relating to that larger framework: the evolving role of UN or other nongovernmental agencies, the warrant in international law for engaging in humanitarian action, the many roles of the media, the political and economic underpinnings of particular crises, or the geopolitical options for early warning, intervention, or prevention. Inevitably and appropriately, however, these subjects are addressed as they impinge upon the circumstances, constraints, and choices faced by those engaged in the medical and public health response.

Four main issues constitute the core topics here: key problems in assessment and intervention from a medical and public health standpoint; mental health consequences and intervention options, both for affected populations and for responders; ethical, legal, and practical dilemmas facing the medical humanitarian aid worker; and opportunities and pitfalls in the relationship between those providing medical and public health relief services and the military forces who are often deployed in these emergency settings. These issues are discussed within a common context defined by war conditions: rapid shifts in needs and access, huge numbers of people requiring help, high levels of personal insecurity, ambiguities in role definition and interagency coordination, and dilemmas or outright conflicts in values and mission.

THE HISTORICAL BACKGROUND

Civilian suffering in war has occurred throughout history. Only in the twentieth century, however, which has added more than its share to wartime's toll of death and destruction,[5] have efforts to mitigate that suffering achieved international prominence and recognition. And only in the last ten or fifteen years has the world community begun to organize efforts to aid civilians in war on a scale to match previous efforts to aid civilians in disaster.

These two transitions have deep roots. The Geneva Conventions, as the core documents of international humanitarian law (IHL), the body of law that relates to the protection of persons, had addressed the rules and principles defining the protection of combatants and prisoners of war but, with the important exception of common article 3, had not prior to 1949 detailed the obligations of warring parties toward civilian populations.[6] In the wake of the massive scale of atrocity and death inflicted upon civilians during World War II, the establishment of the Fourth Geneva Convention in

1949 explicitly provided that protection of civilians be added to the tenets of IHL. Further bitter experience in the anticolonial and revolutionary wars of the post–World War II period led to the strengthening of these protections and an expansion of the definition of war to include conflicts within nation states, provisions established in 1977 as the Two Protocols to the Geneva Conventions. The International Committee of the Red Cross (ICRC), since its founding in 1863, has been charged with monitoring compliance with IHL throughout the world.

A resurgence in regional conflicts and a proliferation of national and international responses, developments with a common origin in the end of the cold war, mark the second transition. For most of the post–World War II era, a concern for national sovereignty and the imposition of superpower interests helped to contain and organize relief efforts along governmental lines. Governments provided international relief for local natural disasters and reserved to the ICRC the mission of humanitarian aid in war. With the waning of the cold war, hostilities long held in check by superpower rivalries have rekindled, often along ethnic or communal lines and often disrupting structures of governmental control. Furthermore, erosion of cold war concerns has permitted access by nongovernmental agencies to more areas of the world and has also encouraged governments to rely on these groups to carry out more flexible and less politically charged relief efforts.[7] In effect a system of subcontracting has developed, whereby governmental grants to NGOs (nongovernmental organizations) have replaced much direct government control and funding of relief work.[8] This shift is particularly evident in medical and public health relief, in that volunteers or professionals under short-term contract with NGOs are increasingly asked to be responsible for providing the emergency response to major crises in population morbidity and mortality.

As a result, more medical and public health relief workers than ever before are working in extreme circumstances, exposed to random and organized violence while attempting to provide medical and public health assistance to huge numbers of stressed peoples in various stages of flight, exhaustion, and privation. Workers are far from their customary supports and often have relatively little training for the demands of the job. It is these people, and the agencies who hire and deploy them, for whom this book is intended.

DEFINITIONS AND DESCRIPTIONS

In 1994, of the thirty-two armed conflicts throughout the world, all were internal, waged over issues of territory, minority status, or power.[9] Depending upon the definition used, the number of these wars has ranged from twenty-five to forty in the years since the end of the cold war.[10] More than 100 million people have been directly involved, living in the arc of crisis that extends from sub-Saharan Africa to the Mideast through the Caucasus across to Central Asia and into South and Southeast Asia.[11] Waged by irregular armies using abundant stores of weapons acquired during the years these countries were considered proxy regimes of either the United States or the Soviet Union, these conflicts increasingly appear to rely on tactics that deliberately target civilians. A political animus infuses these emergencies. Although famine, flood, epidemics, or economic distress may accompany and accentuate the emergency, the defining feature is organized violence, carried on within the boundaries of failed states or collapsed regimes, creating widespread insecurity for local populations and external responders alike.[12,13] Humanitarian crises in the 1990s have included those in Afghanistan, Somalia, Sudan, Bosnia, Rwanda, Chechnya, and Congo/Zaire. The term applies as well to the civil wars and hostilities that ravaged Mozambique, Angola, and Cambodia during the 1970s and 1980s.

As the ebbing of superpower interest in these regions has made access more possible and external assistance more feasible, public and private organizations from around the world have attempted to intervene on behalf of humanitarian aims. From 1983 to 1992 the number of humanitarian aid agencies registered with the U.S. Agency for International Development (AID) grew from 144 to 418.[14] The number of development NGOs in the North registered with the Organization for Economic Cooperation and Development (OECD) grew from 1,600 in 1980 to 2,970 in 1993.[15]

Funding for these efforts comes from private and public sources. Pivotal to supporting this flood of international concern and financial aid are the electronic and print media, who rely on a communications technology that can make the most remote scene immediately and vividly visible to millions of viewers.[16,17,18] According to a UN report on complex emergencies,[19] as of 1996, the last year for which complete data are available, worldwide spending on humanitarian emergencies was estimated at $6.6 billion, having peaked at $7.2 billion in 1994. (This figure does not include costs associated with military support of humanitarian operations, amounting in the United States to $418 million for 1994.) The bulk of this support comes from the OECD countries, channeled through national government programs, UN aid agencies, or nongovernmental organizations. From 1990 to 1994, the amount of OECD aid going to emergency relief efforts in war zones doubled (to 10 percent of all combined development and relief aid), thus encroaching upon funds previously allocated to longer-term development needs.

Many different national and international players from numerous NGOs and agencies now participate in delivering emergency relief and aid to conflict areas. In addition to the relief and development agencies within the UN umbrella, such as UNICEF and UNHCR (the UN High Commissioner for Refugees), major actors in the humanitarian effort include the International Committee of the Red Cross; the umbrella organization for national Red Cross and Red Crescent societies, the International Federation of Red Cross and Red Crescent Societies (IFRC); Médecins sans Frontières (MSF), originating in France but now with many affiliates worldwide; and a number of other European and U.S.-based organizations, such as Save the Children, Oxfam, CARE, Catholic Relief Services, International Rescue Committee, and the American Refugee Committee. Thousands of NGOs are also springing up in countries directly affected by the crises, responding to local or regional needs and initiatives. From decades of work in disaster response, much is now known about the technical aspects of providing medical and public health relief to large populations.[20,21,22] There is also considerable agreement regarding the ethical norms that undergird medical and public health responses to disasters and humanitarian crises. Within the tradition of medical ethics are the principles found in the Hippocratic Oath *(primum non nocere)* and the guidance embedded in the concepts of virtue (tell the truth and lead a life of integrity), social contract (the physician must care for all members of society under all circumstances), and utilitarianism (the physician in emergency situations must strive to maximize the numbers who survive).[23,24]

Recent complex emergencies differ in key respects, however, from traditional disasters. Their scale and intensity are greater than have been seen in natural disasters, and the element of organized armed conflict aimed at segments of the population creates new dilemmas for outside humanitarian relief efforts.

KEY CHARACTERISTICS

Four key characteristics define these changes in scale and intensity: population dislocation; destruction of social networks and ecosystems; insecurity of civilians and noncombatants; and human rights abuses.

Massive population dislocation is present in virtually all CHEs. Forms of population dislocation include forced migration, refugee settlement, internal displacement, and local entrapment. In 1997 the number of world refugees was almost 14 million, and an additional 30 million were displaced within their own countries,[25] resulting in a total of 44 million—or nearly 1 in 100 people in the world—displaced from their homes. Such numbers have not been seen since the end of World War II, when in Europe alone approximately 50 million people had been forced into displaced or refugee status.[26]

CHEs ravage countryside and destroy communities, family networks, and ecosystems. Land is abandoned, crops are laid to waste, livestock starved or slaughtered, towns and infrastructure devastated. Entire villages have disappeared in Bosnia and Rwanda. In Sarajevo and Mogadishu, the cultural heritage of generations has been gutted. Land mines have been strewn throughout these ravaged areas, separating people from their land for the years it will take to clear the fields and roadways.[27,28] Studies of the environmental impact of humanitarian crises have thus far focused only on short-term effects in limited refugee settings.[29,30]

In humanitarian crises, where civil war or some other form of armed conflict is ongoing, the security of civilians and neutral noncombatants is in high jeopardy.[31] In many of these conflicts, the combatants are irregular forces, poorly trained and organized, fighting under unclear or unstable leadership and chains of command. There is either widespread ignorance or rampant disregard of the principles of international humanitarian law that protect access to civilians and define medically neutral safe zones. Civilians are frequently the preferred targets in conflicts based on communal antagonisms or along lines of identity politics,[32] which makes it particularly difficult to persuade the combatants to respect civilian human security rights as defined under the Geneva Conventions. In such situations all population groups are vulnerable, women and children perhaps more vulnerable than others, and external medical relief workers, if not also deliberately targeted, are at least unprotected by customary legal conventions.

Human rights abuses lie at the root of many humanitarian crises. In international law, definitions of atrocities and mass killings conform to commonsense understandings of these words. But recent experience with complex emergencies has forced to the surface two additional terms that have now become familiar to humanitarian workers: ethnic cleansing and genocide. Ethnic cleansing is the phrase used by the Bosnian Serbs to describe their policy of driving Muslim and Croat peoples from certain territories; the policy may involve all forms of intimidation, atrocity, and mass killings, but its intent, according to the Serbs, is not to annihilate a population but to move it into another area. This definition is designed to avoid the designation of genocide, which in international law means the deliberate policy of annihilating an entire population on the basis of identifiable characteristics of ethnicity or race.[33] For one country to apply the term genocide to describe the action of another country carries with it the formal obligation under international law, defined by the 1948 Convention on Genocide, to intervene to put a stop to that action. Reluctance to trigger that obligatory response caused the international community to delay labeling what was occurring in Rwanda as genocide[34] and contributed to an unwillingness to mount an official legal challenge to the Serb use of the term ethnic cleansing.

In the eastern Congo in 1997, a wave of killings of Rwandan Hutu refugees and the local Congolese Hutus alleged to be harboring them has been attributed to Congolese and Rwandan Tutsi forces, prompting calls for an international human rights investigation into possible mass killings or even genocide. Resistance by Laurent Kabila's government in Kinshasa, Zaire, frustrated attempts by the international community to obtain details of these killings and initiate steps to protect remaining refugees and targeted local populations.[35,36]

ASSESSMENT AND RESPONSE: KEY CHALLENGES

The central characteristics of humanitarian crises (mass population dislocation, destruction of community and infrastructure, pervasive insecurity, and gross human rights violations) have mandated substantial revisions in the ways in which the humanitarian community has approached its role of providing emergency aid. Traditional medical relief must be reframed to accommodate great numbers torn from basic life supports, often moving rapidly across different terrains, burdened by a mixture of serious primary health care needs, acute war injuries, and the physical effects of rape and torture. Emergency health workers and their agencies must acquire a developed understanding of the psychological effects of these abusive and bloody experiences. For their own safety and to support the people they serve, relief workers must also become aware of the stress they as workers are experiencing. To behave appropriately in a conflict situation, emergency health responders must understand the international legal and ethical expectations placed upon them and begin to understand the roles and mission of other local and international agents active in the field.[37]

These issues of assessment and response are addressed in detail in the chapters that follow. In terms of medical response, the public health crises for populations caught in complex emergencies are ones that require expertise in a population approach to issues of medical triage and austerity. As discussed in Chapter 1, by Michael Toole, and Chapter 2, by Eric Noji and Brent Burkholder, the emphasis must be on an early and accurate epidemiologic needs assessment, the provision of adequate water and sanitation, and the deployment of personnel who are expert in public health prevention strategies and the introduction of population-based primary care.[38] Building on civilian disaster experience, Susan Briggs and Mark Leong in Chapter 3 outline the classic principles of triage used in the care of those injured in war and civilian mass casualty incidents. In Chapter 4 Jennifer Leaning describes the issues facing humanitarian medical personnel who work in emergency field settings where the local hospitals and local personnel are overwhelmed by war wounded or where refugees arrive with untreated injuries and illness.

Civilian relief activities often must now take place in situations where the military forces of national governments, the UN, or NATO are also active. As described in Chapter 12, by Trueman Sharp, George Luz, and Joel Gaydos, and in Chapter 13, by Frederick Burkle, Jr., the military in recent years has assumed one of three distinct roles in humanitarian crises: providing logistical support (as in Bangladesh in 1991); enforcing the creation of humanitarian corridors (as in the initial phase in Somalia in 1993); or enforcing the terms of a negotiated political settlement (as in the former Yugoslavia in 1996). The practical and political difficulties of deploying the military in either relief or security roles in these crises are debated in these chapters. From the perspective of humanitarian workers, as analyzed in

Chapter 14 by Pierre Perrin, the security and protection provided by military forces is sufficient only to the extent that these forces are perceived by the local warring parties as nonpartisan. If the military is seen as taking sides, then humanitarian workers are also seen as suspect, and their neutral status is at risk. For these reasons, there is a wide difference of opinion among humanitarian aid agencies regarding the usefulness of military forces in complex emergencies.[39,40]

At the same time, it is evident to many in the humanitarian community that nation states and the UN have used the introduction of peacekeeping forces as a means of avoiding international responsibility for the active engagement of the military as an extension of political will. It is argued that a number of humanitarian crises persisted and escalated because effective outside military intervention did not occur (early intervention in Bosnia in 1992, early intervention in Rwanda in April 1994). Relief workers in the former Yugoslavia are particularly bitter about the role the UN played in helping to keep people fed on one day so that they could be shot by snipers the next.[41]

The ethical ambiguities involved in these political choices create role conflicts for humanitarian workers in the field. In Chapters 8 and 9, which approach this issue from different perspectives, Sissela Bok and Aryeh Neier and Jennifer Leaning note that humanitarian workers must be neutral (not party to the conflict, but bound by international law to report or denounce witnessed human rights abuses); must be impartial (distribute goods and services without discrimination); must maintain access and secure protection for their work (and thus not alienate either side). These imperatives do not all sum together neatly or consistently. As relief workers view their dilemma, they may be saving lives only to prolong the conflict; gaining access but eroding principled commitment to neutrality; securing protection but failing to remain impartial.[42]

The escalating technical and programmatic demands on the staff of humanitarian NGOs have not yet been met with sufficient institutional investment in capacity building at all levels both within and among organizations. As described in Chapter 10 by Marc Lindenberg, speaking from the perspective of CARE, and in Chapter 11 by Judith Lee, from her experience with the American Red Cross, entering a war or disaster zone to support a large population that continues to be at risk creates major problems of access, assessment, security, and coordination. The safety of relief personnel and the efficient delivery of goods and services become high and often conflicting priorities. In the rush to provide aid to vast numbers in an insecure political environment, relief agencies must take great care not to be forced into accommodations that lead to inadequate or incomplete outcomes.

The psychological effects of CHEs on victims has not begun to be fathomed.[43,44] We are finding, for both victims and responders exposed to these levels of stress, that resilience cannot be assumed. With regard to the victims, thousands are suffering the effects of rape or the wounds of survived atrocities and torture and thousands of children are orphaned or separated from their parents. The dislocated of all ages are required to endure great personal and community loss and bereavement. The enormity of scale, now involving hundreds of thousands of people at risk of suffering from severe psychological consequences, poses a huge challenge. In Chapter 5, on disaster mental health and CHEs, Brian Flynn reviews from the U.S. experience what is known about the mental health impact of disasters on affected populations, providing insights that may prove applicable in the context of populations forced to endure complex emergencies.

Practical intervention and research in this area is very limited. Chapter 6, in which Richard Mollica draws on several field experiences, describes the current understanding of the trauma story. He analyzes the major problems affecting those exposed to horror and loss, and reviews recommendations for assessment and treatment of individuals and small groups, emphasizing cultural context and coping strategies. The psychological stress on responders working in this context has also begun to make this issue a high priority among most humanitarian agencies. Techniques developed for supporting relief workers during more routine disasters[45] are now starting to be employed, but in this area as well, little has been written. In Chapter 7, Ruth Barron reviews what is known about disaster worker stress and makes recommendations to improve individual worker and overall agency performance in this area.

THE DISCUSSION AHEAD

Each of the subsequent chapters thus addresses a particular feature of the medical and public health approach to complex humanitarian emergencies, noting the ways in which assessment and response may continue to follow or must now depart from the approach taken in more traditional disasters. Where relevant and whenever possible, practical guidance is offered relating to mission definition, priority interventions, training in core competencies, and organizational readiness. A few cautionary guidelines are proposed, and a number of areas are identified where past experience provides an insufficient basis for action.

Improvements in approach and practice must take place in a context of wary respect for the issues that characterize these humanitarian crises: identity politics fueling irregular wars; humanitarian relief substituting for political action; medical and public health response in the midst of war and abuse of human rights. It is evident that the humanitarian agenda for these times must be at once more technical and more infused with moral awareness, more practical and more attentive to the influence of politics, more culturally competent and more constrained by a sense of limits. Medical and public health personnel who respond to these crises enter a domain of perilous complexity. Road maps do not exist, but the possibility of good outcome favors the prepared mind.

I

ASSESSMENT AND INTERVENTION

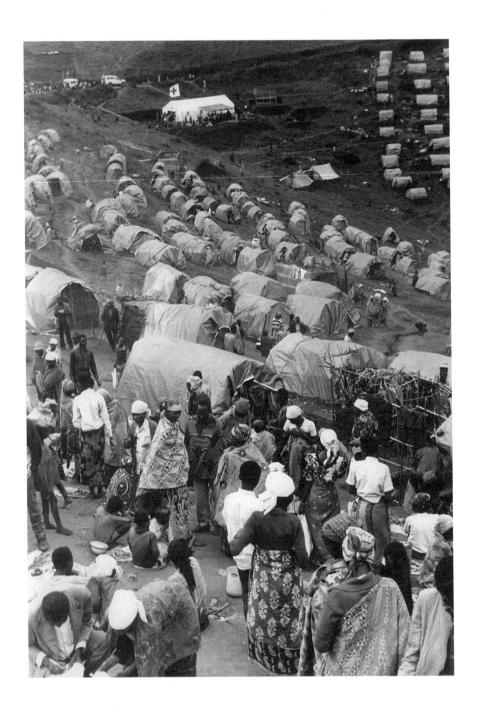

1

THE ROLE OF RAPID ASSESSMENT

michael j. toole

The immediate priorities of assistance programs in the setting of complex humanitarian emergencies are the protection of the affected populations and the reduction of mortality. To be effective, relief programs must be based on assessments conducted early in the emergency that identify the most critical public health threats to the population and the immediate priorities for action. Although the response to disasters is multisectoral, the common goal of reducing mortality requires that an epidemiological evaluation of the situation be a major component of needs assessments. This chapter discusses key components of rapid assessment and the use of this information in establishing priorities and evaluating the effectiveness of relief and assistance programs.

PUBLIC HEALTH CONSEQUENCES

The public health consequences of disasters may be characterized as direct or indirect. In the case of acute, natural disasters such as earthquakes and hurricanes, most of the consequences are direct in the form of deaths and injuries. In the case of complex humanitarian disasters related to armed conflict, the indirect public health impact may be even more significant than the direct impact.

Direct Consequences

The direct public health consequences of armed conflict include death, injury, disability, sexual assault, and psychological stress.

Casualties   Particularly high civilian death rates have been reported in wars in Angola, Ethiopia, Liberia, Mozambique, Somalia, southern Sudan, El Salvador, Guatemala, Afghanistan, Cambodia, Tajikistan, Bosnia and Herzegovina, Chechnya, and Rwanda. Since 1980, approximately 130 armed conflicts have occurred worldwide; 32 of these wars have each caused more than 1,000 battlefield deaths.[1] Most have occurred in Asia, Africa, and Latin America; since 1990, however, four European conflicts—in the former Yugoslavia, Azerbaijan, Georgia, and Chechnya—have caused at least 300,000 deaths. In April 1996, there were at least 22 unresolved armed conflicts in the world.[2] Armed conflicts have increasingly targeted civilian populations; during the first half of this century, approximately 50 percent of war casualties were civilian; this figure rose to approximately 80–90 percent in wars during the 1980s and 1990s.[3]

Land mines   Included in the direct impact of war on civilians has been the devastating effects of land mines. An estimated 100 million anti-personnel land mines have been laid by various armed factions in Afghanistan, Angola, Cambodia, El Salvador, Iraq, Mozambique, Somalia, western Sahara, and other war zones, resulting in a global epidemic of deaths, injuries, and disabilities. As an example of the impact of this problem, approximately 1 in 360 Cambodians is an amputee, largely due to land-mine injuries.

Sexual violence   Systematic sexual violence directed primarily against women has been documented in many modern wars, notably during the war of independence of Bangladesh, and more recently in Somalia, Uganda, Myanmar, and the former Yugoslavia, resulting in a high incidence of severe psychological trauma, unwanted pregnancies, and sexually transmitted diseases that may include HIV infection.

Indirect Consequences

The indirect public health consequences of war are mediated by mass migration, food shortages, hunger, and the destruction of health services, and have been especially severe in developing countries where basic services and food reserves are already inadequate.

Refugees   The global number of refugees fleeing war increased from approximately 5 million in 1980 to more than 20 million during 1994; in 1997, there remained approximately 14 million dependent refugees in the world.[4] In addition, there are an estimated 30 million internally displaced persons worldwide.[5] Death rates among refugees have been extremely high, ranging from 8 to 18 times the normal baseline death rates in Thailand (1979), Sudan (1985), and northern Iraq (1991).[6] In 1994, death rates among Rwandan refugees in Goma, Zaire, were 60 times the baseline rates.[7] Most deaths have occurred among children under five years of age; for example, 65 percent of deaths among Kurdish refugees on the Turkish border occurred in the 17 percent of the population less than five years of age.[8] The most common causes of death have been preventable conditions, such as measles, malnutrition, diarrheal diseases, pneumonia, and malaria, the same conditions that cause most deaths in nonrefugee populations in developing countries.[9] The triad of malnutrition, measles, and diarrhea has been a particularly lethal combination.

Internally displaced populations   The situation among internally displaced populations has generally been even worse, although accurate documentation of public health problems in these groups has been problematic. For example, since 1990, death rates among internally displaced persons in Angola, Liberia, Somalia, and Sudan have been 6–25 times baseline rates.[10] High death rates reflect the prolonged period of deprivation suffered prior to displacement, the often inadequate response by the international community, and problems of gaining access to war-affected communities.

Malnutrition   Acute protein-energy malnutrition, caused by either disrupted food production or inadequate access to food supplies, has been the condition most closely associated with high death rates in these settings. In 1992, widespread looting and banditry deprived millions of Somalis of much-needed food aid. Malnutrition rates were markedly elevated in certain areas of southern Somalia in early 1992, long before the international community launched its massive relief program. By November, death rates among displaced persons in the town of Baidoa had reached 25 times the baseline rates.[11] The intentional use of food deprivation as a weapon has become increasingly common. For example, armed factions on all sides have obstructed food aid deliveries in southern Sudan, resulting in mass hunger and—during 1993—death rates up to fifteen times those reported in nonfamine times.[12]

Although the direct death toll from the war in Bosnia and Herzegovina was high, the indirect public health impact has been less severe than in comparable settings in developing countries. While diarrheal disease and hepatitis incidence rates increased seven- to tenfold in Sarajevo, Tuzla, and Zenica between 1992 and 1994, these rates remained relatively low compared with those documented in African refugee camps.[13] Nevertheless, perinatal and infant mortality rates more than doubled in Bosnia during the first year of the war. Malnutrition rates among children remained low; however, the average adult in Bosnia lost about twelve kilograms during the first two years of the war.[13]

Disruption of health services   The physical destruction of health facilities, the burden of treating war wounded, and the high costs of maintaining military forces have caused disruption of basic health services in most war-affected countries—especially in Mozambique, Afghanistan, Angola, and Bosnia, where much of the destruction has been intentional. In the Bosnian province of Zenica, for example, the proportion of surgical cases related to war injuries rose from 22 percent to 78 percent between April and November 1992, resulting in the cessation of almost all preventive health services.[13] Disrupted prenatal services consequently led to increased rates of spontaneous abortions, premature deliveries, and low birthweight babies.[2]

PUBLIC HEALTH NEEDS ASSESSMENTS

Because countries of asylum are unable to provide relief on the necessary scale, refugees are often dependent on external assistance. Despite the recent increase in the number of European refugees, most of the world's refugees still seek asylum in developing countries, many of which are among the world's poorest; these include Malawi, Guinea, Zaire, Pakistan, Burundi, Ethiopia, and Tanzania. In addition, many internally displaced communities are perceived by their governments as sympathetic to rebel forces and may be intentionally deprived of access to internal relief, increasing the need for external aid. An external assessment is often indicated in order to (1) alert the international community to the severity of the situation; (2) accurately characterize the needs of the affected population; (3) ensure that the type of assistance provided is appropriate; and (4) enable aid to be targeted toward the most vulnerable groups in the population.

Rapid public health assessments evaluate the extent and magnitude of an emergency and alert the international community to its severity. The rapid needs assessment should provide a medium for advocacy to ensure that the response to an emergency is not just one that appears abundant and satisfies the domestic constituents and mass media of donor nations but one that addresses real problems in the affected communities (Box 1.1). Such assessments should be based on sound information collected in an accurate and standardized manner. In truly sudden population displacements, such as the Kurdish exodus from northern Iraq in 1991, the location and mapping of affected communities and the rapid estimation of population size and composition, mortality rates, and nutritional status are high priorities. Assessments critically examine the public health impact of an emergency as well as look at environmental conditions that might lead to future public health problems. On the basis of these findings, assessments review the availability of resources necessary to address key problems and, therefore, by default the need for external resources. Unfortunately, external resources are often sent ahead of the assessment and are sometimes in-

---

Box 1.1 Characteristics of a public health needs assessment for humanitarian crises

---

- Provides medium for response that addresses real problems in affected community
- Based on accurate, standardized data
- Locates and maps affected communities; estimates population size and composition, mortality rates, and nutritional status
- Examines current public health impact of the emergency
- Assesses environmental conditions that might lead to future public health problems
- Reviews availability of resources and need for external resources
- Serves as initial step in development of an ongoing health information system

appropriate. In addition, rapid needs assessments should be the initial step in the establishment of an ongoing health information system.

Needs assessments should ideally be performed by the agencies that will implement relief programs (Box 1.2). Relief agencies need to ensure that their staff members are adequately trained in the collection of accurate and representative information on displaced populations. Rapid assessments should be performed by an interdisciplinary team with skills in nutrition, epidemiology, water and sanitation, logistics, and social sciences. Members of the assessment team should include host country nationals; however, in many recent disasters the participation of government officials has not been appropriate because the government has been part of the cause of the emergency and is hostile to both the people who need assistance and those providing assistance. Local nongovernmental organizations, such as the Red Cross, churches, universities, and human rights groups, may be sources of assessment team members. Even in the most complex of emergencies there are usually local groups who can take part in an assessment. In Somalia, for example, where it was problematic to work with the various armed factions, the Somali Red Crescent continued to function. This group was able to take

---

Box 1.2 Who should perform the needs assessment?

Individuals and/or agencies participating in the preparation of public health needs assessments during a humanitarian crisis should have the following credentials and characteristics:

- Assessments should be performed by those agencies that will implement the relief programs.
- Staff must be adequately trained in collection of accurate and representative data.
- Teams should be interdisciplinary.
- Members of the assessment team should include host country nationals if possible.
- Local NGOs should participate, as appropriate.

an active role in public health assessments and provide the necessary cultural understanding, language skills, and continuity of contact with the affected communities.

One of the major constraints on performing timely public health assessments is the delay in the recognition of evolving humanitarian emergencies by the international community. In many cases, requests for assessment come at a time when significant increases have already occurred in mortality rates and malnutrition prevalence—late indicators of stress in a population. Therefore, it is critical that public health assessments be performed early in the evolution of a crisis in order to measure trends in leading public health indicators. For example, in Armenia, which has suffered the effects of a land blockade by its neighbors for several years, a system of surveillance was established in 1992 that focused on trends in market food prices, consumer purchasing power, household food reserves, birthweights, rates of weight loss in the elderly, communicable disease incidence, and other leading indicators, as well as late indicators such as childhood nutritional status and mortality rates.[14] In addition, a national population survey of food and heating reserves was conducted prior to the winter of 1993–94. The results of this survey enabled the Armenian government and international aid agencies to focus both on the populations most at risk and on the most acutely needed commodities.

Assessment Methods

Rapid epidemiologic assessments are essential to prioritize relief measures in remote, isolated settings where resources and logistics are severely limited. Much useful information on the affected population may be gathered in the capital city from government, United Nations, and nongovernmental organizations prior to commencing the field assessment. At least some team members should be fluent in the language of the affected population, and the majority should be fluent in the national language. If interpreters are used, special care should be taken to ensure that they have the necessary translation skills.

Initial Assessments

Initial assessments rely on observation, key informant interviews, record reviews, and limited community surveys. Systematic observation should follow a predetermined checklist of characteristics, such as population density and composition, family size, environmental conditions (for example, water supply, sanitation, shelter, drainage, and possible vector breeding sites), food availability, and morbidity (for example, malnutrition, dehydration, febrile illnesses, and injuries). Critical issues related to access, security, community organization, sexual violence, and human rights abuses must also be carefully evaluated.

Preexisting Conditions

Community leaders (formal and informal), health workers (traditional and modern), and religious leaders should be interviewed to assess the degree and nature of predisplacement deprivation; preexisting health problems, beliefs, and behaviors; predisplacement health service coverage (for example, vaccination coverage); and relevant cultural attitudes to health services. For example, in the assessment of the public health needs of Rwandan refugees in Zaire, the high measles immunization coverage in prewar Rwanda was useful information and allowed measles immunization to take second place to diarrheal disease control in prioritizing public health interventions. In contrast, the low immunization coverage in Somalia in 1992–93 indicated that mass measles immunization campaigns were a top priority during the nutritional emergency in that country.[11]

Prevailing Health Trends

Record reviews are an integral part of an assessment. Local health facilities may provide useful information on prevalent morbidity, death rates, and the availability of vaccines and other medical supplies. Frequently some form of medical care is being provided, by local health personnel or by international agencies such as the International Committee of the Red Cross or Médecins sans Frontières that have already gone into the area. In a rapid assessment, surveys are usually conducted on convenience samples that do not provide statistically precise estimates of the parameters being measured (for example, mortality rate, malnutrition prevalence). These samples can be chosen in a way that avoids obvious bias, but the results of such surveys provide only an impression of the magnitude of the problem and cannot be used as comparisons with later surveys that employ probability samples. In contrast, probability sampling techniques are based on statistical theory and provide results that are representative of the total population from which the samples are taken. Common types of probability sampling include simple random, systematic, and two-stage cluster sampling.

Survey Methods

Convenience sample surveys may provide approximate information on population composition (age and sex), family size, nutritional status (measuring mid-upper arm circumference), prevalence of diarrheal disease, and vaccination coverage. Maps indicating population density, water points, health facilities, roads, storage facilities, markets, vector breeding sites, and other relevant environmental features are useful assessment tools. After two to three weeks, when time and the appropriate expertise are available, population surveys of nutritional status (measuring weight and height), mortality, and access to relief supplies may be conducted on equal probability samples of the affected community. If adequate trained personnel and measuring equipment are available, a thirty-cluster sample survey of 600 to 900 households may be conducted in a well-defined camp population in two to three days.[7] Such a survey permits estimation of mortality and malnutrition rates without needing to know the exact size of the population.

Assessments are only useful if the findings affect program planning and implementation. Assessment missions need to have authority and credibility among relief agencies, and should be coordinated by a designated lead agency, such as UNHCR, UNICEF, ICRC, or the national disaster coordination body. Essential interventions (for example, provision of potable water, food rations, and vitamin A supplementation) should be established immediately and usually need not await the completion of the assessment. Assessments may provide an opportunity to establish a routine screening program for new arrivals in a camp setting, focusing in particular on identification of acute malnutrition and life-threatening illness in young children. The time needed to perform a rapid assessment will depend on the remoteness of the location, security, ease of access, and the degree of cooperation of local authorities. Rapid assessments may fail if appropriate arrangements for transport, travel permits, and communications are not carefully planned. In most situations, important baseline information may be gathered during a seven- to ten-day period. If a population survey is conducted employing probability sampling, a further three to five days may be required.

Rapid needs assessments should include the establishment of an ongoing public health surveillance system, focusing on mortality (crude, age-, sex-, and cause-specific), nutritional status, morbidity of public health importance, and diseases of epidemic potential. Data generated by public health surveillance should be used to evaluate the effectiveness of relief interventions and to plan or redirect future public health programs. Periodic population surveys may provide important complementary information on nutritional status, mortality, and relief program coverage (for example, immunization or supplementary feeding).

Specific Information

Demography   The initial assessment should include an estimation of the size and demographic composition of the affected population. This will provide essential information to calculate relief needs and to enable the calculation of various mortality and morbidity rates. While women and children commonly make up the majority of refugee populations, there is considerable variation from emergency to emergency. For example, the overwhelming majority of Sudanese refugees fleeing to western Ethiopia in 1988 were young boys. The assessment of the scope and demographic composition of a disaster-affected population can be very difficult. One of the technical aspects of assessments that is most imprecise is the estimation of population size. Aerial photographs, maps, sample surveys of household size and composition, and the use of advanced technology such as satellite photographs and the global positioning system may be necessary to determine the size of the population. Greater efforts are needed to ensure the cooperation of agencies with these resources at their disposal. Various methods of estimating population size using mapping exercises are described in the MSF manual on rapid assessment.[15]

Mortality (crude mortality rates)   Death rates are the most specific indicators of the health status of a population, meaning that a community with high death rates cannot be deemed healthy. By the time refugees and displaced persons arrive in the country or region of asylum, most have suffered extensive periods of deprivation and food scarcity. Documenting the death rate early in an emergency will establish a baseline against which later trends may be measured and the effectiveness of assistance programs may be evaluated. In the absence of mortality data, people will tend to evaluate the response in terms of the quantity of relief supplies provided rather than in terms of the impact on the affected population.

In a population of refugees or displaced persons, the crude mortality rate (CMR) may be measured by designating a burial area and employing guards to count burials and, if possible, to administer simple questionnaires on the age, sex, and probable cause of death. Other means of monitoring deaths might include the distribution of burial shrouds to the family of the deceased or the training of community surveillance volunteers. Such systems may not yet have been established at the time of the rapid assessment; therefore, the initial estimate of mortality may be based on counting existing graves, reviewing hospital or camp administration records, or simply interviewing community leaders. The assessment exercise should include the establishment of an improved mortality surveillance system.

In an emergency situation, the CMR is usually expressed as deaths per 10,000 population per day. During nonemergency times, the CMR in a developing country is commonly between 15 and 24 per 1,000 per year, which is equivalent to approximately 0.4 to 0.6 per 10,000 per day. A CMR of more than 1.0 per 10,000 per day is considered elevated, and a rate of more than 2.0 per 10,000 per day is considered critical.[16] Table 1.1 presents crude mortality rates documented in various refugee and displaced populations.[10] The normal trend in mortality among refugee populations is one of gradual improvement, as demonstrated by the evolution of death rates among Kurdish refugees on the Turkish border (Figure 1.1).[8] Nevertheless, this has not always been the case. The death rate among Somali refugees in Ethiopia, for example, steadily increased during the first twelve months after their arrival in 1988 (Figure 1.2).[17] This increase was associated with an increase in acute malnutrition among young children caused by inadequate food rations. Such analyses would not be possible if prompt efforts had not been made to determine baseline death rates. On the Turkey-Iraq border in 1991, for example, an MSF assessment team counted the graves that already existed when the team arrived and divided this number by the number of days since the arrival of the refugees (seven) in order to estimate the average daily number of deaths in the camp. This was divided by the camp population (estimated by mapping and conducting a sample household survey) to calculate the CMR.

Age-specific mortality rates   In emergency situations, age-specific data are usually confined to under five years and over five years of age. In developing countries, under-five mortality rates are normally higher than death rates in older age groups, and this trend has also been observed in emer-

Table 1.1 Estimated average crude mortality rates (deaths per 10,000 per day) in selected refugee and internally displaced populations, 1990–1996

Date	Country of asylum	Country of origin	Crude mortality rate (deaths per 10,000 per day)
Jan.–Dec. 1990	Liberia	Internally displaced	2.4
June 1991	Ethiopia	Somalia	6.7
March–May 1991	Turkey	Iraq	4.2
March–May 1991	Iran	Iraq	2.0
March 1992	Kenya	Somalia	7.4
March 1992	Nepal	Bhutan	3.0
April–Nov. 1992	Somalia (Baidoa)	Internally displaced	16.9
June 1992	Malawi	Mozambique	1.2
April 1992–March 1993	Sudan (Ayod)	Internally displaced	7.7
April 1993	Bosnia (Sarajevo)	Siege situation	1.0
December 1993	Rwanda	Burundi	3.0
July 1994	Zaire	Rwanda	19.7–31.3
May 1995	Angola (Cafunfo)	Internally displaced	8.3
February 1996	Liberia (Bong)	Internally displaced	5.5

Source: M. J. Toole and R. J. Waldman, "The public health aspects of complex emergencies and refugee situations," *Annual Review of Public Health* 1996; 18.

gency situations. Some reports have noted, however, that the relative increase in mortality due to emergency conditions has been less pronounced among children under five years than among older children and adults.[18] Nevertheless, a practical breakdown of age groups for the purpose of assessing mortality continues to be over five and under five years. As the emergency subsides, mortality surveillance data should be disaggregated into the following age groups: less than one year, 1–4 years, 5–14 years, 15–45 years, and over 45 years. Efforts should be made to classify deaths according to the gender of the deceased, because female-specific death rates have been higher than male death rates in some situations.[16]

Reliability of data The most reliable estimates of mortality rates have come from well-defined and secure refugee camps where there is a reason-

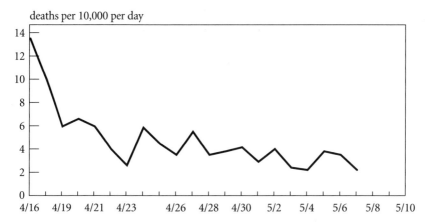

deaths per 10,000 per day

Figure 1.1   Crude mortality rate, Cukurca camp, Turkey-Iraq border, April 16 to May 10, 1991. (MSF, France)

able level of camp organization and a designated agency has had responsibility for the collection of data. The most difficult situations have been those where internally displaced persons have been scattered over a wide area and where surveys could take place only in relatively secure zones. These safe zones may have sometimes acted as magnets for the most severely affected elements of a population; for example, the Somali town of Baidoa was the site for the storage and distribution of massive amounts of relief food in 1992 and became known as the "famine epicenter."[11] It is also possible, however, that the worst-affected communities have been in areas that have been inaccessible to those performing the surveys. In either case, it has proved difficult to extrapolate the findings of surveys on mortality conducted in specific locations to broader populations in conflict-affected countries.

Extensive differences in mortality survey methods have been identified; for example, an evaluation of twenty-three field surveys performed in Somalia between 1991 and 1993 found wide variation in the target populations, sampling strategies, units of measurement, methods of rate calculation, and statistical analysis.[19] Population surveys of mortality should report the proportion of the sampled household members at the beginning of the recall period who died during that period. The average daily mortality rate should then be calculated for the recall period and expressed as deaths per 10,000 per day. Recall periods should be chosen that represent

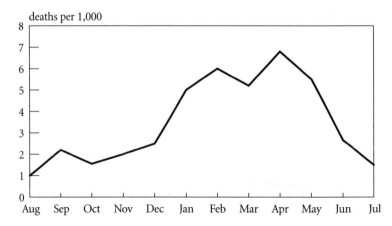

deaths per 1,000

Figure 1.2 Crude mortality rate, Somali refugees, Hartisheik A camp, Ethiopia, 1988–89. (Save the Children Fund; UNHCR; Ethiopian Ministry of Health)

the period of time during which the population has been exposed to emergency conditions. If the period is too long, however, the surveyed families may have difficulty remembering all the deaths that have occurred in the household during that time. If the period is too short, the sample size may need to be too large for a survey to be feasible. If the results are to be compared with mortality rates estimated at an earlier or later time or in other populations, then confidence intervals should be estimated using a formula consistent with the survey sampling method employed. The computer software EpiInfo Version 6 will calculate confidence intervals for surveys using simple random and cluster sampling techniques.

Cause-specific mortality   The most common causes of death in complex emergencies in developing countries have been confined to a small number of conditions: diarrheal diseases, measles, acute respiratory infections, malnutrition, and malaria (Figure 1.3).[16] Surveys should attempt to ascertain the cause of death through the use of standard definitions in questionnaires. Doing so will enable a later evaluation of the effectiveness of disease-specific interventions. These disease definitions need to be based on symptom complexes or terms in the local language that will be readily recognized and understood by the survey population. Precise terms exist in most languages for measles and dysentery; however, definitions of conditions such as watery diarrhea, malaria, pneumonia, and meningitis may require careful development and field testing to ensure their accuracy.

MICHAEL J. TOOLE

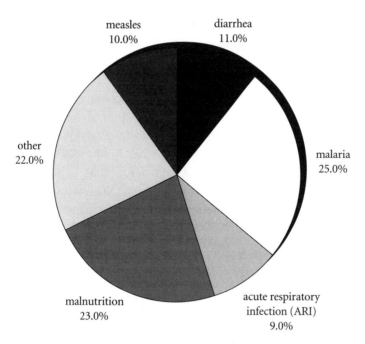

measles
10.0%

diarrhea
11.0%

other
22.0%

malaria
25.0%

malnutrition
23.0%

acute respiratory
infection (ARI)
9.0%

Figure 1.3 Major reported causes of death in children under five years of age for refugee hosting areas in nine districts of Malawi, July 1990. (UNHCR, MSF, IRC)

One objective of a rapid assessment is to ascertain which condition is most likely to be a major problem in a given situation in order to determine the focus of initial relief efforts. If a measles epidemic is highly likely, then efforts should focus on a mass measles immunization campaign; if the incidence of diarrheal diseases is high, then the provision of clean water, sanitation, and oral rehydration therapy will be the top priorities. If acute malnutrition is highly prevalent among young children, then the provision of adequate food rations, supplementary feeding, and therapeutic feeding will be top priorities. Making decisions on priorities is important. Relief agencies may be quickly overwhelmed by the demands of programs such as supplementary feeding which, if not based on a real need, may be implemented at the expense of adequately addressing a more severe threat such as a dysentery outbreak.

The following situations illustrate differing emergency public health priorities. In northern Iraq, the major problem among the 450,000 Kurds displaced on or near the Turkish border in March 1991 was acute diarrheal disease (including cholera) associated with the lack of clean water and sanitation facilities.[8] In Somalia during late 1992, when food supplies were improving, vaccinating children against measles and providing appropriate treatment for diarrhea and dehydration were the most critical public health priorities. At that time, up to 75 percent of deaths were caused by measles and diarrhea.[11] Among Cambodian refugees who passed through endemic areas on their way to camps in eastern Thailand in late 1979, malaria was the overwhelming cause of death.[20] Among refugees in Rwanda, Tanzania, Burundi, and Zaire, bacillary dysentery has been the most important health problem.[7,21] Among Rwandan refugees in Goma in August 1994, approximately 90 percent of deaths were due to one complex of diseases, cholera and dysentery (Figure 1.4). Among Somali refugees in Kenya in 1991, a severe epidemic of illness caused by hepatitis E infection led to many deaths, especially among pregnant women.[22]

Morbidity Through interviews with health workers, reviews of clinic records, and direct observation, rapid assessments should seek to identify those health problems that are most likely to cause high death rates. In particular, the relative importance of measles, bacillary dysentery, cholera and other diarrheal diseases, meningitis., and malaria should be established. It may be necessary to confirm the diagnosis of these conditions with appropriate laboratory tests; therefore, assessment teams need to be adequately prepared to transport the relevant samples of blood, stool, or cerebrospinal fluid to the nearest laboratory. When accurate information on the incidence of these diseases is not available at the time of a rapid assessment, a system of surveillance should be established if any of these diseases is likely to occur in the area. Population surveys tend not to be the most accurate method of collecting morbidity data; immunization coverage data may be helpful, however, especially if vaccination record cards have been distributed.

Nutritional status The level of malnutrition in a population affected by an emergency is often the subject of considerable debate. The issue affects important decisions about the quantity and quality of food rations and the need for supplementary and therapeutic feeding programs. The critical nutritional indicator in an emergency is usually the prevalence of acute malnutrition (low weight for height) among children less than five years of age. Prevalence rates of acute malnutrition among children less than five years of age in various refugee populations have been as high as 50 percent

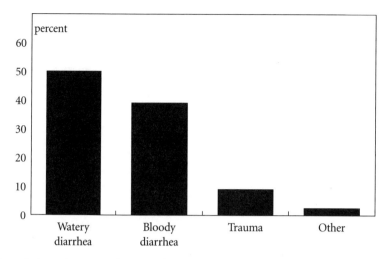

percent

Figure 1.4 Major reported causes of death, Rwandan refugees, all ages, Mugunga camp, Zaire, July–August 1994. (CDC/UNHCR survey)

among Ethiopian refugees in eastern Sudan (1985), 45 percent among Sudanese refugees arriving in Ethiopia during 1990, 29 percent among Somali refugees in Kenya in 1991, and 48 percent among Mozambicans in Zimbabwe (1992).[16] In Somalia and southern Sudan, acute malnutrition rates among displaced persons were as high as 80 percent between 1991 and 1993 (Table 1.2).[10,11,12] In addition to acute protein-energy malnutrition, outbreaks of relatively rare micronutrient deficiency diseases have occurred in certain African refugee populations. Several scurvy epidemics have occurred in refugee populations in Ethiopia, Somalia, and Sudan. One of the largest outbreaks of pellagra since World War II occurred among Mozambican refugees in Malawi in 1990, and an outbreak of beriberi was reported among Bhutanese refugees in Nepal during 1993.[23,24]

Rapid assessments should include an evaluation of acute protein-energy malnutrition among children between six months and five years of age either by measuring the mid-upper arm circumference (MUAC) or weight-for-height.[25] When weight and height are measured, acute malnutrition prevalence is defined as the proportion of children measured with a weight-for-height index less than 80 percent of the reference median or a Z-score of less than -2 (moderately malnourished) and less than 70 percent of the median or a Z-score less than -3 (severely malnourished). (The Z-score

Table 1.2 Prevalence of acute malnutrition among children under five years of age in internally displaced and conflict-affected populations, 1988–1996

Year	Country (region)	Population affected	Prevalence of acute malnutrition (in percent)
1988	Sudan (South Darfur)	80,000	36.0
1992	Southern Somalia	3,000,000	47–75
1993	Sudan (Ame)	47,000	81.0
1994	Sudan (Bahr el Ghazal)[a]	345,000	36.1
1994	Ethiopia (Gode)[a]	35,000	35.6
1994	Afghanistan (Sarashahi)[b]	163,000	18.6
1995	Angola (Cafunfo)[c]	10,000	29.2
1995	Liberia (Goba town, Margibi)[b]	N.A.	11.7
1995	Sierra Leone (Bo)[c]	250,000	19.8
1995	Sudan (Labone)[c]	38,000	22.6
1996	Zaire (Masisi)[b]	100,000	31.0

Note: Acute malnutrition defined either as weight-for-height 2 standard deviations below the reference mean or less than 80 percent of the reference median.
   a. Survey conducted by Médecins sans Frontières (Belgium).
   b. Survey conducted by Médecins sans Frontières (Holland).
   c. Survey conducted by Action Internationale contre la Faim.

equals the number of standard deviations above or below the mean of the WHO/NCHS/CDC reference population.) Children with edema should be classified as severely malnourished. The cutoff point for MUAC used to define acute malnutrition is still controversial and somewhat age-dependent. Field studies indicate that a MUAC between 12.0 and 12.5 centimeters correlates with a weight-for-height Z-score of -2; the lower figure (12.0 centimeters) is more appropriate in children less than two years of age.[25] It is important, however, to perform this evaluation on a representative sample of children. If a mass screening of all children in the population is feasible, this will provide the most reliable estimate of malnutrition prevalence. A thirty-cluster random sample survey of children in this age group should be conducted if the necessary time and expertise are available. Normally an acute malnutrition prevalence of greater than 8 percent is considered severe; greater than 10 percent is critical.[16]

The assessment of the importance of micronutrient deficiency diseases in the early phase of an emergency may be limited to an evaluation of the micronutrient content of available foods. Surveys of clinical deficiency diseases require specialized skills that may not be available. There may be information available locally, however, on how common certain deficiency diseases are. In most developing countries, it is safe to assume that foods available for refugees and displaced persons will probably not contain adequate vitamin A; therefore, routine supplementation with four- to six-monthly capsules is usually indicated for children between one and five years of age.

Vulnerable groups An important element of a rapid assessment is the identification of vulnerable groups, which might include particular ethnic or religious minorities, unaccompanied children, and households headed by women. For example, in the Rwandan refugee population that fled to eastern Zaire in 1994, more than 12,000 unaccompanied children were identified and required specialized care. In the same population, households headed by women were found to have less access to relief items, such as food and shelter material, than households headed by men.[7] Among the Iraqi refugees on the Turkish border in 1991, there were a number of Christians and deserted Iraqi soldiers. Both groups had difficulty gaining access to the relief distribution system and required special efforts to ensure that their needs were met. In other settings, the elderly have been at high risk and have warranted special attention.

Impact of disrupted health services In areas affected by conflict, health facilities are often damaged or destroyed and routine health services disrupted. The first services to be affected are usually routine preventive services, such as child immunization and prenatal care programs. Assessments should seek to identify those services most severely disrupted and those that require urgent rehabilitation. Assessments in Bosnia have attempted to evaluate the impact of the war on health services; for example, in Sarajevo, disruption of reproductive health services led to increases in the rate of pregnancy termination, perinatal death rate, low birthweight rate, and the frequency of congenital abnormalities.[2] Childhood vaccination rates decreased from 90–95 percent before the war to less than 40 percent in 1994.[13]

Existing relief measures No assessment is complete without making sure that the basic elements of a relief program are in place. The key factors that should be assessed early include the adequacy of shelter and access by the affected population to sufficient quantities of clean water, food rations, and sanitation facilities. These parameters should be quantified as much as possible and compared with the standard requirements established by the international community. UNHCR recommends that refugees and displaced persons should have access to at least 15 liters of clean water per person per day (Box 1.3).[26] Food rations should contain an average of 2,100 kilocalories of energy per person per day as well as the basic requirements of protein and essential micronutrients.[27] Sanitation is difficult to establish early in the emergency; however, assessments should evaluate the potential risk of fecal contamination of drinking water supplies, and temporary measures such as designated defecation fields should be established. An early goal for a sanitation program would be the provision of one latrine per twenty persons. Adequate shelter is a priority in all populations but particularly so in cold climates, such as Bosnia, Chechnya, and Georgia. In these settings, inadequate protection from the cold will also increase caloric requirements.

Measles immunization is a major priority in any emergency where the affected population is housed in crowded camps, especially if the measles immunization coverage rate in the population is low. Assessments should include an evaluation of the risk of a measles outbreak and the availability of vaccines, immunization equipment, cold chain facilities, and trained

---

Box 1.3 Standard requirements for basic relief provisions (UNHCR)

Refugees and displaced persons should have access to:

- At least 15 liters of clean water per person per day
- An average of 2,100 kilocalories of energy per person per day (as well as the basic requirements of protein and essential micronutrients)
- One latrine per 20 persons
- Adequate shelter, particularly in cold climates

personnel. If the risk of an outbreak is high, steps should be taken immediately to organize an immunization program aimed initially at young children, who are most at risk of dying from measles.

If diarrheal diseases are determined to be a major problem, the capacity to provide adequate rehydration should be assessed. If cholera is endemic in the area, a surveillance system should be established immediately and a laboratory identified that has the capacity to culture cholera organisms and to test sensitivity to antibiotics. The initial assessment should examine the availability of essential supplies for the management of a cholera outbreak and the readiness of local health personnel. In recent years, epidemic dysentery caused by *Shigella dysenteriae*, type 1, has caused many deaths among refugees and displaced persons in central and southern Africa.[21] Surveillance for this disease should be established early and a laboratory identified to confirm the diagnosis of initial cases. The availability of appropriate antibiotics for the treatment of dysentery should be assessed as an early priority.

If malaria is an endemic problem in the area, information should be gathered on the sensitivity of the parasite to commonly used drugs and the availability of appropriate drugs. Identification and treatment of infected individuals is the first priority in an emergency. The assessment should also examine whether local conditions promote the transmission of malaria and whether environmental interventions such as drainage might decrease transmission. Control of the local vectors through the use of insecticides is expensive and should await a more thorough entomological assessment.

In the so-called meningitis belt of Africa, comprising most of west, central, and east Africa, assessments should determine the risk of a meningitis outbreak in the emergency-affected population. The risk may be increased in crowded camp settings, especially during the dry season. In these situations, the adequacy of meningitis surveillance, availability of a laboratory for confirmation of the diagnosis, preparedness of health personnel, and availability of meningococcal vaccines should all be determined.

The overall organization and coordination of health services should be assessed as well. In emergencies, there is often a tendency to focus on the creation of hospitals and outpatient clinics. In the early phase of the Goma crisis in 1994, for example, there was an understandable emphasis on inpatient and outpatient treatment of patients with cholera and dysentery. Surveys showed, however, that only 50 percent of those who died during the first month of the emergency had managed to seek treatment at fixed health facilities.[7] An outreach program might have enabled sick patients to receive prompt treatment and, where necessary, assisted in the transfer of patients to hospitals. Similarly, some agencies on the Turkish border concentrated on treating diarrhea patients with intravenous therapy in hospitals while neglecting to establish community-based outreach and oral rehydration programs in the camps. The rapid assessment should evaluate the appropriateness of the medical program structure, its capacity to adequately reach the entire population, and the level of participation in the program by the affected communities. A program of community health worker recruitment and training should be an early component of an emergency relief program.

CRITICAL ISSUES

Linking Assessments to Program Planning

Recent observations from refugee populations in Uganda, Tanzania, and Zaire that increases in mortality were higher among older children and adults than among children under five years reinforce the notion that each emergency is different and each requires a thorough needs assessment at the outset, followed by a system of ongoing surveillance.[18] The epidemiology of refugee emergencies has developed as a specialized field. The challenge remains, however, to ensure that this information forms the basis of program planning and resource allocation and that relief programs are managed and coordinated efficiently. Assessments need to be linked to program decision making; otherwise they may be useless exercises ending up as historical records rather than program management tools. The initial assessment should identify early relief priorities, and ongoing surveillance should guide later program decisions. Changing patterns of mortality and morbidity should signal shifts in program priorities as each emergency situation evolves.

Integrating Assessments

Health assessments should not be done in isolation from food, water, or other sectoral assessments. There should ideally be a single, integrated assessment whose goal is to identify the key threats to the well-being of affected communities and the most critical priorities for action to protect those communities and to reduce mortality. There is a critical need for better coordination of information gathering and improved sharing and dissemination of data. There are often multiple, poorly coordinated assessments of an emergency situation; NGOs, military forces, and other organizations should be willing to cooperate with designated lead relief agencies to ensure the most efficient use of information. The relief program for Rwandan refugees in eastern Zaire, in 1994, demonstrated a high level of standardized information collection, dissemination, and use in program management.[7]

Balancing Priorities

During recent emergencies, it has been difficult to balance the need for sound methodology (including representative sampling and reliable survey instruments) with the need for timely information and—more than ever—the protection of personnel. Somalia, southern Sudan, Bosnia-Herzegovina, and Angola have been dramatic examples of this precarious balance. In Somalia, attempts were made to evaluate mortality rates and nutritional status in displaced populations with reasonable scientific precision by conducting population surveys using probability sampling techniques.[11,19] Surveys were curtailed midstream by security incidents, and several epidemiologists had close encounters with armed bandits. Statisticians were faced with difficult decisions on the validity of findings by field staff. The representativeness of survey findings under such conditions is increasingly in doubt.

Establishing Effective Communications

In addition, the findings of field surveys are often poorly understood and need to be explained carefully to program managers, policymakers, and the media. Despite efforts to explain the limitations of the surveys and the difficulties in extrapolating results to large populations, survey results are sometimes misquoted in the media. In assessing the validity of findings, it is useful to compare trends revealed in population surveys with those detected from surveillance data. In southern Sudan, nutrition and mortality assessments have been intrinsically biased because they took place in areas where food distribution acted as a magnet for the displaced and the most severely affected segments of the population. Given the insecurity in areas such as southern Sudan, it is impossible to collect data that are representative of the whole population.

Reconciling Internal and External Priorities

Priorities are inevitably based on the values and judgments of outsiders; however, the affected community's priorities may be quite different from those identified by the relief team. For example, in 1985, some Ethiopian community leaders expressed concern with the focus of Western relief workers on saving the lives of severely malnourished infants rather than putting their efforts into treating the health problems of economically productive adults in the famine-affected population. The use of epidemiologic studies has contributed significantly to a better understanding of the impact of disasters on populations, to more informed decisions on relief priorities, and, one hopes, to the more efficient use of resources and evaluation of relief activities (Box 1.4). The resulting selectivity of services, however, may lead to a sense that relief aid is being imposed by outsiders, reducing the autonomy of a community. Disaster needs assessments must therefore include genuine and objective efforts to listen to the voices and opinions of the affected communities. Although such an approach is encouraged in current assessment guidelines, in the actual chaotic conditions of a disaster it is frequently neglected, and assessments may tend to overemphasize

---

Box 1.4 Key questions for evaluating the effectiveness of relief agency activities

- Are relief agencies meeting regularly?
- Are they collecting and sharing standard health information?
- Have there been efforts to standardize essential drugs, treatment protocols, and vaccination schedules?
- Has the local Ministry of Health been involved in decision making related to public health issues?
- Is there an effective channel of communication to and from the field personnel?

MICHAEL J. TOOLE

quantifiable or measurable parameters. Political realities in the field, conditions imposed by donors on funding, and decisions made on the basis of epidemiological or sociological studies may all lead to situations where assistance programs benefit only certain targeted groups in the population and exclude other needy groups.

CONCLUSION

Health and nutrition data carefully collected in evolving emergency situations allow the public health community to play a crucial role of advocacy in bringing to the attention of key decision makers the plight of the ever growing numbers of civilians affected by war, population displacement, and hunger. Greater attention needs to be given to training relief workers in rapid assessment methods and to developing improved methods of epidemiological evaluation techniques. Nevertheless, more accurate and timely assessments will have limited impact on populations affected by emergencies unless the international community develops a commitment to respond more consistently to the needs identified by those assessments.

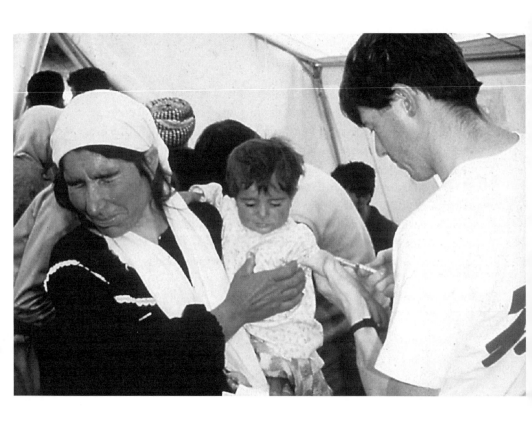

2

PUBLIC HEALTH INTERVENTIONS

eric k. noji

brent t. burkholder

In humanitarian crises, where warring forces tend to target civilians intentionally, civilian populations trapped in areas of conflict have increasingly suffered severe public health consequences, even if they have not been displaced from their homes.[1] For example, death rates increased almost fourfold from 1991 to 1993 during the war in Sarajevo, owing to a combination of direct violence, food shortages, the destruction of public utilities and health facilities, and severe disruption of preventive health services.[2] In other settings, damage to water, sanitation, and health facilities as well as to housing and agriculture may lead to a rapid increase in malnutrition and communicable diseases such as measles, infectious diarrhea, and pneumonia.[3] Remi Russbach, former chief medical officer of the International Committee of the Red Cross, put it aptly: "Today's armed conflicts are essentially wars on public health."[4]

Epidemiologic studies and direct experience in the field have identified the major causes of mortality and morbidity during the acute phase of complex humanitarian emergencies involving refugees or internally displaced populations (see Chapter 1).[5] Much is now known about the provision of health and medical care for refugees and other victim populations and the technical means of delivering such care. It is well understood that adequate food, clean water, shelter, and sanitation will prevent the most serious outbreaks of illness and epidemics.[6] Further, several useful treatment guidelines, standardized drug lists, and essential drugs kits have been developed (Box 2.1).

Discussed here are the major public health issues that arise from large populations massed in conditions of emergency settlement, whether in refugee camps or in urban areas caught in siege or conflict, and the critical public health interventions now understood to have a substantial impact during the first several months of a crisis.

EMERGENCY SETTLEMENTS

General Issues

Refugee camps tend to be crowded and are often located in isolated areas, while internally displaced persons from the countryside often migrate into larger cities where they may blend into the local population or form their own urban tent settlements or shantytowns.[7] If the refugees have had to walk long distances, many will be ill or suffering from malnutrition even before arrival at a camp. For example, both the Hmong tribespeople of Laos in 1976 and Cambodians fleeing the Khmer Rouge in 1979 passed through areas hyperendemic for malaria en route to asylum in Thailand. As a result, the death rate in the Sakaeo camp in eastern Thailand in October 1979 was more than ten times the rate for the surrounding Thai population. Most deaths resulted from malaria or malnutrition.[1,8,9,10]

The poor health of many refugees on arrival, crowded and unsanitary emergency settlement conditions, and difficulty in providing even minimum water, shelter, and food to the displaced population result in elevated mortality rates.[11] Somalia has provided a graphic example of this situation. As a result of civil war in the early 1990s, the country's economy, social and political institutions, and infrastructure were destroyed. Superimposed on the warfare and chaos was a severe and prolonged drought, which began when the rainy season failed in early 1991. Crops planted by the few remaining farmers were devastated; the combination of drought and social disintegration resulted in catastrophic famine. There were massive population migrations of up to 900,000 people out of war-torn rural and urban areas to refugee camps in Kenya, Ethiopia, Djibouti, and Yemen.[12] Many of

Box 2.1 Selected manuals and handbooks on public health assessment and intervention

- Centers for Disease Control and Prevention, "Famine-affected, refugee and displaced populations: recommendations for public health issues," *Morbidity and Mortality Weekly Report* 1992; 41(no. RR-13): 1–76.
- J. C. Desenclos, ed., *Clinical Guidelines: Diagnostic and Treatment Manual,* 2nd ed. (Paris: Médecins sans Frontières, 1992).
- EpiInfo Version 6.0 computer software
- C. Mears and S. Chowdhury, eds., Health Care for Refugees and Displaced People (Oxford: Oxfam, 1994).
- Médecins sans Frontières, *Refugee Health: An Approach to Emergency Situations* (Paris: Médecins sans Frontières, 1997).
- P. Perrin, *Handbook on War and Public Health* (Geneva: International Committee of the Red Cross, 1996).
- R. H. Sandler and T. C. Jones, eds., *Medical Care of Refugees* (New York: Oxford University Press, 1987).
- The Sphere Project, *Humanitarian Charter and Minimum Standards in Disaster Response* (Geneva: Sphere Project, 1998). Web site: www.ifcr.org/pubs/sphere.
- University of Wisconsin Disaster Management Center–UNHCR *Emergency Tools Kit* (Madison: University of Wisconsin Disaster Management Center, 1992).
- World Health Organization (WHO), *The New Emergency Health Kit* (Geneva: WHO, 1990).
- World Health Organization (WHO), *Guidelines for Cholera Control* (Geneva: WHO, 1992).
- World Health Organization (WHO), *Treatment and Prevention of Acute Diarrhea: Practical Guidelines,* 2nd ed. (Geneva: WHO, 1989).
- World Health Organization (WHO), "Clinical management of acute respiratory infections in children," *Bulletin of the World Health Organization* 1981; 59: 707–716.

the refugees traveled on foot over hundreds of kilometers seeking safety and food; many reportedly died of hunger.[13] In early 1992, large numbers of Somali refugees arrived at two camps (Ifo and Leboi) on the Kenya/Somalia border. The high crude death or mortality rates (CDR or CMR) reported among these newly arrived refugees, peaking in February 1992, were due to two major causes:

1. the fatigue and malnutrition of those just arriving (the highest mortality was observed among those who had been on foot);
2. inadequate supplies of potable water (there were only two boreholes in the camps at the time, to service the town's permanent residents and more than 50,000 refugees).

As a result, a significant percentage of the refugee population developed life-threatening dehydration, diarrhea, and dysentery. Eventually boreholes were dug by relief organizations, per capita water supplies increased, and death rates came down dramatically—an excellent illustration of the effectiveness of simple sanitary measures. In another situation in 1984–85, refugees from the Ethiopian province of Tigray walked up to thirty days to reach refugee camps located in eastern Sudan, with insufficient food to sustain them on the long journey. Upon their arrival in Sudan, malnutrition prevalence rates of up to 30 percent were recorded in the camps.[14]

The risk of death is usually highest during the period immediately after refugees arrive in the country of asylum. This was shown in 1992, when more than 150,000 Mozambicans fled to refugee camps in neighboring Zimbabwe and Malawi. During July and August 1992, the crude death rate among Mozambican refugees who had been in Chambuta camp for less than one month was four times the death rate of refugees who had been in the camp between one and three months, and sixteen times the death rate normally reported for nondisplaced populations in Mozambique.[15]

High mortality may occur during emergency migrations even when the affected populations do not exhibit chronic health or nutritional deprivation prior to their exodus. When approximately 500,000 Kurds fled from Iraq toward Turkey in 1991, the majority were stranded in several remote mountain passes between the two countries. The passes ranged from 1,500 to 2,500 meters (5,000 to 8,000 feet) in altitude, and temperatures at night were below freezing. Water sources were limited to melted snow, and food, shelter, and latrines were not available.[16] Despite rapid emergency intervention, in the initial phase of the crisis the Kurds experienced high rates of morbidity and mortality similar to the African cases just described.[17] In contrast to the refugee populations already debilitated from the effects of war, famine, and disease before reaching camp, the Kurds from northern Iraq were a stable population with evidence of prior good health and nutritional conditions.[18,19] In retrospect, the sequence of events leading to the rapid spread of diarrheal disease among the Kurds and resultant high levels of mortality apparently was triggered by the extremely poor conditions in the remote mountain passes during the initial phase of the crisis: low temperature, limited food and shelter, severe overcrowding, poor sanitation, and contaminated water supplies.[20]

Major priorities for refugee well-being soon after arrival in an emergency settlement are food, water, and shelter, in addition to protection from war- or conflict-related trauma.[7,21,22] Because crowded, unsanitary camps may lead to elevated death rates, relief organizations should avoid creating settlements with more than 10,000 people;[23] in practice, however, emergency settlements may swell to far more than 100,000 people and, as already noted, tend to be located in isolated areas that relief organizations have difficulty reaching.[7,24] Even after relief groups are able to gain access to displaced populations, it still may take several weeks for plastic sheeting, latrines, and other construction materials to arrive. In the meantime, refugees make do as best they can, sleeping out in the open air or constructing makeshift tents from whatever materials they can find around them.[11] Until relief agencies can organize borehole or well digging or begin to provide chlorinated water, refugees must often walk great distances for both water and food supplies.

Refugee Camp Settings

Once refugees reach the relative safe haven of camps in neighboring countries, the adverse effects of displacement continue. During the acute phase of emergency relief operations for Ethiopian refugees in Somalia in 1980 and for Ethiopian refugees in Sudan in 1985, death rates were between eighteen and forty-five times greater than the death rates found in the surrounding nonrefugee populations. During the 1992–93 famine in Somalia, mortality rates for displaced persons living in temporary camps were more than twice as high as rates for nondisplaced persons.[25,26]

Children are at exceptionally high risk for increased mortality. For example, death rates among children less than five years of age in Sudanese camps were almost eight times higher than death rates among persons fifteen years of age and older,[1] and in Somalia, mortality rates for these children were two to four times greater than for older persons living in the same communities.[26]

HEALTH ISSUES IN REFUGEE CAMPS

Water-Borne Diseases

Both the site of refugee camps and the local climate have a profound effect on refugees' health. The terrain may be mountainous, swampy, or semi-arid, and very different from the refugees' countries of origin. Refugees are often settled on land not desired by the local population, in harsh border-lands, on urban outskirts, or on virgin land. Firewood may be—or may quickly become—scarce. Supplies of water, particularly ground water, may prove insufficient, especially in the dry season. There may be flooding during the wet season. The slope of the site is important for drainage and water supply. Nearby pools of stagnant water can become breeding grounds for vectors of disease, and other types of terrain may harbor disease-carrying rodents. The spread of the main communicable diseases causing morbidity and mortality in refugee settings—measles, malaria, cholera, dysentery, and respiratory infections—is encouraged by poor environmental conditions: water contaminated by excreta, problems of waste disposal, and close living quarters. The bigger the camps, the more pronounced these effects become.

Epidemics of diarrhea and dysentery have caused high rates of morbidity and mortality in several refugee and displaced populations—for example, among Kurdish refugees in 1991,[20] displaced Somalis in 1992,[26] and Burundian refugees in Rwanda in 1993.[27] In April 1994, the resumption of a long-standing conflict between the Hutus and Tutsis—the two major ethnic groups in Rwanda—resulted in civil war and mass genocide. In early July 1994, as armed strife subsided, an estimated one million Rwandan Hutus fled to Zaire, where they concentrated in several large refugee settlements. The crude mortality rates ranged from 19.5 to 31.2 deaths per 10,000 per day—among the highest recorded in history.[28] Between 6 percent and 10 percent of the refugee population died during the month after arrival in Zaire, a death rate two to three times the highest previously reported rates among refugees in Thailand (1979), Somalia (1980), and Sudan (1985).[6] This high mortality was due almost entirely to the epidemic of diarrheal diseases. The epidemic of cholera among refugees in Goma, Zaire, was remarkable for the rapidity of its spread through the population, the peak being reached just one week after the first case was diagnosed.[28] Cholera cases also occurred elsewhere; for instance, camps in Tanzania experienced an outbreak in December 1994, with a second smaller peak in February 1995. The outbreak was confined to Benaco and Mushura Hill camps, which, at that stage, had a combined population of around 290,000. In all, 1,800 people were infected, of whom 90 died. A comparison of the situations and the responses to the cholera epidemics in the Goma camps with those in the Tanzania camps is useful. Whereas in Goma, 100 percent of the refugees were infected with cholera within two to three weeks, in Benaco and Mushura Hill camps approximately 6 percent of the population was infected with cholera in the space of four months.

Crucial to the successful response to the outbreak in Tanzania was the protection of water sources from contamination, although other factors included:

- good contingency plans for dealing with an outbreak, with each camp having its own dedicated cholera center;
- well-developed programs to mobilize the community, with many community health workers and community awareness groups who promoted early case-finding and referral to the centers;
- a well-motivated population conscious of what had happened five months earlier in Goma;
- good coordination between curative and public health services and among UNHCR, UNICEF, and the NGOs involved.

These measures prevented the explosive epidemic profile that occurred in Goma and enabled the well-developed curative and community services in the Tanzanian camps to operate without becoming overrun.

Given the endemic nature of cholera in the Lake Kivu region, it was virtually inevitable that a cholera epidemic would strike a large population concentration with virtually nonexistent sanitation facilities for proper excreta disposal (as was the case early on in Goma) and utilizing open water sources. Even if the start of the outbreak could not have been delayed, greater preparedness for the movement of refugees into this area could well have slowed the spread of the outbreak (for example, prepositioning more pumping and storage equipment, water tankers, and heavy equipment such as bulldozers) and could have allowed more time for the establishment of oral rehydration treatment centers and their more effective operation. By the third week of the Rwandan refugee influx into camps in eastern Zaire, the international community's response began to have a significant impact. Routine refugee relief measures such as measles immunization, vitamin A supplementation, standard disease treatment protocols, and community outreach programs were established in each camp, and the water distribution system was geared up to provide an average of five to ten liters per person per day. A consensus was quickly reached on standard information to collect (information that was shared among multiple agencies and organizations), and a high level of cooperation and coordination of public health programs was achieved. The relief program in the Goma camps, now based on rapidly acquired health data and effective interventions, was associated with a steep decline in death rates to 5–8 per 10,000 per day by the second month of the crisis.[28]

In summary, long-term solutions for the problem of diarrheal disease control in emergency settlements require time and resources, but the excess mortality associated with diarrheal disease outbreaks may be prevented, or at least mitigated, by prompt implementation of several effective measures that depend more on human than on technological resources. These measures include the organization of chlorination brigades at untreated water sources, the designation of physically isolated defecation fields, community outreach to identify and treat patients outside of clinics, and oral rehydration therapy. In addition, greater emphasis needs to be placed on education about personal hygiene and the provision of soap.

Measles

The spread of measles via respiratory secretions can be a major life-threatening problem among unimmunized people (particularly children) living in crowded camp environments. For example, the measles epidemic in Somalia during the 1992–93 humanitarian crisis was probably greatly exacerbated by the fact that the displaced populations were living in densely settled camps.[29] The need to vaccinate children against measles is one of the most critical public health priorities in refugee settings.[5,26]

Food Shortages and Malnutrition

Nutrition-related diseases in camps are common because refugees are almost entirely dependent on food aid, which is often of insufficient quality or quantity.[30,31] It is mainly in camps that micronutrient deficiencies such as beriberi, pellagra, and scurvy are still widespread.[6,32,33,34]

As Harrell-Bond[35] and a 1985 *Lancet* editorial[36] have pointed out, camp conditions affect physical, mental, and social well-being.[37] The manner in which camps are administered encourages passivity, and the lack of autonomy engenders hopelessness.[38] Camp life is commonly cited as the cause of breakdowns in traditional social networks and coping mechanisms. The camp environment may increase the incidence of domestic violence; it also diminishes refugees' capacity for self-provisioning, affecting nutrition and increasing susceptibility to illness. As an example of the latter situation, restrictions on movement by the local authorities may make it difficult for refugees to gather wild foods—a long-standing survival strategy when communities face food shortages. Restrictions also prevent access to markets where food can be purchased that may provide essential nutritional supplements. Locally consumed resources such as wood for cooking fires become increasingly scarce, and refugee families must search further and further afield from their camps (if allowed to leave the camp for such foraging activities by the authorities).

Local Market Economies

As time goes on, camp residents may begin to develop their own market economies; these may complicate the purchase, distribution, and availability of both food and medical supplies and health services. For example, "market forces" in the camps influence which foods get traded—bulk grains away from the camps; vegetables into the camps. Drug supplies are also freely traded, promoting greater self-medication, drug resistance, and a variety of infections such as skin abscesses from self-injection using dirty needles.

Settlement Options

All of the adverse health consequences of camp life suggest avoiding the establishment of camps wherever possible in favor of dispersed self-settlement. Furthermore, since camps are often in remote locations (or areas of high security risk), humanitarian assistance frequently requires substantial transport investments and the hiring of armed guards for staff protection, resulting in higher per capita costs. Neither refugees (including internally displaced persons) nor the agencies assisting them, however, usually have much control over the locations or environment in which they are obliged to settle.

One successful health program for 700,000 refugees in Somalia achieved sustained improvement in health status by emphasizing preventive interventions, standardizing treatment protocols, implementing an essential drugs policy, and training more than 3,000 refugees as community health workers.[39] Although death rates had been high during the emergency phase of this program (1979–80), the formation of a specialized refugee health unit within the Somali Ministry of Health toward the end of 1980 promoted a unified approach to health care in the camps by the twenty or more foreign, voluntary agencies operating in the country. Priorities were established on the basis of regularly collected data on nutrition, mortality, and morbidity. The hallmark of this program's success was that good health parameters were sustained in the refugee population long after most expatriate relief workers had withdrawn. The program operated successfully until 1988, when it was seriously disrupted by a civil war in the north of Somalia.

In summary, the provision of adequate clean water and sanitation, timely measles immunization, simple treatment of dehydration from diarrhea, supplementary feeding for the malnourished, micronutrient supplements, and the establishment of an adequate public health surveillance system will greatly reduce the health risks associated with the harsh environments of refugee camps (Box 2.2).

URBAN SETTINGS

Increasing numbers of people displaced by war or civil conflict live in a state of urban or dispersed emergency settlement or are crowded into what have

Box 2.2 Elements of the priority response of a coordinated health program for emergency settlements

- Protection from natural and human hazards
- Establishment of census/registration systems
- Provision of adequate quantities of reasonably clean water
- Provision of acceptable foods with recommended nutrient and caloric composition (where it is difficult to ensure that vulnerable groups have access to rations or where high rates of malnutrition exist, supplementary feeding programs should be established)
- Access to adequate shelter
- Well-functioning and culturally appropriate sanitation and hygiene systems (latrines and buckets, chlorine and soap)
- Family tracing (essential for mental health)
- Information and coordination with other vital sectors such as food, transportation, communication, and housing
- Monitoring and evaluation, prompt problem solving
- Provision of medical/health services:
  (a) Public health surveillance (including nutritional surveillance/screening as a part of an emergency health information system)
  (b) Information on the health services that are available
  (c) Measles immunization (later all EPI vaccines)
  (d) Vitamin A provision
  (e) Selective feeding (supplementary and therapeutic) when there are problems with malnutrition
  (f) Basic curative care especially for acute respiratory infections, diarrheas, and malaria
  (g) Referral, supervision, and supply systems
  (h) Training and retraining of health workers from the emergency settlement community to provide basic health care and preventive services
  (i) Promotion of health education activities including education about AIDS and sexually transmitted diseases
  (j) Prenatal and obstetrics services
  (k) Assistance with family planning

become "garrison towns."[40] In such large urban environments, people will often be housed in public buildings and community facilities such as abandoned factories, warehouses, schools, churches, universities, gymnasia, stadia, or community centers. Recent violent conflicts in urban settings that have experienced active shelling have caused extensive damage to water, electricity, sewage, and heating systems, with potentially important public health implications.[41] Three major issues have been identified as particularly critical to the health of people trapped in these urban areas: the extent to which the water supply is disrupted; the extent to which the health system is compromised; and the supports that can be provided to vulnerable subsets of the population.

Water Supply

Water systems have long been military targets, owing to the debilitating and demoralizing effect that the destruction of such systems has on communities under siege. During the Gulf War (1990–91), air strikes rendered Iraqi hydroelectric plants and water pumping stations totally inoperative. In Afghanistan, the traditional irrigation infrastructure was thoroughly demolished at the outset of the conflict.

In Sarajevo and other large cities in Bosnia and Herzegovina, municipal water supplies were destroyed by shelling during the civil war; similar breakdowns in sewage systems and the cross-contamination of piped water supplies led to the widespread contamination of drinking water. These problems were compounded by the lack of electricity and diesel fuel needed to run generators. A household survey in Sarajevo in April 1993 found only an average of 11.3 liters of water per person per day, well below the minimum of 15–20 liters per person per day recommended by the World Health Organization (WHO).[42] Although widespread epidemics of diarrheal disease were avoided, local health department data showed that the incidence of communicable diseases had increased significantly since the beginning of the war. For example, the incidence of hepatitis A increased almost sixfold in Sarajevo, twelvefold in Zenica, and almost fourfold in Tuzla between 1991 and 1993. The incidence of dysentery caused by *Shigella* increased twelvefold and seventeenfold in Sarajevo and Zenica, respectively, during the same period.[2]

Efforts to confront the lack of water and the increase in communicable diseases in urban settings have required creative solutions. In Sarajevo, water was diverted from a brewery to public use and multiple taps were established around the city; constant sniper fire, however, made trips to collect water from these taps extremely dangerous. In order to increase water availability in homes through the city's piped water system, transportable treatment modules were airlifted from the United States and installed in a tunnel in the eastern sector of the city. Although the system took almost one year to become fully operational, it did significantly increase potable water supplies. Local public and political pressure for high-tech (and comparatively expensive) solutions may make similar demands on relief efforts in future urban complex humanitarian emergencies.

Health Systems

The breakdown of routine health services may contribute heavily to the public health impact of humanitarian crises. In Bosnia and Herzegovina changes in morbidity and mortality caused by communicable diseases and malnutrition were relatively moderate compared with emergencies in Africa. The impact of the disruption of medical services due to the war, however, was dramatic. By necessity, existing health resources focused on treating those injured in the war. Fighting in populated areas forced medical staff to flee, prohibited delivery of medical supplies, and damaged many health facilities, including tertiary care hospitals (such as the State Hospital in Sarajevo) and primary care centers throughout the region. In addition, the conflict prevented much of the population from reaching functioning health facilities and prevented public health programs from reaching out into war-affected communities. Consequently, many routine prevention programs, such as prenatal care and child immunization, were sharply curtailed. For example, vaccination coverage for 13- to 25-month-olds in central Bosnia was only 31 percent for measles, 49 percent for polio, and 55 percent for diphtheria and pertussis in July 1993 compared with prewar coverage rates of 90–95 percent.[43]

Vulnerable Populations

Conflict during these emergencies adversely affects the public health of all residents in a besieged urban setting, but may be even more problematic for refugees or displaced persons who flee to these perceived safe enclaves and are often required to live in collective centers. Lacking access to local resources or relatives, members of this group may be even more vulnerable to health and nutrition problems than the besieged residents of the area. Although displaced persons made up only 10 percent of the local population in Sarajevo in 1993, they accounted for 48 percent of reported cases of enterocolitis. Only 15 percent of the displaced lived in collective centers, but almost two-thirds of the cases were among this group, most likely because of problems in providing adequate water to overcrowded buildings.[44] Vaccination surveys at the same time also documented that coverage was lower among children in collective centers compared with either other displaced children or local residents.[43] With limited local support or ability to generate income, this group is almost totally dependent on humanitarian assistance for food as well as for shelter. In general, displaced persons in collective centers did not have higher rates of malnutrition compared with others in Sarajevo; elderly residents of nursing homes, however, were found to be the most vulnerable.[45]

CRITICAL PUBLIC HEALTH INTERVENTIONS IN AUSTERE ENVIRONMENTS

Critical public health interventions in complex emergencies involving mass population movements (refugees or internally displaced persons) or associated with evacuation camp settings focus on environmental health, communicable disease control, immunization, nutrition, maternal and child health, clinical care, and emergency health information systems.

Environmental Health: Water, Sanitation, Hygiene, and Vector Management

Overcrowding and resulting poor water supplies and inadequate hygiene and sanitation are factors known to increase the incidence of diarrhea, malaria, respiratory infections, measles, and other communicable diseases—the prime causes of death and illness in settings of displacement.[6,46] A good system of water supply and excreta disposal must be put into place quickly. No amount of curative health measures can offset the detrimental effects of poor environmental health planning for communities in emergency settlements.

Where camps are unavoidable, appropriate site location, layout, spacing, and type of shelter can mitigate the conditions that lead to the spread of disease.[24] Site planning must be well integrated with the overall environmental health plan, including access to adequate sources of potable water and the collection, disposal, and treatment of excreta and other liquid and solid wastes. The physical characteristics of the site (vegetation, topography, nature of the soil and subsoil, water drainage patterns, and other attributes), together with the sociocultural profile of the displaced population, are important factors that must be taken into account.

Sanitation, waste disposal, and water distribution systems within the emergency settlement community must be equally accessible for all residents. This access is achieved through the installation of an appropriate number of suitably located excreta disposal facilities, such as toilets, latrines, or defecation fields; solid-waste pickup points and water distribution points; and bathing and washing facilities, supplied with soap and supported by effective health education.[47,48]

Water Adequate quantities of relatively clean water are preferable to small amounts of high-quality water.[49] Unfortunately, it is frequently difficult to provide even the minimum 15–20 liters per person per day recommended by WHO to refugee populations. In 1988, for example, the Ethiopian government placed more than 200,000 Somali refugees in the Hartisheik camp, more than 50 kilometers (30 miles) from the nearest natural water source.[31] Water had to be transported daily by a fleet of donated, poorly maintained trucks over rough, dangerous dirt or gravel roads. For much of 1989, refugees were forced to subsist on an average of 3 to 4 liters of water per person per day for all their basic needs (drinking, cooking, and personal hygiene)—about one quarter of the minimum UN standard.[23] Inadequate quantities of water were also a major problem in a northern Somali camp, where a cholera outbreak in 1985 caused almost 1,000 deaths.[33]

Providing buckets with lids to each family and then chlorinating each bucket at the distribution source is labor-intensive but has proved to be an effective prevention step that can be instituted early in an emergency.[50]

Excreta disposal During the early acute phase latrine construction begins, but initial sanitation measures may involve no more than the simple designation of an area for defecation in each camp, segregated from the community's source of potable water.[51,52] The goal of one latrine for every twenty persons is rarely achieved in camp settings.[23]

Vector control   The control of disease vectors such as mosquitoes, flies, rats, and fleas is an important part of an environmental health approach to protecting community members from disease.[53]

Shelter   WHO recommends 30 square meters of space per refugee, plus the necessary land for communal and agricultural activities and livestock, as a minimum overall figure useful in planning camp layout.[54] Of this total space allotment, 3.5 square meters is the absolute minimum floor space per person in emergency shelters.[23] The first priority in areas where large numbers of people are living in damaged urban structures (and in smaller war-affected villages as well) is to diminish as much as possible the penetration of wind and rain into the structure. In these situations, plastic sheeting for roof and window repairs, along with the materials for attaching it to the damaged structures, is often provided by relief organizations.[55] During sieges, most people from within the enclave or "garrison towns" who lose their homes will initially be able to take shelter with friends and relatives.[21] Only when housing losses reach more than about 25 percent will there be a need to find other forms of shelter.[56]

The decision to provide shelter at all can have significant long-term consequences. Simple shelters provided on an emergency basis may unintentionally evolve into permanent shantytowns or squatter settlements and end up attracting many more refugees to the site.

Communicable Disease Control and Epidemic Management

The major reported causes of death among refugees and displaced populations—malnutrition, diarrheal diseases, measles, acute respiratory infections, and malaria—consistently account for 60–95 percent of all reported causes of death.[6] The prevention of high mortality due to communicable disease epidemics in displaced populations relies primarily on the prompt provision of adequate quantities of water, basic sanitation, community outreach, and effective case management of ill patients based on essential drugs and public health surveillance to trigger early appropriate control measures. For example, proper case management of diarrheal diseases using relatively simple measures can reduce case fatality to less than 1 percent even in epidemics of cholera.[57,58]

Immunization

Immunization of children against measles is one of the most important (and cost-effective) preventive measures in emergency-affected populations, particularly those housed in camps.[59] Immunization of refugee children against measles in Thailand in 1979 saved many lives. In Somalia, although measles was an early problem, immunization of the refugee population was effective in preventing outbreaks after 1981. Since infants as young as six months of age frequently contract measles in refugee camp outbreaks and are at greater risk of dying from impaired nutrition, it is recommended that measles immunization programs along with vitamin A supplements in emergency settings target all children from the ages of six months through five years (some would recommend as old as twelve to fourteen). Ideally, one should strive for measles immunization coverage in refugee camp settings of better than 80 percent.[59] Immunization programs should eventually include all antigens recommended by WHO's Expanded Program on Immunization (EPI).

Nutrition

Undernutrition increases the case-fatality rate for measles, diarrheal diseases, and other infectious diseases, and deficiencies of vitamins A and C have been associated with increased childhood mortality in nonrefugee populations.[32,33] Because malnutrition contributes greatly to overall refugee morbidity and mortality, nutritional rehabilitation and maintenance of adequate nutritional levels can be one of the most effective interventions (along with measles immunization) to decrease mortality, particularly for vulnerable groups such as pregnant women, mothers who are breast-feeding, young children, the handicapped, and the elderly.[60] It is more and more common, early in emergency situations, to establish selective feeding centers for malnourished children and pregnant women. Although therapeutic and supplementary feeding programs may be essential for those with the most severe (and potentially life-threatening) degrees of acute malnutrition, it is equally important that the general ration be of satisfactory nutritional quality and caloric content to prevent malnutrition in the first place, and to address the nutritional needs of less severely malnourished children.[61] Monitoring and evaluating available food sources and supplies for quality and quantity are essential (for example, "food-basket" surveys).[62] The highest nutritional priority in the refugee camp setting, however, is the timely and adequate provision of general food rations containing at least 1,900 kilocalories per person per day (some would recommend as high as 2,100–2,400 kcal), and that includes sufficient protein, fat, and micro-nutrients.[61]

Maternal and Child Health (including Reproductive Health)

Maternal and child health care programs may include health education and outreach; prenatal, delivery, and postnatal care; nutritional supplementation; encouragement of breast-feeding; family planning and STD/HIV prevention; and immunization and weight monitoring for infants. Giving responsibility to women heads of households to control the distribution of relief supplies, particularly food, will ensure more equitable apportionment of relief items.

Clinical Care (Curative Medical Services)

Substantial experience shows that medical care in emergency situations should be based on simple, standardized protocols.[63] The Kurdish refugee crisis along the Iraq–Turkey border in the spring of 1991[20] and in refugee camps in eastern Zaire for Rwandan refugees in 1994[28] have reinforced the principle that public health measures (as opposed to curative measures) such as the deployment of community outreach workers to actively seek out cases of cholera and the establishment of oral rehydration therapy (ORT) centers in a refugee camp are critically important in the emergency phase. In Kurdistan, for example, severely malnourished and dehydrated children were sometimes kept in a dark corner of their shelter and were not brought to the clinic unless a community health worker actively sought them out.[20] In the eastern Zaire refugee camps for Rwandans, a high proportion (initially 90 percent) of deaths occurred outside health care facilities, indicating either that health care services were not accessible to a high proportion of severely ill persons or that services at clinic sites were exceeded by demands. This observation emphasizes the need for establishing conveniently accessible community rehydration programs at the beginning

Box 2.3 Typical basic curative care requirements for responding to the needs of residents of emergency settlements

- Treatment of diarrhea (for example, oral rehydration, intravenous fluids, and appropriate antibiotics)
- Treatment of acute respiratory infections
- Treatment of other prevalent conditions (for example, malaria)
- Therapeutic feeding
- Care of wounds
- Psychological counseling or the equivalent

of the emergency phase.[64] Box 2.3 and Figure 2.1 provide lists of basic curative care requirements for refugee camp settings.

The World Health Organization and other organizations such as Médecins sans Frontières have developed basic, field-tested protocols for managing diarrheal disease, respiratory infection, febrile illness, and other common clinical problems that are easily adaptable for emergency situations.[6,57,58,65,66,67] Underlying these basic case management protocols are what have been termed "essential" drug and supply lists.[68] Such standard treatment protocols and basic supplies make it more likely that overall curative care (the overwhelming majority of which will be provided by nonphysicians) will be appropriate and allow the most efficient use of limited resources. Following basic protocols enables physicians' assistants, nurses, and community health workers to provide effective medical care without the need for time-consuming and overly technical interventions. The management of relief supplies, moreover, has been a difficult problem in many disaster efforts.[69] Essential drug and supply lists help ensure that logistic resources are devoted only to needed items.

Emergency Health Information Systems

Accurate public health surveillance activities were rare during refugee emergencies prior to about 1978. One of the first documented uses of "data

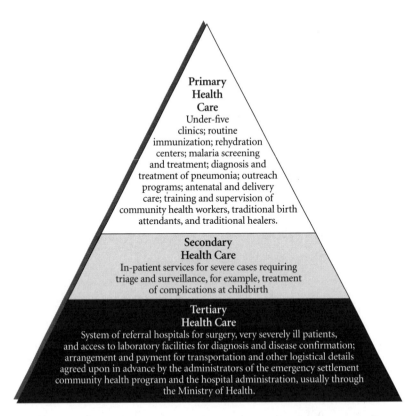

Figure 2.1 The basic model for organizing health service systems in emergency settlements is a three-tiered structure. (Adapted from University of Wisconsin Disaster Management Center, First International Emergency Settlement Conference: New Approaches to New Realities, April 15–19, 1996)

for decision making" in the midst of a refugee crisis occurred in 1978, when 10,000 to 20,000 Burmese refugees in camps in Bangladesh died during an eight-month period.[70] One measure of the technical progress that has been made in managing refugee crises since then is the almost routine establishment of emergency health information systems to monitor the health of populations affected by complex humanitarian emergencies (Box 2.4). Particularly since the early 1990s, humanitarian organizations such as UNHCR and MSF have recognized the importance of a standardized health information system to track disease patterns and to assist in health plan-

Box 2.4 Case study: Cambodian refugee crisis in Thailand, 1979–80

The usefulness of rapid public health surveillance to target a relief effort involving deaths, injuries, and often severe illness was demonstrated in 1979 when 30,000 Cambodians arrived as refugees in Thailand. This group had escaped from the war with neighboring Vietnam, and were exhausted from the fighting, short of food, injured, and heavily infected with malaria when they arrived in the camps located in eastern Thailand. Their high mortality rate was visible to the world when dead bodies were collected each morning for burial. A massive international relief operation was begun, but no information was available early on to determine whether relief efforts should be targeted to children or adults or to malnutrition, immunization, malaria control, treatment of war injuries, or control of epidemic diseases. In the absence of epidemiologic data, many visiting newspeople described the refugees as living in "death camps," a condition they associated with a relief effort that was failing by not immediately preventing deaths. However, public health surveillance activities were soon initiated; their immediate aim was to rapidly identify preventable causes of death and decide on the highest priorities for relief activities. The second aim of surveillance was to monitor mortality and morbidity to ascertain whether the relief effort was having an impact.

Public health surveillance rapidly provided data on the rates of death, identified cerebral malaria as the principal cause of death and serious hospitalization, and led to specific strategies for aggressive treatment. The swift decline in mortality during the first weeks of the effort was directly linked to a relief effort that had correctly targeted the chief preventable causes of death. The collection of simple data on the daily number and presumed cause of deaths and admissions to the hospital, the use of "quick and dirty" field surveys targeted to the specific questions of relief, and the preparation of a brief weekly surveillance report made the relief effort responsive to the priority health needs in the camp and provided reliable information for donor organizations and the press.

ning and evaluation. Epidemiologists are now routinely called upon by these organizations to establish basic mortality and morbidity surveillance systems and to conduct health and nutrition surveys during the acute emergency phase to assess program effectiveness and the need for further public health interventions.[71]

All components of an emergency health information system should be analyzed in an integrated fashion. A single element examined alone will reveal only a small portion of the entire picture and may be easily misinterpreted. For example, an apparent decrease in malnutrition prevalence should be interpreted in the context of childhood mortality rates.[72] In the 1991 Kurdish refugee crisis, the overall prevalence of wasting was misleadingly low, since many of the youngest and most severely affected children—those with the lowest weight-for-height status—had already died.[20]

The use of health information to guide refugee program decision making will be facilitated if targets and critical indicators are established at the beginning. Agencies responding to humanitarian crises currently lack a mechanism to evaluate the effectiveness of the health response and outcome of refugee relief organizations.[73] How do such organizations evaluate whether the relief operation is succeeding or failing? Just as emergency managers monitor the early warning signs that may indicate a potential emergency situation, they should stay abreast of those indicators or "measures of effectiveness" that may point to a reduction in emergency needs (Table 2.1). Five basic categories of data (indicators or measures of effectiveness) are useful for monitoring and evaluating emergency relief programs:[74]

1. Mortality
   - crude mortality rate (deaths/10,000/day)
   - under five mortality rate
2. Morbidity
   - serious communicable diseases (cases/month)
   - nutrition-related diseases
3. Nutritional status
   - screening of new arrivals by mid-upper arm circumference
   - periodic surveys by weight-for-height
4. Public health activities
   - immunizations
   - feeding center attendance
   - numbers of outpatients, inpatient admissions, referrals
5. Vital sectors
   - food distributions, rations
   - water and sanitation
   - shelter, blankets, clothing, domestic utensils, cooking fuel

Table 2.1 Life-threatening conditions and emergency indicators (adapted from UNHCR-EMTP workshop notebook materials)

Crude mortality rate	Rate in many developed countries	0.3/10,000/day
	Rate in many developing countries	0.5/10,000/day
	Relief program under control	< 1.0/10,000/day
	Relief program in serious trouble	> 1.0/10,000/day
	Emergency: out of control	> 2.0/10,000/day
	Famine, major catastrophe	> 5.0/10,000/day
Under 5 mortality rate	Rate in many developing countries	1.0/10,000/day
	Emergency phase under control	< 2.0/10,000/day
	Emergency phase: serious situation	> 2.0/10,000/day
	Emergency phase: out of control	> 4.0/10,000/day
Lack of clean water	Min. "survival" allocation (few days)	7 liters/person/day
	Min. maintenance allocation (few weeks to months)	15–20 liters/ person/day
Lack of food	Min. "survival" allocation	1,900 kcal/person/day[a]

Malnutrition	More than 1 percent of the under 5 population of children severely malnourished or more than 10 percent moderately malnourished
	Presence of scurvy, pellagra, beri-beri, and avitaminosis-A outbreaks
	For children under 5 the indicators for severe malnourishment are:
	MUAC[b] less than 12.5 cm
	WFH[c] ratios less than 70 percent of reference median CDC/WHO
	WFH Z-score −3 standard deviations below reference mean
	For children under 5 the indicators of moderate malnourishment are:
	MUAC between 12.5 and 13.5 cm
	WFH or WFL ratios between 70 and 80 percent
	WFH or WFL[d] Z-score −2 through −3 standard deviations below reference mean
	and/or edema
Lack of ap-propriate shelter	"Appropriate" shelter is dependent on the immediate environment. Protection from wind, rain, freezing temperatures, and direct sunlight is universally applicable.
	Minimum shelter area 3.5 sq.m/person
	Minimum total site area 30.0 sq.m/person
Lack of sanitation	Poor excreta and waste disposal

Source: Compiled by University of Wisconsin Disaster Management Center–UNHCR Emergency Tools Series, 1992.

a. In cold climates increase minimums by 1%/degree C for every degree below 20 C.

b. Mid-upper arm circumference.   c. Weight-for-height.   d. Weight-for-length.

Refugee relief programs should be systematically evaluated, not merely for their quantity and content, but for their impact and effectiveness.[75] See Box 2.5 for examples of questions that are useful to address in evaluations of refugee health programs.

Box 2.5 Questions that should be addressed in evaluations of refugee health programs

---

1. Appropriateness and cost-effectiveness of the response:

- What were the actual needs of the population?
- How were they assessed?
- Were the assessments accurate?
- Were the needs of the affected population actually addressed by the intervention's design?
- To what extent did the actual response(s) meet the needs of the affected population?
- Were the responses appropriate given needs and resources?
- How might such a response be better designed in the future to meet those needs?

2. Coverage and coherence of the response:

- How were beneficiaries in the affected population identified/targeted?
- What were the principle gaps in the response?
- Were attempts made to fill those gaps? If not, why not?
- Were the various responses adequately coordinated?
- What were the results when they were/were not coordinated?
- How might the response be redesigned to ensure coherence among the various actors and responses?

3. Connectedness and impact of the response:

- What was the impact of the response on mortality and malnutrition rates, security and protection, restoration of coping mechanisms?
- How did the relief effort affect longer-term recovery efforts?
- How might future responses be redesigned to ensure connectedness between the relief program and longer-term recovery needs?

Source: University of Wisconsin Disaster Management Center, *First International Emergency Settlement Conference: New Approaches to New Realities, April 15–19, 1996* (Madison: University of Wisconsin Disaster Management Center, 1996).

Important questions concerning health aspects of refugee relief services and the appropriateness of critical interventions in complex humanitarian emergencies remain unanswered. Operational research is needed to identify the most effective methods of providing adequate micronutrients to refugees, improved mortality and morbidity surveillance, better case management of malaria and dysentery, better methods of treating chronic infectious diseases such as tuberculosis, effective prevention of hepatitis E, HIV/AIDS, and sexually transmitted diseases, and improved delivery of reproductive health services. Finally, it would be useful for relief organizations to conduct prevention and cost-effectiveness analyses of relief operations in the health sector. (The "Joint Evaluation of Emergency Assistance to Rwanda" [1996] provides an important example of the use of cost-effectiveness as one criteria in the evaluation of an emergency operation.)[76]

SUMMARY

In the complicated, unpredictable, and often dangerous environment of current humanitarian crises, there can be no single, perfect formula for mounting an effective and appropriate public health response. Every situation is unique in terms of its political, environmental, cultural, economic, and public health context; what works in Angola may not work in Rwanda or Bosnia or Kosovo. What has been discussed here are principles of practice that are relevant to every complex humanitarian emergency (Box 2.6).

Obstacles to instituting these core urgent relief measures in any complex emergency include issues of access to the population in need, whether they have refugee or internally displaced status, and timely coordination of a multisectoral international response. These issues are in turn dependent upon the local political context, the physical terrain, the numbers of people seeking refuge, the pace at which they arrive, and the managerial capacities and resources of the relief community. If these obstacles are not surmounted within an appropriate timeframe, the outcome will be at first a renewed imposition of hardship upon people who have already suffered in the circumstances that had led to their flight and seeking of refuge. Longer delays in providing core priority relief meaures, such as water, shelter, or food, will lead to a measurable increase in rates of morbidity and mortality from exposure, dehydration, and disease.

Box 2.6 Ten critical emergency relief measures

Although every complex emergency is different and the relative prioritization of emergency health interventions may vary, a core of urgent relief measures is fundamental:

1. Rapidly assess the health status of the affected population

2. Establish disease surveillance and a health information system

3. Immunize all children aged six months to five years (some would recommend as old as fourteen) against measles, and provide vitamin A in situations of malnutrition

4. Institute diarrhea control programs

5. Provide elementary sanitation and clean water

6. Provide adequate shelter, clothes, and blankets

7. Ensure at least 1,900 kcal of food per person per day

8. Establish curative services that follow standard treatment protocols and are based on essential drug lists, and that provide basic coverage to the community as a whole

9. Organize human resources to ensure one community health expert per 1,000 population

10. Coordinate activities of local authorities, national agencies, international agencies, and nongovernmental organizations

Source: Adapted from T. W. Sharp, "Conflict-related complex emergencies," in P. W. Kelley, ed., *Military Preventive Medicine—Mobilization and Deployment,* Textbook of Military Medicine series (Washington, D.C.: Borden Institute, 1997).

Once these absolutely basic life supports have been provided, with some minimal reach that extends to all members of the population, certain public health interventions must be instituted to

1. ensure that rations contain adequate caloric and micronutrient content and are equitably distributed;

2. ensure that sufficient quantities of relatively clean water are available;

3. establish a medical care regime that maintains
   (a) a focus on community outreach (such as oral rehydration outposts to manage dehydrated diarrhea patients),
   (b) effective case management of common life-threatening diseases, such as malaria and pneumonia, and
   (c) disease prevention (for example, measles immunization);
4. institute a basic health information system that includes mortality and nutritional surveillance.

These key measures must take place in the context of providing an overall measure of security, safety, and dignity for the population in need. It is essential that law and order be maintained, including disarming all elements of the population and introducing other measures to prevent outbreaks of violence against individuals or groups. People who enter emergency settlements will need to be registered and many, as in the situation of the Kosovar refugees, may need to be issued identity papers. Often families will have been separated and the institution of sensitive and competent tracing capacities will help support all other public health, including mental health, interventions. Community mental health measures must be introduced with attention to cultural, religious, and other group preferences.

Public health intervention in humanitarian crises is a graded, prioritized response where success lies in adherence to a set of practice principles that are applied in a timely manner, in an appropriate sequence, and with attention to the expressed needs and interests of the affected population.

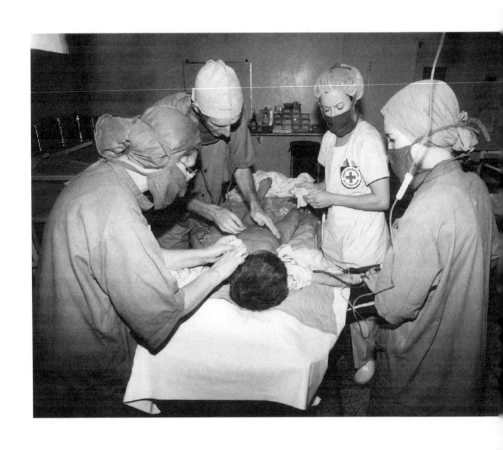

3

CLASSIC CONCEPTS IN DISASTER MEDICAL RESPONSE

susan m. briggs

mark leong

Complex humanitarian emergencies, events involving large population movement, armed conflict, and human rights abuses, present unique challenges to medical responders. In terms of complexity, scale, and the imbalance of needs over resources, CHEs are at one end of the spectrum of disasters that the response community must now address.[1] An assessment of these challenges begins with a discussion of classic civilian disaster medical response deployed in the setting of natural and technological disasters that afflict rich as well as poor societies. These disasters, in some instances, have precipitated population migration, economic crisis, food scarcity, or famine.[2] The new element introduced by CHEs, from the perspective of disaster responders, is the sweeping social and political turmoil that characterizes these emergencies and the resulting great increase in the numbers of people affected and dislocated. The issues of regional disorder and regionwide distress make CHEs special cases in the wide range of contingencies disaster responders have been trained to address.

CIVILIAN DISASTER RESPONSE: MASS CASUALTY INCIDENTS

Organized civilian medical response to natural and technological disasters has developed as a function and as a field of expertise during the last twenty-five years.[3] This development has evolved as a reaction to devastating experiences with earthquakes, volcanoes, hurricanes, nuclear power plant accidents, mass fires and floods, building collapses, terrorist bombings, and large-scale airplane and train disasters. A consistent medical approach to these events, based on an understanding of their common features and of the response expertise they require, has gradually become accepted practice both in the United States and in Europe.[4,5] Within this approach is the core strategy for immediate response to acute mass casualties (traumatic injuries, burns, toxic exposures, and metabolic emergencies). This strategy, called the Mass Casualty Incident (MCI) response,[6,7] has the primary objective of reducing or mitigating the mortality and morbidity caused by the disaster. MCIs have been defined as events resulting in a number of victims large enough to disrupt the normal course of emergency and health care services of the affected community. Use of the term MCI implies a limited geographic and demographic scope.

In general, and more securely in the past, the term MCI has also connoted a certain positive equilibrium between needs and resources. In civilian disasters occurring in the developed world, where trained medical personnel, transport, and well-equipped facilities can be summoned to an organized response in a timely fashion, response planners have expected that all victims will receive appropriate care. But as disaster responders have now formed teams to proceed to catastrophes occurring in developing countries, where local resources are often inadequate to meet primary health care needs, let alone the burden of casualties imposed by a major disaster, medical responders to these overseas MCIs have seen need outstrip supply. Such situations have been seen most dramatically in disasters such as the volcano and mudslides in Armero, Colombia, in 1985[8] and in the response to the earthquake in Soviet Armenia in 1988.[9] These disasters and many others demonstrate that civilian MCI responders are beginning to come up against what the world's military have long called an "austere environment," a setting where resources, transport, access, or other aspects of the physical, social, and economic environment impose severe constraints on the adequacy of immediate care that can be delivered to the population in need.[10] This concept of austerity is dynamic, depending upon numbers and kinds of victims and local conditions.

As the scenarios the MCI response is called upon to address become more complex and intense, the gap between the classic MCI in a highly developed urban area and what the humanitarian community now calls complex humanitarian emergencies continues to close. Terrorism, involving chemical, biological, or nuclear weapons, is capable of destroying response capacity and producing casualties in numbers that would overwhelm any resources that do persist.[11,12] Contingency planning for a major terrorist disaster in a large U.S. city invokes most aspects of a military austere environment. Although a general description of a terrorist disaster in New York City might look very different from that of a medical station in Kigali, Rwanda, in the midst of the 1994 genocide, in terms of key MCI features there are many similarities: victims more numerous than resources to support them, inadequate infrastructure and supply lines, and dangerous and insecure sites for whatever delivery of care can be organized.

KEY FEATURES OF THE MCI RESPONSE

The MCI response comprises four basic elements:

- search and rescue;
- triage and initial stabilization;
- definitive medical care;
- evacuation.

Rapid, objective medical assessment by experienced personnel will allow initial medical responders to select which of these four key elements is appropriate in the acute phase of the disaster response to achieve the primary objective. It is crucial to recognize that these four elements, and all other aspects of disaster medical response, are sustained and maintained by a system of nonmedical inputs that provide essential infrastructure, supplies, and security. These elements include establishing logistic supply lines for food, water, and other material and equipment, maintaining security, sanitation measures and disease control, and repairing or building core communications and transportation systems (Box 3.1).

Search and Rescue

The past decade has seen an increase in the incidence of disasters of all kinds, establishing a demand for professionals skilled in search and rescue techniques. The rapidity of the medical response, particularly when the disaster involves victims of collapsed structures, is key to the critical reduc-

Box 3.1 Essential nonmedical elements in disaster response

- Ensuring adequacy and safety of food, water, and shelter
- Implementing sanitation measures to prevent and/or contain endemic diseases likely to have an impact on the delivery of medical care
- Implementing security measures to ensure the safety of both the disaster responders and people seeking care
- Establishing adequate lines of communication among disaster responders, both medical and nonmedical
- Establishing significant transportation capacities to facilitate achievement of the primary objective

tion in mortality and morbidity. Review of major earthquakes throughout the world has shown that the success of extricating live survivors drops off dramatically 24 hours after the quake.[13]

The immediate search and rescue resource in disasters is the local population. In disasters involving large numbers of victims trapped in collapsed structures, the local response may be unsophisticated and haphazard, and may lack the technical equipment and expertise to facilitate extrication. Many countries have developed specialized search and rescue teams as an integral part of their national disaster plan. The search and rescue units include:

- a cadre of medical specialists;
- technical specialists knowledgeable in hazardous materials, structural engineering, heavy equipment, and technical search methodology (such as sensitive listening devices and remote cameras);
- trained canines and their handlers.

Members of search and rescue teams receive specialized training in "confined space environments." In the United States, specialized search and rescue teams are developed, trained, and mobilized under the authority of the Federal Emergency Management Agency (FEMA). The Oklahoma and World Trade Center bombings are recent U.S. examples of effective use of these search and rescue teams; earlier instances of deployment of such teams, from the United States and elsewhere, occurred with the 1988 earthquake in Soviet Armenia and the Iranian earthquake of 1990.

Triage and Initial Stabilization

Triage is arguably the most important mission of any medical response, whether in the setting of a disaster of limited scope or in a complex one of wide scale such as that seen in humanitarian crises. The concept of disaster medical triage is based upon the assumption of a potential imbalance between the health needs produced by large numbers of casualties and the available medical resources.[14] In classic MCIs of limited geographic and demographic scope, triage functions as an analytic sorting process that has as its objective to "do the greatest good for the individual patient."[15,16,17,18] The focus is on efficiency; adequate resources for each patient are presumed available, provided these resources are appropriately deployed (Box 3.2).

By contrast, in MCIs, whether as a response to major natural disasters in the developing world or to terrorist bombings in urban societies, the objective of triage becomes to "do the greatest good for the greatest number of people."[19] This version of triage, often called "field medical triage," is characterized not only by the urgency of victim status and the severity of injury but also by the availability of health care resources, which in turn will directly influence the likelihood of victim survival. Field medical triage is widely taught within military medicine, because austere environments (where need grossly outstrips resources) are envisioned as a given feature of serious combat settings. (Recent U.S. military engagements, however, have

---

Box 3.2 Conventional civilian triage priorities

- Identification and evaluation of the severity and urgency of the patient's injuries
- Initiation of immediate critical interventions to stabilize the patient at the site of injury (control of airway, breathing, and circulation and extrication if necessary)
- Transport of the patient to the appropriate treatment facility for further evaluation and definitive care of injuries requiring specialized care (burns, trauma, pediatric expertise)

---

been supported by such robust evacuation transport and medic intervention that most survivable military casualties have been brought to sites of adequate care within time frames essential for salvage.)[20,21]

Field medical triage (Box 3.3) is recognized as a concept but is infrequently required in practice for most civilian disaster responders. Most civilian disaster medical plans are still drawn up under the twin assumptions that the disaster will not occur in an austere environment (or will not result in the creation of one) and that resources, including trained personnel and equipment, will always be adequate to meet the demand. These assumptions are coming under increasing pressure as previous experience from large-scale disaster response is analyzed and as anticipatory plans for terrorist attacks are being developed.

Two factors will drive first responders toward the practice of field triage.

First, in most large-scale disasters that have occurred throughout the

---

Box 3.3 Field medical triage priorities

- Prioritize and categorize casualties so that they can receive timely rescue, treatment, and evacuation in an orderly fashion
- Optimize the use of available medical, nursing, and emergency personnel at the disaster site
- Optimize the use of available logistic support and equipment

The factors that will worsen the imbalance between medical need and the resources required to meet that need include:

- Lack of an appropriate number and type of medical, nursing, or emergency personnel
- Lack of access by rescuers and emergency medical personnel to the disaster site
- Lack of access by rescuers and emergency personnel to the casualties at the disaster site (because of extrication issues, exposure to hazards)
- Shortages of medical equipment and supplies
- Limited availability of evacuation assets (for example, transport capacity such as ambulances, helicopters)
- Inadequate physical and functional integrity of medical facilities

---

world, the first responders are members of the local population, who are almost always forced to begin a rescue effort with few resources and with a disproportionate number of casualties.

Second, in disasters of sudden onset, whether natural disasters such as earthquakes or terrorist bombings, the absence of warning and the potential for the event to cause immediate injury or death to large numbers of people can at best evoke only a reactive medical response, not only among the first responders but also among the professionals who are first at the scene. This response, in its early stages, may not be sufficient to provide adequate medical care to all casualties. Gradual onset disasters (for example, hurricanes and certain kinds of floods) allow for a more organized, planned medical response. In settings where a certain volume of casualties is always expected as a regular occurrence, or where casualties occur later in the event or in some sequence as the event progresses, a more sophisticated and fully supported triage system can be employed.

Field medical triage must be conducted at three levels.

On-site (Level 1) triage   Level 1 triage involves the rapid categorization of victims "where they are lying" or at a collection site (triage site). The objective is the rapid identification of victims with potentially severe injuries needing immediate medical care, which can be delivered either at a temporary field stabilization facility or at an established medical facility. Personnel are typically first responders from the local population and/or emergency medical personnel if available. Patients are classified as acute or urgent. Simplified color coding to designate acute (red) and nonacute (green) status may be done at the Level 1 triage site if resources are available.

Medical (Level 2) triage   The goal of Level 2 triage is the rapid categorization of victims at a casualty collection site by the most experienced available medical personnel (advanced medical post), with the objective of swiftly identifying the level of medical care needed. Triage at this level should be provided by medical personnel available at the disaster site who have experience in triage and disaster management. To be able to "do the greatest good for the greatest number of people," the individuals in charge of Level 2 triage must be able to prioritize the casualties for medical treatment and evacuation. Knowledge of the medical consequences of various types of injuries and mechanisms of injury, especially those dealing with burn, blast, or crush injuries or with injuries from exposure to chemical, biological, or nuclear weapons, is essential. This knowledge guides the decision-making process by which to assess probability of survival based on the severity of the injury and the availability of resources.

Color-coded casualty triage tags are often used at this level to classify patients.

Red (urgent): This classification includes patients who require immediate life-saving interventions (airway, breathing, hemorrhage control). Many patients classified as red or urgent in conventional civilian triage will be classified as yellow (delayed or expectant) in complex humanitarian emergencies because they have no chance of survival owing to the severity of injuries and the limited nature of medical resources.

Yellow (delayed or expectant): This classification includes two very different populations: (1) patients who do not require immediate life-saving intervention and for whom treatment may be delayed, with the expectation of full recovery; and (2) patients who are not expected to survive owing to the severity of the injuries in that austere environment (defined by either limited medical resources at the disaster site or inaccessible, destroyed, or unsafe surroundings, or both).

Green (minor): Individuals who require minimal or no medical care; nonurgent.

Black (deceased).

The casualty collection sites should be located so as not to increase casualties, but to treat them. Important characteristics of the casualty collection site (Level 1 and Level 2 triage) are

- proximity to the site of the disaster;
- safety from hazards and upwind location from site of the disaster in contaminated environments;
- protection from climatic conditions;
- easy visibility for disaster victims;
- convenient egress routes if possible (air and land evacuation).

Evacuation (Level 3)   Level 3 triage assigns priorities to disaster victims for transfer to existing or adapted health care facilities. The objective at this level is to facilitate transfer to appropriate health care facilities by the most appropriate method (air or land evacuation) depending on the severity of injury and the available resources. The personnel involved are the same as for Level 2 medical triage.

Triage is a dynamic process. Patients and casualties must be assessed by a triage officer every few hours. The application of critical field interventions at timely phases in the evolution of an individual patient's care can decrease the urgency for definitive medical treatment. In the best case, as additional disaster resources become available, patients may be retriaged according to the severity of their injuries. As more personnel, equipment, and supplies arrive at the disaster scene, patients initially assigned to the delayed treatment category (yellow) on the basis of limited medical capabilities may, perhaps, be reassigned to an urgent category (red) and receive essential life-saving medical interventions.[22]

In the more grim circumstances that often apply in CHEs, the large number of casualties may force a decision to place many patients in the category for delayed treatment (yellow) and also may eliminate any possibility of the development of evacuation (Level 3) triage. In CHEs, where there may be many seriously injured patients in need of sophisticated medical treatment that cannot be provided within the field setting and where resources are completely expended on emergency relief, evacuation out of the region is usually not a realistic option.

Definitive Medical Care

In military medicine and classic civilian field disaster care (or MCIs), requirements for definitive medical care will vary widely depending on the magnitude and epidemiology of the disaster.[23,24] Both small-scale and large-scale disasters, as well as CHEs, may require the mobilization of specialty medical teams (for example, trauma, burns, critical care, pediatrics) to participate in the field medical response. These teams may work from facilities in the host country. Alternatively, the evacuation of disaster victims to regional facilities outside of the disaster area may be required. Disaster plans must prepare for potentially "contaminated" victims of a disaster as well as mass casualties.[25,26]

Evacuation

Disaster victims may be evacuated by land or air. As part of the predisaster planning process, therefore, officials should identify what resources are lacking in their country or region and develop transportation options in advance for the evacuation of specific injuries. The predisaster evacuation plans can then be more easily adapted to the unique geographical features of specific disasters.

The numbers of people injured or made ill in various phases of recent humanitarian crises, however, would have overwhelmed any evacuation plan that might have been developed. Entire populations in distress cannot be evacuated, while proposals for the evacuation of individuals or particular groups can lead to serious political and ethical dilemmas.[27]

APPLICATION OF CLASSIC DISASTER RESPONSE APPROACH IN HUMANITARIAN CRISES

The discussion thus far has suggested that the basic MCI model is undergoing expansion and redefinition for reasons not directly related to the increasingly urgent demands placed on disaster providers by complex humanitarian emergencies, and that difficult adaptations of civilian triage categories and practice are already being required by international attempts to respond to major natural disasters or to terrorist incidents using weapons of mass lethality. The fundamental issues in application are less the resilience or flexibility of the model than the philosophical, political, and economic choices that must be made were the model to be applied.

The civilian disaster response in MCIs presumes the capacity to establish a coherent and unified chain of command and a consensus on needs assessment and outcome objectives. In recent experience with large-scale disasters, particularly those involving international efforts, these aims have not been uniformly achieved. There is, however, agreement among all disaster professionals that these capacities are essential to the organization and delivery of an effective response.[28] Substantial efforts in training, monitoring, and review of actions in the field now take place in all agencies and units set up for disaster response.

A significant impediment to application of the MCI model in the medical response to complex humanitarian emergencies is the lack of an efficient, timely, international system of disaster medical response that can assemble, train, and integrate disaster personnel and resources.[29] This has impeded response to disasters of smaller scale, as experience over the last twenty-five years has demonstrated.[30] Without such a preexisting system, attempts to coordinate, let alone link, command structures in medical response to CHEs will continue to prove difficult and incomplete.

Medical preparedness, however, is an expensive, time-consuming, and ongoing effort. Arguably, the resources required to improve preparedness beyond our current state of readiness might better be marshaled and directed toward the enormous work of preventing these vast crises in the first instance. Given the many large issues at stake in these emergencies, it is thus not surprising that the political will to establish and fund an integrated international medical response system is lacking.

The other major impediment is the absence of agreement among the many responding agencies regarding objectives during a humanitarian crisis. An axiom of civilian disaster response is that the objectives of the medical response must be defined before committing medical personnel and supplies.[31] In civilian disasters, the primary objective, even in disasters with extremes in imbalance between need and resources, is to mitigate the associated mortality and morbidity. In response to complex humanitarian emergencies, however, depending upon which organization or international agency is involved, secondary objectives (for example, the restoration of the health status of the affected population) or tertiary objectives (for example, the promotion of a higher level of health status than that attained prior to the emergency) can be at work.[32] The varied relief and development agendas of different actors, including local and national authorities, can result in different approaches to initial medical response in the field, configuration and deployment of resources, level of care delivered, and duration of the assistance effort. To find the cost-effective balance between reliance on ad hoc arrangements of diverse responders for providing that care and an investment in coordination and training of a network of providers is a task that lies ahead.

CONCLUSION

Humanitarian crises present unique and sometimes insurmountable challenges to disaster medical responders. Austere conditions, mass casualties, and food and water shortages characterize many contemporary complex emergencies. The features that combine to prevent the development of a routine and systematic acute phase medical response, however, are as much political and economic as they are practical. There is nothing in the theory or potential practice of civilian disaster medicine that could not encompass an adequate response to complex humanitarian emergencies. The response would require, however, a level of international commitment, coordination, and funding that is not yet in reach.

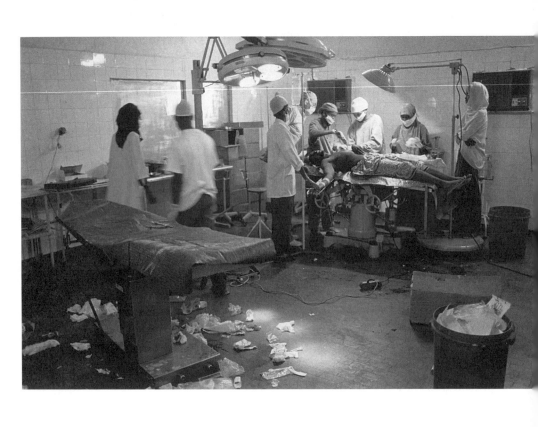

4

EMERGENCY CARE

jennifer leaning

In the last twenty years, thousands of expatriate medical and surgical relief workers have been deployed to provide emergency medical care in the war zones of Africa, Asia, Central Europe, and Latin America. Their field experience is only now beginning to be reported in the medical literature.[1–13] Evident in these early reports are four main themes:

1. the physical and political environment defined by humanitarian crises imposes distinctive burdens and demands on all members of the medical team;
2. the medical function of triage is forced into closer linkage with ongoing medical treatment issues than in civilian mass casualty or military medical care;
3. medical treatment in these settings requires substantial modification in content and application when compared with standard approaches used in developed countries;
4. training and supervision of medical professionals who aspire to work in these settings must pay explicit attention to these newly recognized challenges.

Chapters 1 and 2 address the ways in which public health and primary medical care are adapting to meet the needs of large populations, often refugee or displaced, caught up and swept along in civil and regional wars. The body of knowledge to which Toole, Noji, and Burkholder refer and that they have helped create is now recognized and established. This chapter examines the problem of providing emergency care to individuals who have sustained injuries, either as combatants, targeted civilians, or civilian bystanders, and who assemble or accumulate in large numbers under austere war conditions.

Most practitioners who have acquired significant experience in delivering care under these conditions have not yet recorded their observations in systematic and retrievable ways. Some of the knowledge gained to date is reflected in training manuals, preparedness kits, and training courses.[14–19] There remains a gap, however, between what physicians seasoned in these settings know and can transmit through face-to-face interactions, or in meetings and training sessions, and what the general medical, humanitarian, or policy community has yet to come to understand. The discussion that follows is intended to acknowledge this crucial area of medical practice and to identify a few key issues.

THE WAR ENVIRONMENT

The physical and political environment of humanitarian crises defines a setting in which emergency care must take place that differs considerably from that in which civilian and military medical personnel from the developed world have acquired their training and developed their cognitive and psychological patterns of practice.[20,21] The locations are more isolated, the facilities meager, the infrastructure shattered, the pace more chaotic, and the work conditions unstable, hostile, or at times personally dangerous.[22] This fraught environment has the potential to distract and exhaust all practitioners immersed in it and particularly those who have been trained to focus on patients in circumstances of comparative discipline, support, and routine.

Geography

Emergency care in these recent civil or regional wars often takes place in facilities located within or near the zone of active ongoing conflict. Three location patterns have been seen:

1. an urban site in an area under siege or in the midst of battle, where preexisting medical facilities may still be standing but are at risk of sudden attack or intermittent damage; and where first aid and definitive care must be delivered at the same site with no chance to evacuate patients;
2. a new rural site established along a route of population flight or within a refugee camp where wounded people collect or to which they are brought for first aid and later evacuation;
3. a new or modified site established in a town or village adjacent to areas of heavy fighting or heavily mined countryside, to which injured patients walk or are carried by some form of transport for first aid and definitive care.

Practicalities dictate this proximity to battle zones. Transport capacities are extremely limited (Sarajevo had some ambulance capacity for much of the three-year siege period, but it was an exception),[23] so the medical facilities must remain near the scene of injury occurrence in order to reduce transport time (via jeep, cart, or hand-carry). Further, building materials and human capital are sufficiently scarce that people must make do with the structures they have, so in urban battle areas with standing hospitals and clinics these sites are used as medical facilities unless they are in actual line of sustained fire. Finally, the tactics of these wars, unless focused on siege, often lead to rapid shifts in positions without stable front lines or rear staging areas, where medical outposts have traditionally been placed. Thus medical teams in first aid roles can find their physical sites closely encroached upon or even overrun by hostilities.

Neutral Space

Hospitals and medical facilities of all kinds that deliver medical care in the midst of war are protected entities within the definitions of the Geneva Conventions. All medical personnel, buildings, infrastructure supports, transport, supplies, and equipment are considered, under international humanitarian law, neutral assets that must not be interfered with or infringed upon by any party to the conflict. The neutrality of this medical function is to be respected by all concerned, thus allowing medical providers to take care of all civilians and all combatants from whatever side according to priorities defined by medical need only.

This neutral status is rarely granted to medical facilities in complex humanitarian emergencies.[24] The military leadership and rank-and-file soldiers in these conflicts have in most cases not heard of the Geneva Conventions, and those who have often openly scorn them. The principles of international humanitarian law that are designed to protect civilians in war do not meet the purposes of armed groups, whose intent is either to target civilians and terrorize them into flight from home and land or to eliminate them as a community or people.[25]

Further eroding the reality of neutral space is the fact that these facilities often treat civilians and combatants at the same time. Few of the armies engaged in these regional conflicts have a fully developed separate medical unit and chain of medical support, so that injured soldiers are instead brought to the nearest medical facility by their armed comrades. On many occasions throughout these conflicts, physicians and nurses have been ordered at gunpoint to give preference to one soldier over another; in some settings soldiers have threatened or killed injured combatants or civilians presumed to come from the "other" side.[26]

Finally, hospitals or medical facilities located in an area held for any length of time by one party to the conflict are considered to be allied with the politics of that regime. To some extent it is necessary for those who staff and supply the facility to maintain reasonable relations with the faction that controls that geographic area. The presumption that arises in a context where the rules and principles of IHL are not understood or endorsed, however, is that this practical accommodation represents a conscious political expression of affiliation. This presumption, in turn, places health care personnel at risk whenever they are forced to travel to an area held by the other faction or when they encounter combatants from the other side.

Capacities

Most, if not all, medical facilities established in these areas prior to the onset of recent wars were designed to deliver primary and community health care, not technically advanced or high-volume trauma care (Box 4.1). With the outbreak of war, the casualty areas have been hastily reorganized or enlarged, but resource constraints prevent much building of new operating

There is electricity for most of the time in the hospital. However, fuel for the emergency generator is not always available. Throughout the hospital, there are dangerous situations with respect to the electrical supply. All of the wall lights next to each other are broken. Many are hanging from the wall by their wiring within easy reach of children in bed below them. A similar situation exists with respect to wall sockets. In one ward we saw a cable running across the ward with bare wires at a junction in the middle of the ward made using surgical tape. Most of the lighting is provided by bare light bulbs.

The infrastructure of the plumbing system is present, but all toilets were filthy. There were instances of faecal material in sinks and on floors. There was a small number of filthy showers producing only cold water. There was no hot running water available in the hospital.

The paint is peeling from the walls and, apart from the orthopaedic ward, the hospital has received no decorative attention for more than 20 years. Many of the windows are broken and boarded up. The central heating system is not functioning and with the impending winter, kerosene fires [heaters] will be used in each ward area.

There is a library/conference room in which, during morning hand-overs, female doctors are separated from their male colleagues by a sheet hanging from the ceiling. None of the books in the library were published after 1982. There are no audio-visual aids.

There is an X-ray department containing a machine more than forty years old. There is no radiological screening for the staff or for the relatives who attend with their children. . . .

(continued)

theaters or recruitment of additional trained staff. Direct damage and scarcities brought by the fighting diminish essential supports: medical transport, electricity, fuel for generators, spare parts, supplies, equipment, pharmaceuticals. The local medical staff are often forced to flee to avoid getting caught up in hostile partisan politics or to accompany their families to safety. Those that remain often work without secure income, adequate food, or shelter.

Newly established sites, to the extent that they are built or maintained by

There is a casualty department/reception area without any facilities except 4 filthy and decrepit beds . . .

This ward like other parts of the hospital could be described as an accumulation of despair in which kind and caring doctors and nurses were overwhelmed by the environment and lack of facilities and beset by worries about their own families and how they could provide for them. The doctors and nurses were also aware that if their own children became ill this would represent the best available standard of care in their country.

There are two operating theatres. Only one has a functioning light. The oxygen supply had run out and a ten-year-old child was undergoing a laporotamy for peritonitis under ketamine anaesthesia. She was only lightly anaesthetised (she was moaning and moving). The doctors had no monitoring and were worried that if they gave too much anaesthetic she might die from suppression of respiration. There were no facilities to provide assisted ventilation. The surgeons were highly skilled. They used disposable gloves provided by ICRC but reused them as often as possible.

Source: D. Southall, "Report on the Indira Gandhi Children's Hospital," October 1997; reprinted by permission of the author.

outside relief agencies, contain rudimentary utility supports (generators for electricity, limited by fuel supplies) and packaged supplies and equipment. Organizations with substantial experience in maintaining robust supply lines include the ICRC and MSF. Military medical units, in the rare and brief instances they have been deployed for humanitarian purposes to assist in the care of civilian casualties (U.S. military in northern Kurdistan, Israeli army units in Goma, and British military in Rwanda, for instance), also deliver impressive field hospital capacities. Reliable access to these sites is often a major problem from the perspective of resupply and staff rotation, however, since road and air transport can be interrupted by weather or political hostilities.

These strained medical facilities are always working at the margins of what is possible. During periods of protracted fighting or when forced to accommodate rapid influxes of refugees, the resources are not sufficient to cope with the heavy burden of casualties and illness. Systematic reviews of these crisis points have not yet been written, but observational reports and series studies from specific sites[1–13] consistently describe the cognitive and ethical burdens of triage and medical management that these resource crises impose.

TRIAGE

In Chapter 3, Briggs and Leong outline the classic model of medical disaster response (the civilian MCI model adapted from military medicine). Most medical providers attached to NGOs or to military units working in complex emergencies have been trained in this approach. The perspective, grounded in modern experience, that except in the most unusual and infrequently encountered situations, resources, if properly organized, can be marshaled to meet the needs of all those injured in battle or disaster, is fundamental. Equally fundamental is the reliance on what the term "resources" entails: a robust and highly developed chain of care, a structure of interlocking levels of care capacity sustained by a system of assessment, referral, and transport that safely carries patients to the level appropriate to provide a definitive response to their medical need.[27,28]

The austere environment of humanitarian crises undermines both of these tenets and in turn necessitates important shifts in the function of medical triage.[29–31] Triage and medical treatment often take place at the same site and are conducted by the same team. The chain of care is very short. First-responder stabilization at the scene is often rudimentary or nonexistent. Casualties are brought, or bring themselves, unsorted and unstabilized, to the receiving location. Here the role of triage is "to bring order out of chaos" and at high volume requires unflappable categorizing skills more than deep medical knowledge.[32] Medical response is directed at the survivors of traumatic field conditions. The first step of triage in these settings is also the first in a sequence of medical management decisions that the medical team must revisit continuously until the patient leaves or dies.

1. The only available medical resources are under the direction of the medical triage and treatment team; there is rarely a possibility of systematic evacuation back to a rear zone of higher capacity.
2. Triage becomes the process of deciding upon the priority with which the team itself will take care of the patients. The medical

staff sorts patients not with an eye toward evacuation but with an eye toward what its own current and short-term management capacities are and are likely to be in the days ahead.

3. Immediate stabilization is provided to those patients whom the team will have the capacity to support.

4. The surgical interventions performed are restrictively determined by the skills of available personnel, the extent of postoperative care required, and the need to conserve scarce medications and equipment. Under these restrictive conditions, it may be decided not to perform a procedure that in other circumstances would be considered necessary and definitive or to stage interventions in a manner unfamiliar to surgeons accustomed to work in a high-technology setting.

Triage is known to be a most intellectually and psychologically taxing activity.[33,34] In the conditions described here, when triage becomes an integral part of daily and hourly medical management decisions, the stress is augmented by having to face a fresh volume of unsorted patients each day whose needs conflict with the time and resources required by those present from preceding days. At a certain point of overload, the triage priorities are set to a higher threshold: those who might have been salvaged in days when the team was not working at maximum output are now deliberately not stabilized, in the recognition that there is a physical limit to the medical resources available.

This narrative describes the normative practice of triage in austere settings. What actually happens may vary considerably in practice, depending upon how members of the medical team can maintain the discipline required to make these decisions or on whether external political or military parties intervene in the triage process. Departures from the triage course outlined above may thus occur when medical personnel try to stabilize people for whom there is no sustainable care in the days that follow; or when medical personnel in the face of heavy volume continue to practice triage at the setpoint defined for lower volumes, in which case there are many more patients alive and occupying beds than can be taken care of adequately; or when it is politically impossible to consign patients to an expectant or palliative category and so salvage efforts are undertaken on a basis that is not medical.

MEDICAL TREATMENT ISSUES

A number of important accommodations are necessary for a medical team to deliver appropriate, effective, and humane care in the setting of complex emergencies. The challenges to be met can be described as a combination of technical issues relating to the content and application of medical care and cultural, social, and ethical issues that arise from practicing in alien and often insecure surroundings.

Technical Concerns

Effective medical interventions in these field conditions differ considerably from what expatriate medical personnel are accustomed to employ in their own societies. Although reported experience guides the use of a standard approach to a few key medical conditions arising in field situations, such as oral rehydration therapy and intravenous fluids for cholera, there are many areas where definitive guidance is lacking or significant practice variation still exists:

1. Definitive guidance is still lacking for the austere field treatment of seizures, tetanus, and a range of metabolic and infectious emergencies;
2. Despite the published experience of the ICRC, variation can still be seen in the field management of injuries caused by high-velocity bullets and land mines;
3. Guidance is lacking and field experience still unrecorded regarding the management of some conditions rarely seen in the developed world, such as mid-labor obstetric catastrophes.

A number of senior medical practitioners in the humanitarian medical community are deeply steeped in these issues. Within their own organizations, they have succeeded in transmitting this education to colleagues. For instance, the ICRC approach to traumatic injury has been distilled to a few basic principles relating to fracture fixation, amputation techniques, use of blood transfusions, management of penetrating abdominal injury, and infrastructure requirements.[35–37] As another example, MSF has developed manuals and training regimes for its medical staff that include practical issues of patient assessment and management, such as diagnostic shortcuts based on epidemiological probability, prudent feeding options, choices in pain control, fluid management, and use of standard antibiotics.[38] This body of clinical knowledge relating to field management and surgical practice has not yet, however, been transferred into the medical community at large, still the source of most volunteer medical personnel in humanitarian relief.

Absent this information, as is quietly acknowledged within the humanitarian community, there is now a most uneven state of field competence among emergency medical responders in humanitarian crises, a situation that causes waste, inefficiency, and probably suboptimal outcomes.

Cultural, Social, and Ethical Concerns

Medical professionals taking care of patients in the setting of humanitarian crises work in channels of meaning and implication that few have been trained to understand or sort out.

Culture and religion are known to influence the ways in which people define health, express pain, select among treatment options, deal with grief.[39] The diversity of populations engulfed in complex humanitarian emergencies presents an unmet challenge to expatriate emergency medical responders, who out of ignorance may mistake silence for absence of pain, control for absence of sorrow, and who may not recognize that strong religious scruples are preventing a patient from agreeing to a clinically indicated amputation of a limb.

This practice world is also laden with moral dilemmas and with the cumulative burden of having to make choices among no good options.[40]

1. Because the physical settings of clinics and hospitals are often insecure at night, medical personnel often leave at dusk and do not return for twelve hours. This exit places at risk those patients who may require more intensive monitoring or an emergency intervention during the night. Expanding the number of expatriate staff to provide twenty-four-hour coverage or training local staff are two possible interventions.
2. Expatriate personnel usually have access to a better supply of food and more equipped accommodation than local relief and health workers. In conditions of real scarcity, this privileged access becomes a matter of comment and difficulty. A good

argument can be made that a key responsibility of the relief organization is to keep its personnel in an effective state of performance. Field staff have not been prepared, however, to deal with the moral dissonance that their relative comfort engenders.

3. Evacuation of patients who have attracted the world's attention can sometimes be accomplished in order to promote their individual chances of securing definitive care in the developed world. This option arouses hot and unresolved debate over issues of equity and preference among families and local institutions.[41,42,43]

4. Although this work attracts some of the best and most accomplished medical people in the world, it also wears down everyone over time. Further, a few medical people have been drawn in whose credentials or attitudes are not exemplary. Among the more corrosive factors in the functioning of medical relief teams is the presence of someone who is burned out or who is not making appropriate and humane decisions in terms of patient care. (See Chapter 7.)

5. Erosion of neutral space and resultant personal jeopardy are frequent aspects of humanitarian crises for medical responders. It is very difficult to think clearly and to maintain physical stamina when one is angry, afraid, or anxious about one's own safety. (See Chapter 7.) The recent experience with providing medical relief to refugees in eastern Zaire/Congo and Tanzania would suggest the need for medical NGOs to define in advance, in a coordinated fashion, a tolerance threshold for such encroachment on neutral space above which the teams would pull out.

6. Humanitarian work, including medical relief, now often takes place in contexts where the authorities and many of the patients have committed serious human rights abuses. Although individual medical professionals react differently to this problem, most find it psychologically debilitating to engage in the daily ameliorative acts of medical practice if the underlying political and legal issues are not also being addressed and rectified. For some who see the issue most starkly, working in a space that is not just non-neutral but also morally contaminated becomes unsustainable over time. (See Chapter 9.)

TRAINING AND RECRUITMENT

These issues of environment, triage, and medical treatment combine to define a new realm of medical practice and career commitment. In Europe and Japan, a growing number of postgraduate physicians and nurses are pursuing paths in medical relief, disaster medicine and humanitarian assistance. This trend is beginning to be discernible in the United States as well. The pace of institutional recognition and response to this development has been slow, reflecting a number of factors that are difficult to weigh in terms of relative importance, since none have been systematically assessed.

Observations and lessons from the field are still infrequently reported in the medical literature, in part because career advancement in this practice is less dependent upon publishing articles, in part because it is more difficult to persuade medical journals that these reports have scientific merit and professional relevance, and in part because returning volunteer practitioners are exhausted and must plunge into new jobs.

Organizations that have developed field medicine training manuals and emergency trauma field apprenticeships tend, without incentives to do otherwise, to focus their attention on internal needs. Moreover, resources for addressing gaps in knowledge, educational materials, and training are in general more difficult to secure from governments and donors than funds for service delivery.

The recipients of this emergency medical care have not yet stated their views and preferences. In this silence lies significant information, which, if solicited or expressed, might influence the ways in which the developed world responds to their needs and suffering.

The pedagogical mission in medicine is to transmit knowledge and skills that will promote improvements in practice and research.[44] Several important initiatives are now under way within the NGO community to identify best practices and to disseminate knowledge relating to refugee public health and the overall delivery of humanitarian relief.[45] Similar efforts could be organized for the subject area of emergency medical care in these crises. The basis now exists for a serious attempt, on the part of seasoned engaged clinicians to develop rigorous practical training programs and best practice guidelines for the entire humanitarian community. Such an attempt, requiring a relatively modest effort and expenditure, would support the aspirations and morale of current emergency medical responders, strengthen preparation of the next wave of personnel, and improve the emergency medical care that is delivered in these humanitarian crises laced with war.

For as long as migration and conflict continue to define world patterns of distress, medical response to these crises will continue to consume resources, preoccupy some subset of the medical profession, and exert an influence on the immediate health outcomes of hundreds of thousands of people who are injured in these events. It is an investment in the future to begin to make sure that this influence is as beneficial as we can make it.

II

MENTAL HEALTH

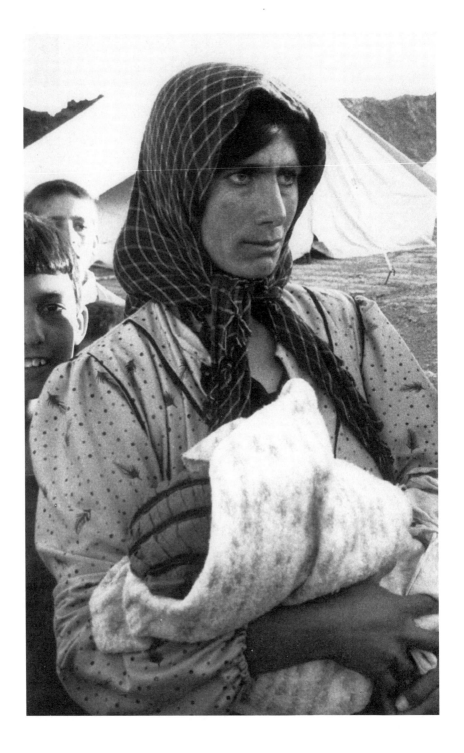

5

DISASTER MENTAL HEALTH:
THE U.S. EXPERIENCE AND BEYOND

brian w. flynn

At any given time, efforts are under way around the world to deal with the psychological sequelae of disasters and of humanitarian crises. The organized response to natural and technological disasters in the United States provides a perspective that can enrich the emerging world dialogue about disaster mental health.

DISASTER MENTAL HEALTH IN CONTEXT

The current state of research and practice in disaster mental health, including the mental health consequences of complex humanitarian emergencies, is a function of the relative newness of this field and of the changing intellectual context from which our understanding is emerging. Prior to the 1970s, generally speaking, the psychological consequences of disaster were viewed and treated from a psychoanalytic perspective (Box 5.1).

Beginning in the 1970s, a number of factors have contributed to the development of the field and continue to influence it today. Several key changes provide a framework for understanding this evolution: increased knowledge of the biological components of mental illness; the expansion of community-based care; the erosion of the stigma associated with mental

PRIOR TO 1970	1970 TO PRESENT
Psychological consequences of disaster viewed and treated from a psychoanalytic perspective	Improved understanding of biological factors in Post-Traumatic Stress Disorder (PTSD), depression, anxiety, etc.; availability of effective psychotropic medications
Hospitalization for difficult mental health problems	Expansion of community-based care and coordinated service systems
Social stigma attached to mental health problems	Erosion of negative attitudes and "normalization" of psychological problems

illness; and the appreciation of stress-related trauma that emerged from the Vietnam War.

The Biological Components of Mental Illness

The 1970s initiated a period of rapid and continuing development of our understanding of the biological factors that play a critical part in mental illness and in acute and chronic stress. Today, knowledge about the biological components of post traumatic stress disorder (PTSD), depression, anxiety, and other mental health problems is growing at a dramatic pace. The availability of effective psychotropic medications and our understanding of the appropriate application of these drugs is evolving steadily.

Community Mental Health

Prior to the mid-1960s, most mental health problems that were not easily dealt with in the office of a mental health professional often resulted in hospitalization. The 1960s saw the dramatic expansion of community-based care, the key conceptual components of which include the treatment of people close to where they live, an increasing understanding of the role of environment and support in coping with mental health problems, the acknowledgment of the role of natural care givers, and the importance of coordinated service systems. Many of these concepts are now central to U.S. disaster mental health response.

Stigma

Although stigma attached to experiencing, acknowledging, and seeking treatment for psychological problems still flourishes in some parts of the world, these negative attitudes began to erode in the mid-1960s. The "normalization" of psychological problems continues today and has been a significant factor in allowing people to understand the psychological sequelae of disasters and to accept, if not seek out, assistance.

The Vietnam War

Probably more than any other single event, the Vietnam War raised awareness within the U.S. mental health community of the effects of traumatic stress. Prior to this war, mental health professionals treating victims of trauma had little understanding of this condition. They had inadequate diagnostic categories and were faced with a large number of people clearly in need of help who could not, or would not, be helped by the established treatment system. What has emerged—and continues to emerge—from this post-Vietnam individual, family, and societal struggle is an acknowledgment and an understanding of the terrible, debilitating effects of traumatic exposure, a better understanding of the role of social support in trauma recovery (and its exacerbation in the absence of such support), and an appreciation for the long-term nature of recovery from trauma. The introduction of the diagnosis of PTSD and of acute traumatic stress both occurred in the post-Vietnam era.

PSYCHOLOGICAL RESPONSE TO DISASTER: FINDINGS FROM THE RESEARCH LITERATURE

Difficulties and Limitations

Much of the existing general disaster research does not address health effects. Further, the few early studies that look at health effects do not examine psychological issues. The lack of focus on mental health concerns in disaster research was observed nearly a quarter century ago by Kinston and Rosser[1] who, by way of illustration, point out that there was a seventeen-year delay before a systematic and detailed study of the psychological and social effects of the atomic bombing of Hiroshima was undertaken.

From the perspective of the service planner or provider, the research in disaster mental health provides frustratingly little systematic information. A few researchers have looked at the psychological impact of nuclear war and have raised important comments about the ways in which psychological response to natural disasters, to war, and to toxic technological emergencies have similar and overlapping features. Thompson,[2] in a chapter focused primarily on the psychological impact of nuclear war, discusses at length what is known about mental health reactions to natural disasters. Lifton, Markusen, and Austin[3] discuss psychological sequelae of natural disasters (especially the flooding in Buffalo Creek, West Virginia), the atomic bombings of Hiroshima and Nagasaki, other war situations, and Nazi concentration camps.

Conducting research in disaster mental health is difficult.[4,5] Several recent reviews of the literature[4,6,7,8] note that research is plagued by methodological problems, including difficulty obtaining adequate controls and getting both pre- and post-measures, and by many intervening variables. Solomon[9] describes a number of challenges in conducting disaster research, including defining the disaster, defining the stressors, identifying consequences, addressing the wide variety of community and other social mediators, and measuring the impact of interventions. There is no consistent definition of disaster "exposure." As a further complication, both victims and relief organizations often resist investigation.[1]

Most of the research has focused on pathological outcomes and on people who seek care, rather than on community-based assessments of entire exposed populations. This orientation provides only part of the picture, as is clear from both the research and the service sectors. Many people have neutral or even positive outcomes following disaster exposure.[10,11,12,13]

Contemporary research, however, has not focused on these latter two groups. Research to date focuses almost exclusively on clinical symptomatology and the development of psychopathology. Moreover, there is virtually no body of quality-controlled research on the impact of mental health interventions (positive or not) following disasters.

Findings to Date

Perhaps the single most comprehensive review of the research has been compiled by Green and Solomon,[14] who find that symptoms seem to increase as a function of exposure, particularly if the exposure involves a life threat, loss of loved ones, property loss, significant community disruption, or exposure to death. The authors note, however, that we lack a consistent and agreed-upon definition of exposure.

Nature of Exposure

The little research that compares disaster exposure with other types of psychological trauma seems to suggest that there are fewer symptoms following natural disasters than there are after other types of traumatic events, particularly events involving victimization. Victimization refers to a wide variety of experiences, such as those resulting from physical assault, terrorist incidents, torture, and other crimes. Reports following the Oklahoma City bombing, submitted by the crisis counseling program funded through the Center for Mental Health Services of the U.S. Public Health Service, have indicated that victims, their families, and emergency response personnel experienced more serious and longer-lasting psychological symptomatology than was seen following the 1993 flooding in the Midwest.

The research addressing psychological symptoms after natural versus human-caused disasters nevertheless notes that although the nature of the similarities and differences is not fully understood, there are more similarities than differences. Bromet[15] presents a good overview of technological disasters in the context of an analysis of research following the Three Mile Island nuclear power plant accident, and Butcher and Dunn[16] describe not only the primary trauma of aircraft disasters for survivors and families of victims but also the secondary trauma of dealing with news media and "ambulance-chasing" attorneys. With technological disasters involving radiation or other toxic emissions or spills, illness may emerge over long periods of time and space, making the "event" more difficult to see, to identify, to understand, and to structure cognitively. In a particularly thoughtful article, Erickson speculates about a number of factors that make these types of events both different from natural disasters and more psychologically unmanageable: a general perception that radiation and various toxins are seen as more threatening than other disaster agents; the lack of a predictable script with a beginning, middle, and end; and the absence of a tangible aspect to the destructive agent, which often cannot be smelled, tasted, or touched.[17]

Persistence of Symptoms

Green and Solomon's review of the research is relatively consistent in reporting post-exposure increases in lifetime rates of depression, anxiety, and post-traumatic stress disorder. Rates vary widely in various studies, particularly for PTSD (5–23 percent). In addition, there are observed increases in several definable behaviors such as medical visits, visits to mental health practitioners and clinics, sick leave, sleep disturbance, and concentration difficulties.

Longitudinal research in this area is rare. One particularly well controlled study of survivors of the 1972 Buffalo Creek dam collapse in West Virginia showed significant symptomatology as late as fourteen years after the event.[18] In an earlier study of this same incident, Lifton and Olson observed significant symptomatology (including intrusive images of death, fear of crowds, sleep disorders, and nightmares) twenty-seven to thirty months following the flood.[19] A study of suicide within four years after natural disasters in the United States between 1982 and 1989 revealed a marked increase in rates after floods, hurricanes, and earthquakes.[20]

Other studies of natural disasters seem to show that symptoms decrease over time.[21,22] Possible exceptions to symptom abatement include anger and hostility following human-caused disasters, which may stay the same or actually increase over time. This phenomenon may be a result of prolonged litigation, which sometimes prevents victims and survivors from proceeding with their lives and may cause conflict between what is in an individual's best legal interest and what is in his or her best psychological interest.

The intensity and duration of the visual impact of the disaster may influence the collective psychological impact on a community. An event that leaves little visual impact denies the community a common reference point. Survivors often report that "everyone seems to have forgotten the flood" when the damage is not dramatic. When damage is dramatic and visible for long periods of time, as it was following Hurricane Andrew in Florida, constant negative stimuli may affect not only individuals but the larger community as well. Green,[23] Bolin,[24] and Myers[25] describe factors relevant to understanding how event characteristics influence psychological response (Box 5.2).

Demographic Factors

Gender and age   Research into personal characteristics as they relate to disaster symptomatology (Box 5.3) produces mixed findings in nearly all areas, including gender[26,27] and age.[28,29,30] Some studies indicate little differential on the basis of gender; others indicate that women may be more vulnerable. Research suggests that middle-aged people may be at particular

---

Box 5.2 Factors affecting psychological response

- Exposure to threat
- Exposure to physical harm or injury
- Exposure to the grotesque
- Sudden violent loss of a loved one
- Witnessing or learning of the violent death of a loved one
- Learning of exposure to a noxious agent
- Causing death or severe harm to another
- Exposure to intentional injury or harm
- Lack of warning
- Abrupt contrast of the scene (for example, airplane debris and bodies raining down on a peaceful neighborhood)
- Uncertain duration of the event
- Time of occurrence (disasters occurring at night are more disturbing than ones occurring during the day)
- Scope of the event (the more deaths, injuries, and damage there are, the greater the psychological impact)
- Human error
- Properties of the post-disaster environment (weather conditions, poor living conditions, frustration)

Box 5.3 Demographics and post-disaster symptomatology

GENDER	• Women may be more vulnerable than men
AGE	• Middle-aged people may be at particular risk because of increased responsibilities
	• Children have limited coping history, lack a "temporal sense"
	• Elderly have successful coping skills, but limited horizon and impaired health status may increase risk for disaster-related stress
PRIOR MENTAL HEALTH HISTORY	• Mentally ill often do well soon after disaster; risks increase over time
FAMILY AND COMMUNITY CHARACTERISTICS	• Family discord and individual parental pathology may contribute to PTSD in children
	• Single parents at higher risk
	• Married women may be at higher risk than married men because of multiple expectations
	• Community cohesiveness has positive effect

risk because, at least in American society, they may have simultaneous responsibilities for themselves, for their children, and for aging parents. Following a disaster, therefore, they may experience increased demands from all sides. The mental health service experience shows very dramatically that children have difficulty following disaster, primarily because of their limited understanding of what is happening, their lack of experience, and their immature coping skills. They are often unable to process cognitively the complex events that dominate their lives following disaster, and they lack a "temporal sense" to inform them that the experience will not go on indefinitely.

The service field also identifies the elderly as a risk group, because although they have a longer history of successful coping and can recover dramatically when they are helped to reestablish those coping strategies and skills, much of the recovery assistance, so valuable to younger people in rebuilding their lives following disasters, has little relevance to older people. Elderly people who have lost a home that was paid for and that was their major fiscal legacy to their children are seldom comforted by being able to obtain a low-interest mortgage toward the purchase of a new house. In addition, the elderly may have impaired health status that places them at risk for disaster-related stress.

Race and ethnicity   Green and Solomon also find that race and ethnicity yield mixed results,[14] as do educational level and the existence of prior psychological problems. Issues of race and ethnicity tend to become difficult to differentiate clearly from factors such as socioeconomic status, availability and intactness of support systems, and historical help-seeking behavior.

Prior Mental Health History

Experience in the mental health services sector suggests that people in communities who have severe and persistent mental illness often do very well in the early days following a disaster (as do most people). Only later do they present significantly increased risk, resulting primarily from the decomposition of the community support system upon which they rely heavily.[31]

Family and Community Characteristics

Research on the importance of social and community mediators[14] indicates that the immediate social environment can be extraordinarily important in predicting individual outcomes. For example, how a mother responds to a disaster may be far more important than the actual disaster exposure that her child experiences. With respect to other family characteristics, family discord and individual parental pathology seem to be contributing factors to PTSD in children. Single parents are at higher risk primarily because they may suffer the loss of their emotional support system following a disaster.

Findings on marital status show that, for women, being married may pose an increased risk factor. One interpretation of this finding is that women in Western culture frequently play many draining and time-consuming roles, such as caregiver, provider, spouse, and parent, and thus when disaster strikes, these multiple roles make heightened demands on married women that may place them at increased risk. Ironically, because of these very characteristics of family life, married men appear to do better.

Community cohesiveness following a disaster seems to have a positive effect on individual response and may have an impact on those members of the community who did not experience direct disaster loss. A tornado may rip through a town but not every home is lost. Nonetheless, the basic fabric of the community may be seriously compromised and there may be serious adverse psychological impact on all those who live in the town, including those who were not directly affected.

PSYCHOLOGICAL RESPONSE TO DISASTERS: FINDINGS BASED ON EXPERIENCE AND OBSERVATION

Because of deficiencies in research, much of what we know (or, more accurately, believe) about sound disaster mental health services comes largely from experience and from published but nonempirical observation. Consideration of the following factors may be helpful to those planning for, or providing, disaster mental health response.

Types, Phases, and Symptoms of Psychological Response

Types   In his study of the Buffalo Creek, West Virginia, dam failure[19] Lifton describes two types of trauma that occur following disaster:

- individual trauma, defined as "a blow to the psyche that breaks through one's defenses so suddenly and with such brutal force that one cannot react to it effectively";
- collective trauma, defined as "a blow to the basic tissues of social life that damages the bonds attaching people together and impairs the prevailing sense of community."

Phases   The psychological impact of disasters occurs in stages or phases (Box 5.4). What happens to people psychologically is very different six days after a disaster than it is after six months, and this affects the services they need. People go through a predictable sequence of phases, but this progression is not linear and is significantly affected by the nature of the event and what is happening in an individual's community. A one-time event may

Box 5.4 Phases of psychological response

- Warning

- Alarm

- Stun reaction followed by heroism

- Inventory and rescue (affective extremes)

- "Honeymoon" period (appreciation, relief, gratitude)

- Anger and disillusionment

- Resolution

have a different impact from one with a high probability (real or perceived) of recurrence a day, a week, or a month later. Several discussions of disaster phases are available.[1,2,24,32,33,34,35] All of these descriptions are variations on a similar theme that incorporates the following pattern.

When and if warning occurs, psychological defenses are activated and people respond in a wide variety of ways consistent with their coping style and social context. This phase is sometimes followed by an alarm that usually heightens anxiety, resulting in various psychophysiological reactions. At the moment of impact there is frequently a relatively short stun reaction. During this phase, we sometimes hear of deeds involving great heroism. Following impact there is usually an inventory and rescue phase in which people may experience many affective extremes, depending on their experience and loss. Joy, relief, fear, grief, and other very individualized responses are typically seen at this time. Communities and individuals frequently enter a "honeymoon" period at this point, during which there are expressions of appreciation, relief, and gratitude for the sparing of those people and community elements not killed or destroyed.

Following this "relief" period, there is almost always a period of anger and disillusionment. People come to appreciate fully the magnitude of their losses; recovery does not occur with the rapidity expected; and people be-

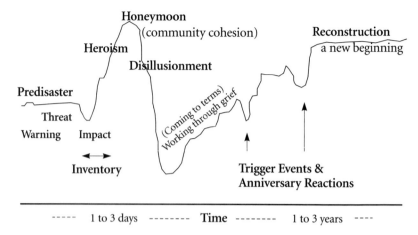

Figure 5.1 Phases of psychological response to disaster. (Myers and Zunin[36])

come angry with insurance companies and relief agencies for failing to meet expectations. Finally, there is typically a resolution phase in which people incorporate the disaster experience and loss and move ahead with their lives. Some are left with the psychological scars of the experience; some change little from the way they were prior to the disaster; and some appear to become stronger and better able to cope in the future. Figure 5.1 is a graphic depiction of the stages of psychological response developed by Myers and Zunin.[36]

Symptoms of Disaster-Related Stress

Descriptions of the symptoms of major disaster-related conditions such as PTSD, major depressive episodes, and acute stress disorder are easily available and are well known to most mental health practitioners.[37] What may be less apparent to disaster survivors and to those who serve them are the signs of disaster-related stress that frequently exist at a subsyndromal level (Box 5.5).[38] Longer-term signs may include decreased job or school performance, marital problems, and recurring nightmares. A comprehensive discussion of disaster symptomatology is provided by Wilkinson and Vera.[39] In a particularly good description of psychological sequelae following the Buffalo Creek disaster, Lifton and Olson describe psychic numbing (the diminished capacity for feelings of all types) and the impairment of post-disaster

Box 5.5 Symptoms of disaster-related stress (PTSD, major depressive episodes, acute stress disorder, etc.)

PHYSICAL
- Increased heartbeat and blood pressure
- Nausea
- Sweating or chills
- Tics
- Fine motor tremors
- Headaches
- Lower back pain
- Feeling a "lump in the throat"
- Exaggerated startle response
- Fatigue
- Decreased resistance to infection

BEHAVIORAL
- Change in general activity level
- Decreased efficiency
- Difficulty communicating effectively
- Inability to rest
- Changes in eating or sleep patterns
- Changes in patterns of intimacy or sexuality
- Increased use of alcohol/tobacco/drugs
- Social withdrawal
- Proneness to accidents

(continued)

Box 5.5 (continued)

COGNITIVE	• Reduced attention span
	• Concentration difficulties
	• Difficulty making decisions
	• Tunnel vision
	• Anomia
	• Slowness of thinking
	• Blaming
	• Inability to stop thinking about the disaster
EMOTIONAL	• Crying easily
	• Mood swings
	• Inappropriate affect
	• Feeling invulnerable
	• Anxiety, anger, irritability
	• Guilt or "survivor guilt" (see Lifton and Olson[19] for an excellent discussion of this phenomenon)
	• Hopelessness, apathy

relationships. Here, victims carrying an unfocused rage are in need of nurturing but are suspicious of those who provide it.[19]

Important Moderators of Response

Exposure   Exposure has many meanings. As noted above, the magnitude of exposure appears to be consistently correlated with the severity of psychological response. One does not have to experience or be damaged by an event directly, however, to have a significant psychological response to it. Those who view disasters on television are often quite disturbed by what they see. Those who respond directly to disasters, such as police, medical workers, and fire and rescue personnel, as well as those people who come from afar to assist, often experience serious stress. Families who take in their family members who have been made homeless by disaster frequently become secondary psychological casualties. In addition, survivor guilt is a phenomenon demonstrating that one does not even have to be in the vicinity of a disaster to experience serious reactions.

Multiple stressors   The disaster itself is often only the first stressor. Dealing with relief agencies (particularly governmental agencies), loss of a job, loss of community status, or a changed sociocultural mix in the community are all experiences that may occur following a disaster and may actually be more significant, over time, than exposure to the disaster agent itself. Acknowledging the relationship between psychological health and physical health is important. Those who have been injured in a disaster event may face prolonged medical interventions and may experience protracted periods of treatment and rehabilitation. Diminished health status is a key risk factor in the development of psychological symptomatology.[40] In cases in which the disaster agent involves chemical, biological, or nuclear exposure, the potential for unknown health effects on the person exposed, or on his or her children, is a particularly significant stressor.

COMPONENTS OF DISASTER MENTAL HEALTH INTERVENTION

Three main elements make up an effective disaster mental health intervention: appropriate training and supervision, appropriate overall organization of the service delivery, and an appropriate content and approach to intervention.

Training

Proper training is essential for work in disaster mental health. Very few mental health professionals emerge from educational programs trained to do this type of work. Many concepts and techniques that are appropriate in traditional mental health services simply do not apply in disaster work. Methods that rely on the reflective and insight-oriented techniques of psychotherapy, in particular, are often not seen as helpful by disaster survivors. Survivors, at least in the period immediately following a disaster, need very concrete, explicit, and directive help. This type of intervention frequently runs contrary to traditional mental health training. Because many people do not turn to mental health professionals following disasters, it is critical that training be provided not only for mental health service providers but also for others to whom disaster survivors turn for assistance, such as school personnel, clergy, primary care physicians, or community elders. To target this training requires knowledge of and sensitivity to the natural caregiving patterns of communities.

Experience in the U.S. crisis counseling program, at the federal level, has consistently shown that a blend of professionals and trained non-professionals is the most effective provider mix. In disaster mental health, disaster survivors are primarily dealing with normal people, responding normally, to very abnormal situations. Although the involvement of mental health professionals is critical, much of the frontline work does not require the full armamentarium of a mental health professional. Trained nonprofessionals who are mature, comfortable with an outreach model, knowledgeable about the community and its culture, and aware of community resources can perform much of this work very well. In the context of refugee situations, Hiegel[41] describes the use of indigenous caregivers in Thai border camps.

For this mixture of professionals and nonprofessionals to work, three components are required:

1. nonprofessional workers must be well trained and supervised throughout the program period;
2. nonprofessional workers must be supervised by mental health professionals;
3. nonprofessionals must have easy access to a smoothly functioning referral system to handle those cases that are beyond their level of training. Components of such a referral system should include an established number of quickly available referral sources and a minimum of procedural barriers to care.

The provision of services in nonclinical settings such as disaster sites or refugee camps requires a number of special considerations that should be a part of any training: licensure, confidentiality, and research.

Licensure issues A provider of services licensed in the jurisdiction should be aware of how the licensing authority interprets the legal limits and standards of care in disaster settings. Providers should be aware that their licenses may not be valid for providing services in other jurisdictions.

Confidentiality   Because a formal treatment relationship does not usually exist in disaster situations or in humanitarian crises, confidentiality laws may not apply. It is usually prudent, when appropriate, to inform those being seen of the service provider's intentions with regard to confidentiality and of any limits on the confidentiality of individual information and/or legal protections.

Research   Service providers are often tempted to conduct research while providing assistance or to use individual information in research-related activities following the event. They do so at great risk. Seldom have disaster victims given informed consent in these situations, and the concerns of such human subjects have almost never been addressed in the literature. Solomon[9] discusses a variety of issues regarding the protection of research respondents and suggests that initial contact (for research purposes) be postponed until acute stress has subsided and victims are able to make reasoned choices about research participation. In addition, mixing service and research agendas in disaster situations has led to serious political problems when sponsoring or support agencies feel that access has been abused or manipulated and when victims/survivors feel that they have been used rather than served.

In the rush to provide services to those desperately in need, legal issues have historically been overlooked. As the response to humanitarian and natural disasters becomes more planned and formal (and less ad hoc and spontaneous), clarification of legal issues must become part of planning and preparedness.

Organization of Services Provided

Important characteristics of the service system include outreach, consultation, and education.

Outreach   Programs must be outreach oriented. Mental health professionals who wait for people to come to them and who see people only in their offices are likely to experience little or no disaster-related work. Services are best provided where people work, live, or gather (for example, schools, churches, homes, and shelters).

Consultation   Appropriate interventions, in addition to counseling, include consultation with other civic institutions or organizations involved in the immediate or longer-term recovery period. City councils, village elders, or development agencies all make decisions having an impact on people's lives, and all may need guidance regarding how the disaster has affected the psychological health of the community.

Education Targeted education, for example to primary care physicians,[42] is important, and information geared toward the general public is also essential. Contrary to reported disaster experience outside disaster mental health, many in the mental health community have found the media invaluable in helping individuals understand what they are going through and how and where to get help. Following disasters, members of the media are frequently seeking stories that provide a unique or unusual side of the disaster experience. They are often very willing to feature accounts of what people are experiencing psychologically and how they can be helped. Care must be taken to ensure that comments by mental health professionals do not reveal specifics about individuals but remain generic. Television stations are often willing to develop and air public service announcements regarding psychological sequelae and services.

Interventions

If the research with respect to psychological consequences of disasters is incomplete, the research on effective interventions is nearly nonexistent.

Box 5.6 Successful disaster mental health intervention strategies

---

- Assume victims have coping skills and ability
- Help people understand that what they are experiencing is normal
- Engage in directive caregiving
- Assist people in organizing and prioritizing tasks to reduce stress
- Listen actively to repeated accounts of a survivor's experience
- Discourage blame
- Help survivors set realistic expectations for recovery
- Establish working referral system, including local and outside service providers

---

Ursano, Fullerton, and Norwood[43] provide a useful model for incorporating patient care, community consultation, and preventive medicine.

Early service experience[34] and current practice point to several important counseling intervention characteristics (Box 5.6). These factors have not, however, been formally measured and evaluated. Testing of these intervention characteristics (which have guided much disaster and emergency response) is sorely needed as trauma mental health grows as a recognized field.

Assumed competence   The guiding principle of disaster mental health, that survivors are demonstrating a normal response to abnormal situations, is very important. It should be assumed, until shown otherwise, that people have the skills and ability to cope (given information, support, and assistance) with what they have experienced. This approach differs from that of many traditional mental health interventions where the first goal is to provide a diagnosis. Disaster workers are aided by the fact that most adults have already experienced some type of difficult traumatic event in their lives and have come through psychologically intact. Eliciting this history, detailing previous coping mechanisms, and trying to reestablish those mechanisms can be a great help.

Normalization   Helping people understand that what they are experiencing is normal is, in itself, a significant intervention. Experienced disaster mental health workers have all heard people make statements such as, "I can deal much better with this now that I know I am not going crazy," or, "I really didn't associate what I am experiencing now with what happened to me in that hurricane six months ago. Now that I understand what is going on, I can cope better."

Directive care giving   Many people respond well to very directive care giving following a disaster. Most disaster survivors are not looking for insight or assistance with existential issues. They want concrete assistance with specific types of problems. Furthermore, a crisis counselor may have the opportunity to see a person only once or twice. Because most mental health professionals have not been trained to be directive, the disaster crisis counselor needs to rethink approaches to individuals and find clear and innovative ways to provide what is often very proscriptive guidance to disaster survivors.

Help in organizing tasks   Assistance in organizing tasks is an example of nontraditional assistance. There are enormous numbers of tasks to be accomplished after one has lost a home or been forced to flee one's community. People can be stressed to the point of immobilization by the immensity and complexity of the problems they face. A significant role for helpers, in the psychological sense, is to assist people in organizing and prioritizing what needs to be done. This type of assistance is a significant stress reducer.

Active and repeated listening Listening to repeated accounts of a survivor's experience often has a very therapeutic effect. Active listening to what happened is a way to normalize the experience. Repeated telling of the trauma story affords increasing control over it.

Discouraging blame Discouraging blame is important in assisting survivors as they progress through the phases of disaster response. The progression is slowed when people become fixated on who is to blame and who is responsible for the loss they have incurred. There may be important differences between natural and human-caused disasters in this area.

Realistic expectations Keeping expectations reasonable is important. In well-intended but naive efforts to comfort, many people make promises to disaster survivors: "things will be back to normal soon"; "pretty soon you won't even remember how traumatic this experience was." Many of these promises are never realized. Besides breeding distrust, promising what cannot be fulfilled can jeopardize an entire program of services. Beyond initial outreach most intervention programs count on word-of-mouth referral to reach communities. Credibility is critical. Good programming (as with any good health or mental health intervention) relies heavily upon trust based on the provider's clarity and credibility about what can be accomplished within a certain time frame. People often expect to be restored more quickly and more fully than reality permits.

Referral The establishment of a working referral system is important. Disaster service programs need established referral systems with resources that include health professionals, mental health professionals, and social services. Much early disaster response and recovery service is provided by individuals and groups who come to assist from outside the disaster area. Even those who are from the area may be engaged in disaster recovery activities on a time-limited basis. It is crucial that planners and providers of mental health services understand that often others will have to cope with work that is left unfinished when mental health interventions cease or become constricted. As both a clinical and a political matter, those who assist in mental health interventions must work in a close and sensitive way with those who will remain when outside services stop.

If services are being provided by trained nonprofessionals, referral is usually necessary when someone is demonstrating signs associated with a serious psychiatric condition (for example, suicidal ideation, delusions or hallucinations, immobility, compulsive ritualistic behavior, or disorientation). A sound schema for evaluating suicide potential in disaster situations is described by Wilkinson and Vera.[39] The mechanism of referral should be established early by the individual or group organizing the mental health effort.

Potential referral sources should be briefed on the type of experience the person has undergone, and it is often helpful to include potential referral sources in any or all training opportunities. Care must be taken to make referrals in a culturally competent manner, understanding that there are enormous differences in the ways various ethnic groups understand and cope with psychiatric problems.

At the point when formal referrals are made, payment for services typically becomes an issue. The cost of services, the sources and requirements for payment, and the ability of the person being referred to make payment should all be considered.

Cultural considerations The importance of cultural factors is frequently magnified in disasters of all kinds, where the recipients of care may come from various cultural backgrounds, may find themselves in a culture different from their own, and where the providers of care may be of a different racial, ethnic, and cultural background. Different cultures view mental health problems in different ways. The attitudes of some groups may be very closely tied to religious and spiritual beliefs. In some cultures mental illness is a source of shame; in others there may not be a well-defined or obvious conceptualization of mental health problems. Cultural groups also vary considerably in the way they cope with psychological problems. In most Western cultures, for example, talking about one's problems is encouraged. In many Asian groups, talking to others about one's problems is often considered inappropriate.

The provider of mental health services must understand both the individual and the cultural history of those being served in order to improve both the accuracy of the diagnosis and the appropriateness of the intervention. Martin[44] points out that trauma and stress among refugees is often cumulative. Prior to becoming refugees they may have experienced violence, sexual abuse, and other traumas that continue when they become displaced. He recommends that outsiders help refugees run their own programs.

The importance of cultural variables can be seen in two examples.

In the early 1980s the United States experienced one of its largest acute immigration emergencies. Approximately 125,000 Cubans left the port of Marial bound for the United States. At the same time, a large number of Haitian refugees arrived. The two groups were very different in nearly all respects. When it became apparent that the Marial population contained many people with physical and mental health problems as well as many individuals from Cuban prisons, the immigrants were detained in a series of camps within the United States. Because of the unclear immigration status of the Haitian refugees, large numbers were similarly detained for extended periods.

During this period, the Cuban Haitian Mental Health Unit at the National Institute of Mental Health was given the task of ensuring the appropriate mental health care of both the Marial Cubans and the Haitians.

Significant numbers of the detained Cubans arrived at the camp infirmaries with dramatic, but superficial, non-life-threatening, self-inflicted injuries (for example, large superficial abdominal lacerations or subcutaneous injection of cleaning fluid). At first, these were treated as cases with a significant psychiatric component and were initially diagnosed as suicide attempts. In reality, the situation was more complex and often less psychiatrically significant. Providers soon learned that there was a widespread sense among the entrants, based on their experience in Cuba, that in order to obtain care or gain admission to a health care facility, their presenting problem needed to be very dramatic. In addition, it became clear that the infirmaries within the camps were seen by the entrants as the safest places to be and were often the only facilities that were air conditioned. Without insight into cultural history and background, providers might easily have overdiagnosed or overinterpreted behavior that might in other settings be indicative of psychological disorder.

In another camp, housing Haitians exclusively, a young man who had been discussing suicide told a personal story that was both unexpected and sad. He readily admitted that he was seriously considering killing himself. He had a wife and young children in Haiti and had financed his passage to the United States by obtaining funds from a loan shark. His original plan, like that of generations before him, was to obtain work in his new country, pay off the loan, and then bring his family to join him. He, with so many others, had been detained immediately upon arrival and was unable to begin repaying the loan. He had been in the camp nearly a year, and his future was very uncertain. He received word from home that the loan shark was threatening to kill members of his family if the loan was not repaid. He believed that if he were dead, word of this fact would get back to the loan shark, who would realize there was no possibility of repayment and therefore leave his family alone. There was a frightening and compelling logic to his plan. Although there were clearly serious psychological elements in understanding this man's plight and determining how to assist him, his story emphasizes the importance of obtaining an in-depth understanding of the individual and collective histories of those being served. In this case, intervention needed to focus far more on cognitive strategies than on affective change.

RECOMMENDATIONS FOR IMPROVING DISASTER RESEARCH AND SERVICE

The field of disaster mental health faces a number of cross-cutting issues and challenges.

Linking Services, Training, and Research

Few mental health training programs in the United States include formal disaster curricula. Only a few (for example, the University of South Dakota) have specific courses and programs. Ideally, services, training, and research should be linked. A number of suggestions can be made to enhance this collaboration.

- Academic training programs should recognize the importance of disaster mental health and develop courses appropriate to the field.
- Providers of continuing education should offer expanded opportunities in disaster mental health.

- Organizations funding disaster research should place high priority on proposals seeking to explore topics related to disaster service.
- Organizations funding disaster research should encourage research into the efficacy of various disaster mental health interventions and into the evaluation of disaster service programs. The service community has many beliefs and considerable experience stemming from a long history in practice, but there is a desperate need for good applied research and program evaluation to assess the efficacy of various interventions.
- Organizations and individuals involved in providing services in disasters and complex humanitarian emergencies should more broadly disseminate and publish their experiences, with careful attention to the identification of areas where research is needed.
- The knowledge base about mental health, in addition to mental illness, needs dramatic expansion. Most mental health professionals are trained to diagnose and treat people with mental disorders. Disaster mental health services are not primarily concerned with mental disorders or mental illness, about which we know an increasing amount. The focus in disasters is on mental health— what makes and keeps people healthy—about which we know little. The mental health field needs to be asking many more questions about the nature of resiliency and psychological well-being.

Structural Considerations

If disaster mental health services are to function optimally, stable organizational and political structures must support and house them. Even the United States, with its comparatively vast public and private sector resources, gives scant support to the community-based disaster mental health response. U.S. federal programs operate through the states, where mental health authorities have many competing priorities. Unless a state experiences frequent disasters, planning and preparedness for such emergencies is at best a secondary consideration.

Furthermore, the role of community mental health in the United States was far more comprehensive in past decades than it is now, as changes in health care finance and organization have forced the public mental health system to deal almost exclusively with people who have serious and persistent mental illness. The traditional programs of consultation, education, comprehensive outpatient services, school services, and services for the elderly are largely gone, and it is difficult for community mental health centers to mount the comprehensive programs for the general population that are appropriate with disaster mental health programs. Attention to the philosophical, political, and fiscal context into which all disaster mental health planning and service must fit is essential, regardless of where in the world the need arises.

Disseminating and Applying Knowledge, Experience, and Information

Despite significant gaps, the disaster mental health community has acquired significant knowledge and expertise in assessing and responding to psychological aspects of disasters. Through Internet access and widespread international consultation, these insights can be shared and the knowledge base expanded.

The Internet contains an increasing amount of disaster-related information. (Quality control, however, as with all Internet resources, is a significant problem.) The Emergency Services and Disaster Relief Branch (ESDRB) at the U.S. Center for Mental Health Services has established a Web site, <http//www.mentalhealth.org>, where a growing amount of information is available. That Web site also provides links to other disaster-related Web sites. In addition, ESDRB is developing a periodic newsletter (available as hard copy and electronically) that will report both significant highlights from disaster service programs and emerging research findings.

Consultation is another important way to share knowledge. International organizations should be encouraged to promote consultative opportunities and exchange programs in this area. In addition to U.S. governmental resources, the American Red Cross has developed disaster mental health expertise and provides assistance in the field. The International Federation of Red Cross and Red Crescent Societies is beginning to provide this service internationally. Several agencies within the UN system (UNICEF and UNHCR in particular) are developing methods and resources for responding to the enormous mental health needs of populations entrusted to their care.

The United States has been very fortunate in its disaster response experience compared with other parts of the world. Natural disasters for the most part have been less destructive in the United States than they have been elsewhere; immigration and refugee emergencies have been infrequent and comparatively minor; there has always been a governmental and volunteer network capable of timely and comprehensive response. In many other areas of the world, either there has been no functioning health or mental health system to build upon in times of disaster, or the collapse of government has itself been an integral part of the disaster, war, or humanitarian crisis. It is crucial that the local and international response to these crises include the integration of mental health with the relief and development effort. The rapid deployment of experts in the field of disaster mental health as part of response activities would be a first step toward ensuring that psychological issues are not forgotten in the crush of other, more visible, and usually more dramatic needs.

POSTSCRIPT: THE ESDRB CRISIS COUNSELING AND TRAINING PROGRAM

While the structure of governmental response to the psychological sequelae of major disasters has not been a major focus of this chapter, a limited description of one country's methodology may be of interest. The Emergency Services and Disaster Relief Branch of the U.S. Public Health Service oversees a major grant program, funded by the Federal Emergency Management Agency (FEMA). This program, part of the legislation directing FEMA's operation and entitled the Crisis Counseling and Training Program, makes available grants to states to provide crisis counseling and educational services following presidentially declared disasters. Services are provided for approximately a year following the disaster event and can be continued longer when needs continue to overwhelm local resources.

The program's efforts to respond to psychological needs following major disasters have grown dramatically over the twenty-two years since it was established. In fiscal year 1994, it spent approximately $60 million assisting with the psychological sequelae of disasters; in fiscal year 1995 that figure was approximately $30 million. Other nations may find a similar program useful as a mechanism for the rapid and consistent addressing of the psychosocial sequelae following disasters, and may find it possible to adapt the concept to other structures of government. A concise yet comprehensive description of governmental and organizational roles in disaster plus a review of many issues regarding a sound disaster mental health response can be found in *Disaster Response and Recovery: A Handbook for Mental Health Professionals.*[38]

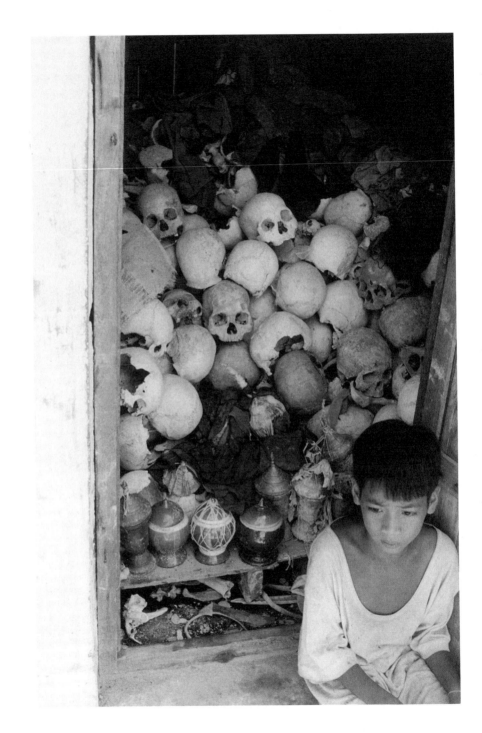

6

MENTAL HEALTH AND PSYCHOSOCIAL EFFECTS OF MASS VIOLENCE

richard f. mollica

The last fifty years have witnessed unremitting violence generated by human beings against one another and causing physical destruction and human suffering of extraordinary proportions.[1-5] Models of humanitarian emergency relief developed since the last world war have repeated patterns of material assistance that, though effective in the emergency phase, have been unproven in long-term situations such as in the Middle East and Asia.[6] International development agencies aimed at reconstructing societies devastated by mass violence now have the heroic task of creating some resemblance of normal economic behavior in over sixty nations.[7] The magnitude of social and physical destruction that exists today and the reality of an interdependent global community demands that new models emerge for the prevention of mass violence as well as for the recovery of nations affected by mass violence. Although this chapter will not focus on the causes and prevention of man-made disasters, it will, by providing new insights into the assessment of traumatic outcomes, indirectly contribute to a partial understanding of those forces in the post-violence phase that set the stage for future rounds of violence. The goal of this chapter is to present a public health framework for evaluating and implementing policy aimed at the recovery of traumatized populations. Special attention will be given to the mental health and psychosocial effects of mass violence as demonstrated by recent scientific evaluations revealing the magnitude of personal and socioeconomic damage that until recently has only been described through anecdotal and biographical reports.

THE PROBLEM OF TAXONOMY

A passage from the late French philosopher Michel Foucault succinctly demonstrates the changing role of classification systems in assigning meaning to our everyday experience. Foucault quotes a "certain Chinese encyclopedia" in which it is written that "animals are divided into: (a) belonging to the emperor, (b) embalmed, (c) tame, (d) suckling pigs, (e) sirens, (f) fabulous, (g) stray dogs, (h) included in the present classification, (i) frenzied, (j) innumerable, (k) drawn with a very fine camelhair brush, (l) et cetera, (m) having just broken the water pitcher, (n) that from a long way off look like flies. In the wonderment of this taxonomy, the thing we apprehend in one great leap, the thing that, by means of the fable, is demonstrated as the exotic charm of another system of thought, is the limitation of our own, the stark impossibility of thinking that."[8]

Until the last quarter-century, public health specialists have been unable to "name" the human suffering associated with mass violence. The mental health impact of the genocidal experience of Cambodian society under the Khmer Rouge regime (1975–1979) and the subsequent confinement of almost 400,000 Cambodian men, women and children on the Thai-Cambodian border remained undocumented for over a decade.[9] Similar acknowledgment of the emotional suffering of Rwanda's entire population remains at the periphery of international policy.[10] The neglect, ignorance, and sometimes outright denial of the mental health sequelae of mass violence is a complex sociohistorical reality beyond the scope of this discussion. In Western society our definition of trauma begins with the early Greek term *traumatikos*. This term refers to a wound or an external bodily injury. Until recently, the psychosocial wounds of traumatized persons and communities have been relatively invisible. We have had no terms for defining or measuring these wounds and have limited ourselves to descriptions of the physical manifestations of violence. This invisibility of the mental health sequelae of violence is most likely due to a number of factors.

- Most mental health sequelae do not have a readily apparent physical manifestation or an easily identifiable lesion such as that seen in serious war injuries.
- The mental health sequelae of violence have been shown to be associated with high morbidity and relatively low mortality. Negative psychosocial effects of psychiatric morbidity even in severe cases have been difficult to describe; no models have been able to establish linkages between the human suffering of war and economic productivity.
- The marginalization of mental health outcomes has been partially stimulated by unexamined and unproven public health attitudes that believe that survivors of violence would prefer not to reveal in public their traumatic life experiences.
- The claim is made that assessing the traumatic experiences of individuals creates additional upset and emotional distress, which can interfere with the natural healing of trauma over time.
- There is a desire to protect the survivor from the stigma associated with psychiatric labeling and treatment.

In recent years, clinical investigations of the psychosocial impact of mass violence on Nazi Holocaust[11] and torture survivors,[12] refugees and displaced persons,[13] and Vietnam and other combat veterans have discounted all of the above misconceptions for these clinical populations. Validation of the diagnosis of post-traumatic stress disorder has generated standardized diagnostic criteria for the first time for evaluating trauma-related psychiatric illness.[14] The cultural adaptation of PTSD in non-Western populations and the ability to assess traumatic life experiences in detail through semistructured interviews have resulted in a new wave of population-based research.[15] For the first time, the psychosocial morbidity associated with cumulative trauma is being measured in traumatized populations throughout the world.

THE CENTRALITY OF THE TRAUMA STORY

The measurement and assessment of traumatic outcomes associated with mass violence poses a conceptual, and possibly an ethical, dilemma. How can public health officials proceed with their assessments of traumatic outcomes without trivializing the horrific and brutalizing life experiences of those affected by violence? In principle, a taxonomy of traumatic outcomes must be centered in the life history of affected individuals and their families and communities. How do we make a transition from the deeply personal nature of a survivor's trauma story to an empirical and less subjective approach or approaches?[16] The public health planner faces an enigma extending from measurement through planning similar to that facing the clinician in his or her diagnosis and treatment of the trauma survivor. Neither the planner nor the clinician wants to lose the essential humanity and dignity of traumatized patients by denying them their reactions to brutalizing and unjust life experiences. Clearly, our new insights into human suffering gained through the measurement of the mental health and psychosocial impact of mass violence have resulted in an expansion of the original definition of *traumatikos*. The physical wound has been extended inward to include internal psychological harm and outward to include social damage to families, neighborhoods, and communities.

Paradoxically, the objectifying nature of the trauma story's universal anatomy or component features provides the bridge necessary for shifting from the core meaning of individuals' traumatic life experiences to the various therapeutic approaches of the doctor, psychologist, and international public health planner. Over the past decade, the oral history of Cambodian-American women archived at the Schlesinger Library for the History of Women in America has led to a number of insights into the major components of the trauma story. Phenomenologically, each of the life histories has within it four stories (Figure 6.1).

The first story or component is the factual accounting of the events. In each oral history the brutality that the Cambodian women experienced under the Pol Pot regime was made explicit. Life under the Khmer Rouge had its similarities for these women in spite of their different ages and social backgrounds. The following quote from SP illustrates the brutalizing violence that all systematically experienced.

> From that time, for two or three month my littlest daughter start to getting very, very sick. She had diarrhea. Here I am, luckily that I have the soldier that would have a crush on me or what, and I don't know, would come to visit me—and begging him anything just to get the medicine for my children. On that time he did give me penicillin. I don't think it would heal, but it better than nothing. And I give it to her. Her condition getting weaker and weaker.

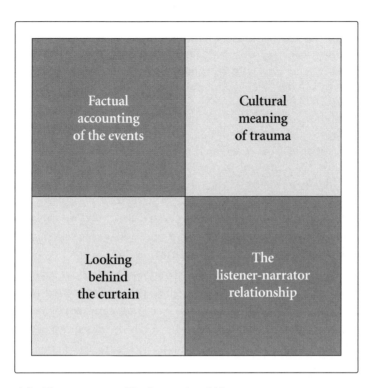

Factual accounting of the events	Cultural meaning of trauma
Looking behind the curtain	The listener-narrator relationship

Figure 6.1   The trauma story: The four stories within a story.

The food getting lower and lower. So does myself getting weaker and weaker. To watch my daughter, it's start to . . . you know she more like . . . She miss her home, she miss her toys, she miss her food, and she start to complain and talk day and night all the time. Somebody told me to burn marijuana, put in a sugar to make her sleep, not to talk too much. They'd give it to her. It does help. To me, until now I think I blame myself for that. Maybe I give her too much. She sleep, and one day I woke up, and she just getting so soft and just couldn't say anything. The diarrhea is still on, the food's not being—we still had some food left for her to eat, but she couldn't eat. She still want her bread, she still want her toy. Everything is start to getting less and less. One day when I—on that time I asked my mother to take care of her, you know, instead of go to work. I go to work, I work for two. It's for my mother and for myself, because I won't have to take care of my little girl. And I go not too far from her, like from here to the corner, and I hear my mother call me. I come over. Here my daughter, she is gone. It just . . . I don't know how to say, because I saw everybody in my family had come, and that time it just shock. She one of the girl would, the bride family would laugh or cry. She just died, her eye open. She's not completely died when I come over and hold her. She look at my face, and she love to touch my breast. Before she put it—before her lie down, she's gone. My father, my brother want to cry, but they have no chance. My father run over here, so does my brother. My sister, my little sister and my son didn't know what going on. And they come back from the back garden with a beautiful flower and say, "Here for her. She'll probably feel better to see this flower." She's gone. That night I hold my daughter body. Our whole family very, very quiet. Nobody want to say anything. She is the first person who die in the family. Start from her. I saw my father start to change his attitude, like instead of make some kind of joke he lost his sense of humor; also because after my husband lost, he's very, very close to her.

The cultural meaning of trauma has been described in previous reports. The history, meaning, and type of violence experienced differs from society to society. This is not to say that sexual violence is not perceived by all men and women in every society as a deep injury and social degradation. The universality of personal responses, however, may be manifested differently in different cultures and stigmatize the victim to a greater degree in some societies than others.[17] All narrators, however, in revealing their trauma story provide unique cultural insights to the listener of the meaning of their experiences, both good and bad, within their cultural framework. A second story from SP reveals the sanctity of death and burial in traditional Khmer society as well as providing insight into the nature of her arranged marriage.

No. One thing my mother, she has well, a tenant house which went to many family. And my husband mother, she's a widow, and she has three kids, no she has four children, two boys and two little girls. And one day, that I go to collect my rent, and my husband saw me and he like fall in love at the first sight. He tried to find out who that girl is. And one of the tenant say, "Ooh, you can't because she is the landlord daughter." And he said like, "Oh." Then he told his mother and he say like, "I really want to marry the landlord's daughter." And my mother-in-law seem to be like, "She's kindly, but fine," because compared to the class we are different because he's only my tenant and my mother-in-law mother doesn't make much money. My mother she—I'm not calling rich for my family, but you call it little bit more than middle class. Then my mother-in-law decide for better she not going to do it. Because she know my mother would say, "No." For that time, the tenant, the neighbor who know that happen, that know my mother very well, that she know my mother very nice, she not going to care so much about money. She care about how nice a person, is he good, tell my mother-in-law that it's OK, go ahead, and "try before you give up." And my mother-in-law said, "I'm not going to try." And that person bring that toward my mother, that my husband saw me and he really want, you know, to get being serious, what will my mother say? And my mother say it's fine if they come through the, we say the rule, we'll take them then, but my mother said, "I won't embarrass them," she just want to know more about family history. Then my mother-in-law start to come. When my mother-in-law start to come, and we found out like, my father-in-law, she left my father-in-law, my father-in-law have another step-wife; and she got involved with another guy which is more like boyfriend and girl-friend, that which is absolutely wrong for my culture to do that. But to see how handsome my husband is. He's very, very pleasant, very, very polite. My mother said, "Well, we'll try." First time she want my husband to come every weekend, you know just to spend time at home at my house to help my father do little bit thing, and he'd be so in for the history more, little bit. And from time to time, my parent falling in love with him, because he's such a very, very sweet person.

It's horrible. I bury my parent by my own hand. Like I said, you used to put the body in a beautiful clothes, the favorite clothes that the body used to like it before they died, OK? You'd give them a bath, you'd give the body— OK first of all you give the body a bath, right? And you put them beautiful clothes. It's like in here. You put beautiful clothes, you put a little bit of make-up, or sometime you just put beautiful clothes for the body before you put the body in the box. Is that the box? Coffin. You put the body in the coffin the only thing the body used to like, OK. And if the body is the mother of the baby, and the mother die and the baby still alive, sometime you put, like a . . . watermelon with the body to pretend like the baby also. This is what I saw in the person next door. I say, "Why you do that?" because they put like a watermelon with that; because they feel like the soul is not completely peace, because she still miss her children, the baby, the youngest one. So they view the soul . . . it's just a fake baby, pretend like—even you die, you still have the baby with you. But this baby is not you any more, leave it alone. You follow me? After that you put the body in the coffin, and you go to the funeral and you bury it. In Pol Pot regime . . . this is I'm talking about my own experience. When my little girl died, first experience, horrible experience in my family. It's my little girl. She's young. She's the first one. I remember I had a beautiful, a beautiful, how you call . . . not blanket, but it's softer than that. It's more like a blanket, but it's made by silk. It's beautiful. It's a gift from my mother after I get married. I cannot even find a wood to make a coffin for her. So I wrap her in the beautiful fabric, with her nice clothes . . . not very nice, it's just the clothes that she like, you know. My father and my brother bury her. I didn't even go over there, because I cannot go. I don't think I can deal with it. Through my family, I mean I cannot even find a piece of wood to put underneath of the hole. You know what I'm saying, because when you dig the ground, it's kind of get wet underneath. Even though, you have no choice. You have to put your parent over there anyway, because you cannot even find anything else to do. Luckily, like my mother I been wrap her in the beautiful clothes that she have. And I didn't even find the mother anything. It's a horrible thing after I bury her for two or three days, somebody tell me that, this is still a nightmare for me until, how they say, like the wolf been go through the whole thing because they didn't dig her high enough—not deep enough. They didn't bury her deep enough. How do you feel if you were me? She is the favorite person in your life. She die, you thought she's in peace. Even the body cannot stay in peace.

Looking behind the curtain reveals the transformation of value systems of survivors of mass violence. Cultural customs and beliefs that were readily accepted by survivors are destroyed by their new insights into a conventional world destroyed by torture and violence. As the violence they survived destroys their old ways of thinking and behaving, many get to look behind the curtain of their previous ordinary life and find something new. SP's third story illustrates this point.

Right, yeah. But one thing is, I think being a human being, you have to love in your heart. You don't have love, you not a human being. Life is create by happiness, sad, exciting, unexciting, boring; that is create to be life. Sometime when the life getting so disgust, I figured out that is to my—this is what this life going to be. I mean, you have to miss everything to become life. For me, it's always one after another. Last week I taking care of my insurance, I take care of my mortgage, all of the sudden feel, OK, I seem to can be relax right now, and all of the sudden, one of the guy hit my car, OK. And I searching out, I found here insurance which is problem I been taking care of. When I go to work, I got flat tire. And I figured out, why me? I mean, God don't you dare get enough? But this is life. You always have something to interrupt, but you always have something to look forward to. But I never chose if I happen to live, to reborn again and know my past life and my life right now, I never want to be alone. Never. It just kind of very scary situation to be lonesome, but I never want to marry with a, you know, unstable married also, because . . . according to what I been through, according to what I brought up, it's just . . . love is just one for one, one person for one person. I don't think I have that kind of love in this country, or maybe I didn't look hard enough. But . . . I see so many people the way they cheating, the way . . . maybe she's right. Instead of get married again, she settle down for being single. But there are no meaning. To be single for what? For be alone and stay home all the time, going to work all the time, for what? I have no answer for that, but the thing is I just hope someday my life would be different, a little bit more excited, instead of be so dark like that. Don't you think?

Finally, the trauma story does not exist unless it is told to the listener. Public health planners, for example, may not appreciate the mental health sequelae of violence if they have not heard the trauma story. Neither the trauma story nor its traumatic outcomes exist unless there is communication between narrator and listener. This reasoning may suggest, of course, a rather naive understanding of the relationship of the doctor, the public health planner, or the policymaker to the trauma story. Trauma survivors are always telling their trauma story to everyone, especially those with whom they are most intimate. However, the trauma story may only exist disguised in bits and pieces. The signs of the survivors' stories are everywhere; because traumatic life experiences affect their health, identity, personality, and feelings.

THE IMPACT OF TRAUMA: CAUSES AND CONSEQUENCES

The survivor's trauma story is not a buried treasure waiting to be discovered. It is a set of phenomena that allows the doctor, public health planner, and policy official, each with his or her own methodology and goals, the possibility of measuring and interpreting traumatic outcomes. Figure 6.2 suggests the ways in which the trauma story can be identified in traumatic events and the major traumatic outcomes of violence: psychiatric symptoms, functional limitations, and disability. Figure 6.3 reveals the basic epidemiologic model of causes and consequences linking traumatic experiences to traumatic outcomes.[18] Until recently, almost all research associating trauma to traumatic outcomes has been based on clinical populations, people who present with complaints in a clinical setting. Since the pioneering community studies of Eitinger and his colleagues[19,20,21] demonstrating the long-term mortality and morbidity of Nazi Holocaust survivors over time, clinical studies have demonstrated strong associations between trauma in various survivor groups with physical illness and with psychiatric symptomatology (especially depression and PTSD).[22] Recent community surveys have linked trauma to functional impairments.[23] Few longitudinal studies exist that would be capable of elucidating the direction of the causal arrows in Figure 6.3 or the natural history of recovery. Dose-

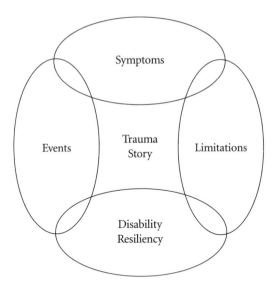

Figure 6.2 The centrality of the trauma story.

effect relationships between cumulative trauma and traumatic outcomes
have been fairly limited in establishing causality linked to violence because
of lack of knowledge of the potency of individual trauma events and the
cross-sectional design of almost all surveys.[18]

Fortunately, major advances in the cultural validation of survey instruments in non-Western and non-English-speaking populations have allowed reliable and valid measures to be used successfully to assess each
point of the triadic relationship of trauma–symptoms–functional limitations.[24,25,26] The traumatic experiences of survivors are different in different
cultures and geopolitical environments. For example, under the Khmer
Rouge many individuals were tortured by having plastic bags placed over
their heads. In contrast, this form of torture did not occur in Bosnia. Tortured individuals have experienced horrifying events unique to their conflict. It is critical to recognize that the cultural meaning of trauma varies
from situation to situation.[27,28] While all cultures have methods for categorizing symptoms of emotional distress, it is still uncertain whether the
symptoms defined by the clinical criteria for the Western diagnosis of post-
traumatic stress disorder are universal.[15] Recent scientific assessments of
Cambodian and Vietnamese populations strongly suggest the relevance of
PTSD in defining trauma-related symptoms in these groups. [29,30] While the

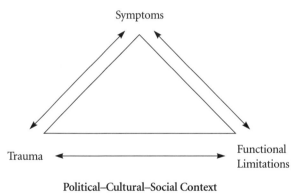

Figure 6.3   Causes and consequences.

criterion validity for PTSD may be accurate, it is unknown whether the construct validity for PTSD is meaningful in societies unfamiliar with its definition and therapeutic usefulness.[31] The cultural relevance of PTSD has been comprehensively reviewed in numerous reports.[15]

The sociocultural contextualization of functional limitations poses the greatest difficulty for assessment.[32] Since functional limitations are primarily related to an individual's ability to master his or her life situation, interact with family, friends, and neighbors, and maintain social responsibilities and obligations, the manifestation of each of these domains is especially culturally dependent. In addition, social expectations related to functional status change for age, gender, social class, and marital status in different cultures. Knowledge of the political, cultural and social context for each point of the triangle in Figure 6.3 is essential for evaluating traumatic events and traumatic outcomes.

Three Major Dimensions of Analysis

Figure 6.4 demonstrates how the triadic relationships described above can be applied to three major approaches—medical, personal, and public health—in assessing traumatic outcomes. Unfortunately, in many previous discussions, competition among these models has not allowed for a comparison of the value of each approach.

All of these approaches assume that traumatic life experiences, especially the horrific experience of mass violence,[33] have a major impact on the medical, personal, and public health aspects of traumatic outcomes. The term

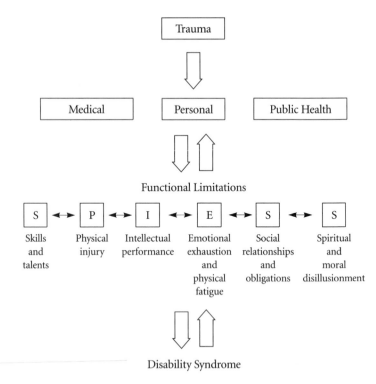

Figure 6.4 Three major approaches in assessing traumatic outcomes.

"symptom," illustrated in Figure 6.3 and usually used to describe psychiatric symptoms and diagnoses, is expanded to include other types of "symptoms" related to traumatic outcomes as defined by the practitioners of the medical, personal, and public health approaches. The medical approach primarily identifies those physical injuries and medical illnesses caused by mass violence and torture. The personal approach describes the myriad ways in which psychologists, writers, and social scientists reveal the human aspects of personal suffering; often this approach is viewed as revealing the "inner life" of the traumatized person. Only the public health approach shows the medical and psychiatric illnesses manifested by entire populations, leaving the individual effects of violence to the clinical attention of the doctor-patient relationship. These approaches overlap with one another, of course, and ideally they are aware of the contributions made by each to the assessment of traumatic outcomes. For example, the symptoms of depression, which is often associated with traumatic life experiences, may be diagnosed as a psychiatric disorder by the medical approach, understood as a world view of despair and hopelessness by the personal approach, and measured as to the prevalence of depressive symptomatology in an entire traumatized population by the public health approach.

In Figure 6.4 the row labeled functional limitations separates the psychosocial disruptions caused by violence (and quite possibly mediated through symptoms) from symptoms as described above. The delineation of functional limitations from medical and psychiatric symptoms has been a major methodological achievement of health outcomes research over the past decade.[34,35,36] In Figure 6.4, functional limitations are expressed by the letters SPIESS. These elements represent the most basic aspects of physical functioning and social relationships. Each element of SPIESS affects the capacity of the trauma survivor to cope with his or her post-traumatic environment. Why are we now emphasizing the importance of functional limitations as a major traumatic outcome of mass violence?[37] While most survivors of mass violence and torture develop traumatic symptoms, it is not known whether or not they become functionally impaired to the degree that their personal life and economic productivity suffers. Evidence of high prevalence rates of PTSD in refugee populations, for example, has not convinced policy planners of their need to respond to what they consider a normally occurring violence-related outcome. Only until symptoms in each of the three approaches are linked to functional status will evidence be generated capable of producing therapeutic interventions and new public policies.

A comprehensive assessment of functional limitations covers a range of items.[38,39] Skills and talents—the individual's abilities to master his or her everyday life—are often severely affected by mass violence. Survivors often state that they are no longer capable of achieving the same level of competence in their work that they had prior to the violence. Physical injury associated with combat and war injuries such as land-mine amputations and blindness is common (and ongoing) in many post-conflict environments. Intellectual performance, especially deterioration in memory and the ability to learn new tasks and ideas, is associated with brain injury, starvation, and the secondary cognitive sequelae of PTSD and depression. Chronic fatigue and mental exhaustion are frequently found in populations experiencing long-standing conflicts. It has become evident that those exposed to mass violence and torture can experience problems in all of their social relationships. This result can be due to a new lack of trust of others caused by violence, the sense of shame and uncleanliness caused by sexual abuse, or the killing and/or disappearance of family members and friends. Normal social obligations, including neighborliness, community activities, and trust in both local government agencies and national policy, can be severely compromised, which in turn makes reconstruction efforts extremely difficult. At the core of spiritual and moral disillusionment is a loss of faith in social justice and a rejection of the belief that rewards are fairly associated with decent human behavior. Existential states of despair and hopelessness associated with the destruction of normal everyday life by terrible and brutalizing violence challenge the religious faith of many. Currently, little is known of the functional limitations associated with mass violence.

The last level of Figure 6.4 describes the disability status of the survivor. A disability syndrome describes the trauma survivor's ability to perform in five areas:

1. basic activities of independent living;
2. economic self-sufficiency and work;
3. family support;
4. community action;
5. political participation.

Although each of these elements of the survivor's capacity to work and participate in rebuilding family and community is essential to reconstruction efforts, almost no knowledge exists on the relationship between trauma and these terminal endpoints of traumatic outcomes. An important caveat related to the issue of disability, however, can be made. It is evident that in many traumatic situations (Figure 6.5) individuals with high levels of trauma, symptoms, and functional limitations can be highly productive members of their societies. The reverse situation is also true. The personal characteristics of individuals as well as the availability of resources and opportunities within a post-traumatic environment have an enormous impact on a survivor's coping strategies and productivity regardless of his or her traumatic life experience. Many survivors are capable of overcoming horrifying life experiences; it is essential for any recovery activity to learn to strengthen those factors associated with resiliency.

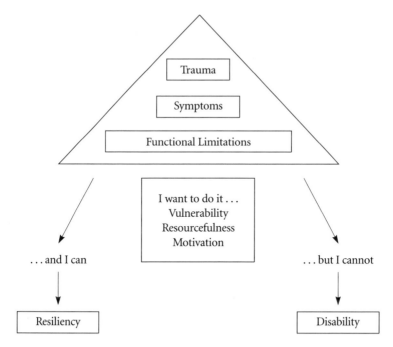

Figure 6.5 The paradox of survival.

Methods of Each Trauma Approach

Table 6.1 summarizes the three approaches to assessing traumatic outcomes. Each approach has its own methodology for identifying traumatic outcomes. The disability syndrome identified by each approach has not been included, however, because it has been impossible for the practitioners of each approach to clearly identify their criteria for establishing disability. Although the practitioner of a particular method may be able to identify traumatic outcomes related to symptoms and functioning, the ability of survivors to perform socially and economically productive activities is most likely more influenced by political factors and work-related opportunities than by prior traumatic life experiences. Current political realities affecting work opportunities, however, may have also caused the survivor's initial traumatic experiences.

The three approaches are described under the categories technique/analysis, diagnosis, and functional limitations. Extensive and thorough investigations of the medical sequelae of mass violence, especially torture, have

Table 6.1 Traumatic outcomes: Assessment approaches

	Medical	Personal	Public Health
Technique/ analysis	Review of systems Physical exam	Oral and life history Testimony	Surveys Interviews
Diagnoses/ specific symptoms	All organ systems affected	Transformation of the subjective feelings of identity and well-being	Brain injury PTSD Depression
Functional limitations	Skills and talents Physical injury Emotional/ physical exhaustion	Emotional/ physical exhaustion Social relationship Spiritual disillusionment	Skills and talents Intellectual performance Emotional exhaustion Social relationships

been well described.[12] Chilean psychologists working with torture survivors have described the approach called "testimony."[40] The oral and life history technique used with Khmer Rouge survivors has been previously presented. Although it is generally accepted that mass violence and torture can greatly distort an individual's inner concept of identity and well-being and profoundly disrupt social relationships, the theoretical literature on personal outcomes remains broad and unfocused. The public health investigation of traumatized populations is still in its infancy. Except for the original studies by Eitinger, only recently have large-scale population studies of combat veterans, Nazi Holocaust survivors, and refugees been attempted.[23,41,42] The results are revealing the prevalence of psychiatric morbidity and related risk factors of major public health importance.

CONCLUSION

Despite centuries of violence that have created suffering for millions of persons, the identification of traumatic outcomes has been ignored, neglected, and even denied by those responsible for the recovery of these communities. New scientific studies of traumatized populations reveal high rates of mental health sequelae previously unknown. The trauma story of every survivor can be identified within each of three major approaches to the assessment of traumatic outcomes: medical, personal, and public health. Although the functional limitations of survivors can be assessed by each approach, the relationship of trauma to economic and social productivity remains elusive. International policy planners are still in need of an estimate of a theoretical construct and empirical case studies that link trauma to symptoms and functioning. Despite the limitations of current research, new measures are emerging that for the first time are capable of describing traumatic outcomes in traumatic populations throughout the world.

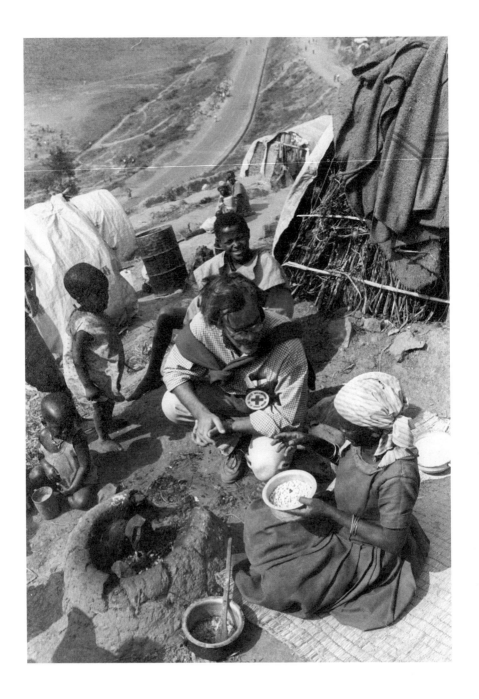

7

PSYCHOLOGICAL TRAUMA
AND RELIEF WORKERS

ruth a. barron

Manifestations of human psychological trauma from any source have tremendous commonality. Behaviors, symptoms, and distortions of affective capacities are similar for individuals exposed to a wide variety of overwhelming events. To begin to appreciate the potential vulnerability of relief workers in humanitarian crises, it is instructive to review key points in the historical recognition of psychological trauma. First, this recognition had its early roots in attempts in this century to address the issue of combat stress. Second, psychoanalytic theory played an influential role in first elucidating and then obscuring the victimization origins of the phenomenon we now call psychological trauma. An understanding of the context in which victimization came to be studied will permit a more solid entry into studies of the stress reactions of disaster victims and rescue workers.

HISTORICAL RECOGNITION OF PSYCHOLOGICAL TRAUMA

Sustained recognition of the psychological basis for traumatic stress is relatively recent. Isolated descriptions of military casualties with the now familiar symptom complex of traumatic stress exist from the time of antiquity. The theoretical understanding that these symptoms had a psychological origin developed only in the 1920s, however, with the focus of early psychoanalysts on World War I combatants. World War II was the first war in which psychological understanding of combat stress symptomatology was used from the outset to identify and treat the significant numbers of such casualties.[1] Although much was learned from the data collected about human responses to extreme and cumulative stress in World War II, these insights largely stayed within the military and were not widely recognized elsewhere. Not until the Vietnam War was the multifaceted way in which trauma can affect soldiers, families, communities, and an entire country brought home to American soil.

In her landmark book, *Trauma and Recovery*, Herman explains the episodic nature of the study of psychological trauma as a function of society's intermittent ability to examine the difficult controversies it engenders. She notes that the exploration of traumatic reality requires a social context and a political movement to legitimate it. For this reason, the study of war trauma can occur only in a context that challenges the sacrifice of young men in war.[2] One can follow the advances made in war trauma beginning with the transient antiwar movement in World War I, continuing within military and professional groups as World War II brought thousands to the battlefield to fight the "good war," and then moving into U.S. public consciousness during and after the Vietnam War.

One of the difficulties in accepting the psychological underside of soldier performance in war was the fact that the understanding of war neurosis or combat stress came unmistakably from the discovery of the roots of hysteria in psychological trauma noted at the turn of the century by Freud and Breuer as well as by Janet. Both groups of investigators determined that the bodily symptoms of hysteria were tied to intensely distressing events that had been removed from the subject's conscious memory. While Freud asserted that hysteria could befall the "clearest intellect" and "greatest character," Janet believed it to be a sign of psychological weakness. Both sets of researchers were studying women patients, for whom the disturbing events at the root of their symptoms were childhood sexual assaults.[3] Freud's initial conclusions that actual sexual abuse formed the core of hysteria were widely rejected, and he eventually recanted this deduction. Rejection of the reality of such widespread individual experience persisted for the next eighty years. Herman explores how initial social interest in the lives and rights of women at the turn of the century was dissipated as history turned away from where the psychoanalytic investigations had led. Society could not accept the traumatic reality. Lacking social or political support, Freud changed his theory, pronouncing as fantasy the distressing "events" recounted by his patients.[4]

So it is that combatants have had a difficult time in seeking to have their psychological pain understood. Soldiers who could not perform on the battlefield or became symptomatic after the cumulative toll of war were tarred by the brush of feminine frailty, weakness of character, and perhaps questions about their sexuality. Using Herman's paradigm, one can see that the ability to unmask the traumatic nature and true horror of war occurred only in the context of the women's liberation movement in the 1970s,[5] when concepts of sexuality were open for revision and issues of human rights for the unprotected came into mass awareness. Only then could society be receptive to learning about the victimization of women and children. Women could have power and standing; men could pay attention to their emotional needs; children could be seen to need greater protection.

In the United States during the 1970s and 1980s, lessons learned from military psychiatry, Vietnam War veterans, Holocaust survivors, and women and children victims of traumatic abuse raised consciousness and catalyzed inquiry into the experiences of victims of disaster. It became apparent that each of these groups of people had been victimized by being caught up in an agonizing event; that the trauma suffered related to the event rather than to an inherent weakness in the victim. There was less necessity to "make the victim worthy of his fate."[6] In fact, as victims gained power in the eyes of society and in their own eyes and struggled to free themselves from their trauma, they came to be called "survivor," rather than solely victims.

Cobb and Lindemann described the emotional sequelae of the 1942 Cocoanut Grove Fire in Boston by detailing the experience of grief and loss and the typical symptoms of the survivors.[7] This paper characterized the three key aspects of what was much later to become codified (in 1980) as post-traumatic stress disorder: avoidance; reexperiencing; and somatic distress.[8] In the wake of the high death rate of significant others who had accompanied these individuals to the Cocoanut Grove nightclub, Lindemann and Cobb, who treated survivors, observed that those who

> show no signs of grief during the period of convalescence for their somatic injuries are likely to have disabling disturbances at a later period. Prophylac-

tic care is most important here. The patient must be allowed to carry through his grief reaction at the optimal time without undue delay; he must be assisted in his efforts to extricate himself from the bondage to the deceased, to be prepared to face the task of social readjustment when he leaves the hospital.[9]

In 1944, Lindemann published a signal paper entitled "Symptomatology and Management of Acute Grief."[10] There he connected reactions to war casualties with disaster trauma, discussed the spectrum of normal and pathological grief reactions, and pointed out the phenomenon of delayed grief reaction.

Further progress in understanding the psychological impact of overwhelming events was made as critical thinkers wrote about the emotional impact of observed disasters in specific tragic circumstances. Lifton explored the emotional disabilities of the hibakusha, Japan's survivors of the atomic bomb explosions on Hiroshima and Nagasaki. His book, *Death in Life,* published in 1967, characterizes the survivor syndrome that distances hibakusha from normal social life and from normal experience of emotion. Lifton found key motifs in his detailed interviews with these victims. He saw the "imprint of death" as the most fundamental theme. Being immersed in death experiences can lead victims in different directions: to a heightened fear of death; to a feeling of invulnerability to it; and/or to a fascination with the scenes of death. A profound sense of guilt is a typical reaction of survivors. Lifton uses the term "death guilt" to refer to the agony of survivors that their life was spared at the expense of someone else. Further thoughts often include the sense that the "other" would have been more worthy of survival. To protect themselves against these devastating thoughts, victims (unconsciously) employ a kind of psychic closing off. Lifton's phrase for this bedrock symptom of traumatic injury is "psychic numbing."[11]

DEFINITION OF POST-TRAUMATIC STRESS DISORDER

The work of Lifton, Herman, and others studying extreme events contributed directly to the recognition of post-traumatic stress disorder and its first iteration in the 1980 *Diagnostic and Statistical Manual of Mental Disorders* (DSM-III) of the American Psychiatric Association. Although the defining features of PTSD have been refined and an acute syndrome has been added, this 1980 statement articulated the elemental aspects of the human response to psychic trauma to a wide professional and public audience. It may seem impossible now, as recognition of psychological injury continues to expand and deepen, to imagine that public understanding could ever again retrench into denial. The entity itself may, however, carry in its own defining features the seeds of a later social amnesia; if its implications again appear to be too threatening, forces within society may drive the genie back into its bottle.[12]

Key diagnostic criteria for adult PTSD (Box 7.1) include the following (emphasis on key words added):

A. The person has been exposed to a traumatic event in which both of the following were present:
   (1) the person experienced, witnessed, or was confronted with an event or events that involved actual or threatened death or serious injury, or a threat to the physical integrity of self or others
   (2) the person's response involved intense fear, helplessness, or horror

B. The traumatic event is persistently *reexperienced* in one (or more) of the following ways:
   (1) recurrent and intrusive distressing recollections of the event, including images, thoughts, or perceptions
   (2) recurrent distressing dreams of the event
   (3) acting or feeling as if the traumatic event were recurring (includes a sense of reliving the experience, illusions, hallucinations, and dissociative flashback episodes, including those that occur on awakening or when intoxicated)
   (4) intense psychological distress at exposure to internal or external cues that symbolize or resemble an aspect of the traumatic event
   (5) physiological reactivity on exposure to internal or external cues that symbolize or resemble an aspect of the traumatic event

C. Persistent *avoidance* of stimuli associated with the trauma and *numbing* of general responsiveness (not present before the trauma), as indicated by three or more of the following:
   (1) efforts to avoid thoughts, feelings, or conversations associated with the trauma
   (2) efforts to avoid activities, places, or people that arouse recollections of the trauma
   (3) inability to recall an important aspect of the trauma
   (4) marked diminished interest or participation in significant activities
   (5) feeling of detachment or estrangement from others
   (6) restricted range of affect (e.g., unable to have loving feelings)

Box 7.1 Key diagnostic criteria for adult post-traumatic stress disorder (acute, chronic, or delayed onset)

- Exposure to event or events that involved actual or threatened death or serious injury to self or others
- Response involved intense fear, helplessness, or horror
- Persistent reexperiencing of event
- Acting or feeling as if the traumatic event were recurring
- Intense physiological/psychological distress at exposure to symbolic cues
- Persistent avoidance of stimuli associated with the trauma
- Numbing of general responsiveness
- Persistent symptoms of increased arousal not present before the trauma
- Duration of disturbing symptoms exceeds one month
- Disturbance causes clinically significant distress or impairment in social, occupational, or other important areas of functioning

(7) sense of a foreshortened future (e.g., does not expect to have a career, marriage, children, or a normal life span)

D. Persistent symptoms of *increased arousal* (not present before the trauma), as indicated by two (or more) of the following:
(1) difficulty falling asleep or staying asleep
(2) irritability or outbursts of anger
(3) difficulty concentrating
(4) hypervigilance
(5) exaggerated startle response

E. Duration of the disturbing symptoms is more than 1 month.

F. The disturbance causes clinically significant distress or impairment in social, occupational, or other important areas of functioning.

Specify if:
Acute: if duration of symptoms is less than 3 months
Chronic: if duration of symptoms is 3 months or more

With Delayed Onset: if onset of symptoms is at least 6 months after the stressor[13]

After PTSD was described, a more immediate Acute Stress Disorder was delineated. This symptom complex occurs within a month of exposure to the event, lasts at least two days, and persists only up to one month.

Acute Stress Disorder includes at least one symptom from the three symptom clusters in PTSD as well as dissociative symptoms such as being in a daze, feeling detached from one's body, and having no memory of the traumatic event.[14]

The addition of this "lighter" PTSD diagnosis helps underscore the fact that these so-called disorders have both normative and pathological aspects. It is important to appreciate this point before turning to the issue of what has been described as "vicarious trauma" in aid workers.[15] That an individual meets the criteria for diagnosis denotes that he or she is suffering a constellation of symptoms from a prior traumatic event, not that the response denotes core pathology. In time, the symptom complex can become entrenched and unmistakably pathological. These are disorders, but the dis-order is caused by immersion in extreme external circumstance.

STRESS AND POST-TRAUMATIC STRESS DISORDER

The disaster literature accumulating over the past thirty years has increasingly included awareness of the psychological vulnerability of rescue workers. This recognition of stress and trauma among workers has profited from the social forces that have allowed greater acknowledgment of the pain endured by others and that have moved to lighten the stigma attached to having emotional difficulties in the wake of an overwhelming event. For many years there has been a significant turnover of individuals in their jobs as rescue workers. Much of the disaster literature in the 1970s and 1980s that addressed worker reactions pointed to the need of workers for ongoing stress management in order to continue to be fully functional in their roles.[16] Those initially studied were emergency workers: police, firemen, EMTs. Portraits of relief workers in natural and human-caused disasters emerged as sociologists and then mental health professionals studied specific disasters. Late in the day, and only in the wake of the most recent humanitarian crises, with their unprecedented mix of horrors, have we heard reports of unparalleled levels of mortality and psychological morbidity among international aid workers.

Relief workers are subject to a common variety of stresses, some of which they share with general workers, some of which are a product of their professional roles in intense settings, and some of which are shared with primary victims of disaster. The issue of when a particular reaction is felt to be normal and when it is judged pathological makes a frequent appearance in discussions of worker stress. Many stress reactions are seen as normal if their magnitude is appropriate to the stressor and if they are short-lived. Pathological responses may reflect the type or intensity of symptoms or may relate to their enduring nature. The level of pathology does not necessarily correlate with the worker's appreciation of his or her own distress.

Appraisal of Threat

In order to understand the influences on an individual's perception and experience of distress or trauma, a consideration of stress and trauma on opposite ends of a continuum is useful. A modicum of anxiety or stress is positive as it allows increased focus and motivation for problem solving.[17] In theory, one might be able to identify and specify the amount of stress to which an individual should be subjected in order to optimize his or her functioning. Additional stress would be expected to decrease function. An interesting point made in the literature is that the subject's appraisal of threat is critical for stress reactions to occur.[18] It follows that if it were possible to intervene to increase the threshold for appraisal of threat, a worker could handle increased levels of threat before function were affected.

Resilience

While early stress research focused on situational or stimulus variables, newer studies view stress as an inner state that is a function of the interaction between the organism and its environment.[19] With a variety of motivations, stress researchers, trauma investigators, and agencies providing emergency and disaster relief have all become interested in exploring individual differences in sensitivity and response to stressors. All other characteristics of disaster settings or stressor variables being equal, the personal factors of the individual are those with which one is left. These factors include the history of the individual's development and character traits that constitute his or her so-called resilience.[20,21] This attribute has drawn increasing focus with the hope that worker recruitment efforts might benefit from a strategically focused screening of applicants.

Apfel and Simon[22] talk about "resiliency variables" in their article on children in war. Their resiliency model has application for aid workers as well as for children, since the common thread is the individual who can manage trauma. The attributes they list may assist aid agencies and institutions in their search for aid workers with "the right stuff":

- resourcefulness;
- curiosity, intellectual mastery, ability to conceptualize;
- flexibility in emotional experience;
- access to autobiographical memory;
- goal for which to live;
- need and ability to help others;
- vision of a moral order.

Little hard data are available on resilience. Conceptualizing resilience not simply as an attribute of an individual but also as a function of his or her relationship to the environment offers further opportunity to protect and support workers. The development of psychological supports typically comes from lessons learned in the field. The Jonestown mass suicide and a high-impact air crash in 1995 stand as examples: the first is a case of a lesson learned; the second, a case of a support offered just outside the traumatizing environment.

Jones studied the effects on personnel involved in the identification and recovery of bodies in the 1978 Jonestown mass suicide.[23] Young people were utilized as helpers even though the disaster setting was one of massive death. Jones was aware of the repeated conclusions in the literature that the handling of dead bodies is especially traumatic for workers in general and that older and more seasoned workers do better with this task.[24] His findings at Jonestown confirmed the high rates of trauma for young people who handle dead bodies. Jones went further in his analysis of the Jonestown efforts and recommended that younger workers be assigned less traumatizing tasks. His detailed findings made it possible for him to advise that if a situation arose in which bringing young people so close to death was unavoidable, pairing them with older, more experienced workers could mitigate some of their distress.

Jones also suggested job rotation and backup to relieve workers on particularly stressful assignments. This recommendation was applied in the next example. Emergency workers involved in the 1995 USAir crash near Pittsburgh had the task of recovering multiple small body parts of victims dispersed over a broad area. They were supported in this work by American Red Cross disaster mental health workers who had been asked (for the first time) to stand by the perimeter of the operation. In that very disturbing setting, disaster mental health workers noted a typical progression of the comments by the rescue crew. In their first contact (after their first shift), when asked how they were doing, rescuers responded that they were "holding up," "hanging in there." On their second contact, crew members reported difficulties. On the third, crew members acknowledged that they were experiencing psychological problems.[25]

In most other recent rescue and aid settings, environmental supports have been much less structured or have been absent altogether. In these situations, the personal resilience of the individual worker stands out. The following example is taken from an International Federation of Red Cross and Red Crescent Societies report[26] on the Rwandan relief operation. It recounts the experience and insights of an Australian doctor and demonstates how a resilient aid worker can extract support even from a forbidding environment. Some of his internal mechanisms for dealing with the horror of the relief situation are apparent in his words contained in the following narrative:

> The day Parker joined the Federation in Goma, 7,000 bodies were collected from Kibumba. He counted 690 on his way to work and found himself in a nightmare. Outside a Federation dispensary a thousand people were waiting, inside he started his day by clearing away the corpses. "The place was running with faeces. Blankets were soaked in it. The stench was indescribable. People kept dying on me. You'd lose someone, clean up their mess and the space would be filled immediately."
>
> For almost three weeks Parker worked amid what he describes as overwhelming death. Bodies were counted by the truckload, 40 loads a day being carted from the camps around Goma. The doctor said, "During the day I created this shell around myself. I said: 'Do what you have to, forget the rest.' Sometimes when I felt like cracking I would go and find some unattended baby and syringe fluid into its mouth. It would suck the syringe and I would feel better. At least here was something I could influence positively."
>
> At the end of three weeks John Parker had a free day. He sat in the Federation compound back in Goma, listened to music on his Walkman, and felt

tears running down his face. "I was scared," he said. "I don't do that, I am not particularly emotional. We had been warned in briefings but I guess nothing could prepare you for Kibumba."

Parker buried his head in his hands so no one could see he was crying. After a quarter of an hour he felt a hand on his shoulder. "It was a nurse. She gave me a cup of tea and a wonderful smile which said: 'I understand what's happening.'

"I wept for 45 minutes. You see, I had to shed all that sadness. Afterwards I felt strong. Isn't it reassuring to know the human body has such a powerful mechanism?"

John Parker still works in Kibumba.

Parker is able to compartmentalize the horrific stimuli and remain functional in his professional role. He employs what stress management experts call positive "self-talk," a deliberate method of coaching himself to focus on his tasks. He is able to find within the chaos an action that is both concrete and symbolic—feeding the baby—to support his sense of moral order and to keep him in his role as a helper. At his first break he takes time to feel some of the pain he has had to bury during his work hours. He is also able to be seen crying and to accept comfort from a peer.

Burnout

Whereas underdiagnosis has been the historical precedent in perceptions of worker trauma, overdiagnosis is now also a risk. Post-traumatic stress is not the only possible understanding of a stressed worker. Beginning at the shallow end of the stress/trauma continuum, a relief worker can react to garden-variety worker stress, such as having difficulty with the boss or being distracted by difficulties at home. More serious or repetitive difficulties are revealed in multiple signs and symptoms affecting work. The term "burnout" has been used to cover a wide spectrum of responses to stressful work. Burnout refers to a process of moving toward emotional exhaustion and poor functioning in the context of all types of work. Many of its signs and symptoms overlap with those rooted in trauma, yet burnout generally implies an incremental or cumulative erosion of worker resources based on multiple relatively minor exposures rather than the result of a single event. Kahill identifies five categories of symptoms associated with burnout. They include many internal feelings of the worker but accent the influence of stress on the job:[27]

1. physical: for example, fatigue, physical exhaustion, sleep difficulties, specific somatic problems such as headache and gastrointestinal disturbances;
2. emotional: for example, irritability, anxiety, depression, guilt, and a sense of helplessness;
3. behavioral: for example, aggression, callousness, pessimism, defensiveness, cynicism, and substance abuse;
4. work-related: for example, quitting the job, absenteeism, tardiness, misuse of work breaks, and poor work performance;
5. interpersonal: for example, withdrawal, poor communication with clients and co-workers, and dehumanizing or intellectualizing clients.

Factors Contributing to Increased Stress

Distinguishing between significant burnout and trauma in disaster workers requires examination of the origins of a worker's distress. This inquiry will generally not be possible until the worker is in a safe place, out of the disaster setting. Fine distinctions as to the origins of poor worker performance are not likely to be of consequence in the middle of an operation, but an off-site investigation is important both for the worker and for the agency. In the field, an assessment will need to be made to determine whether modest interventions can be tried (time off, job rotation) or whether the worker needs to be evacuated.

A worker experiencing secondary trauma is affected by the same key elements as a primary victim. These include variables arising out of:

1. the characteristics of the event;
2. the characteristics of the individual and the group;
3. pre-trauma factors;
4. post-trauma recovery factors.

In a given disaster setting, elements from these categories interact to determine the degree of stress and trauma felt by a worker. Since a disaster is defined as a situation in which resources have been overwhelmed, and a complex humanitarian emergency involves an even broader mix of elements gone awry, we might expect the vulnerability to traumatization to be higher among relief workers in these settings. In their 1994 review of the literature on emergency worker stress, Raphael and Wilson found that 20 percent to 80 percent suffered prolonged stress responses. The themes underlying these stress reactions, although identified within the disaster context, apply as well to humanitarian crises:

1. the force and destruction involved;
2. confrontation with death (massive, gruesome, and mutilating death);
3. feelings of hopelessness ("the helplessness of humanity");
4. feelings of anger (that more was not done, that they are the recipients of survivor anger);
5. significant loss and accompanying grief ("identification sympathy");
6. attachment and relationships ("strong bonds") that develop among rescue team members;
7. elation or "feelings of triumph" among rescue workers;
8. survivor guilt;
9. voyeurism.[28]

FACTORS THAT PLACE WORKERS AT INCREASED RISK OF STRESS

Researchers have noted that disaster workers share specific job and personality attributes that may make them more vulnerable to stress and trauma than the average direct victim (Box 7.2).

Roles

Rescue workers are often in close and protracted contact with the most critical results of a disaster. At times, they must make life and death decisions in the midst of chaos. They are "under pressure to know what to do and must dare to do it."[29] In some relief settings and many humanitarian crises, where the situation is chaotic and personal safety threatened, and in some roles, such as search and rescue, workers may be more vulnerable to psychological disturbance because they have no control over what they might be subject to.[30] In fact, because of their assignments, relief workers may actually spend a greater amount of time within the most difficult zone of the disaster than many of the direct victims.

Situations in which rescue workers are themselves direct victims are not unusual. In such settings, workers may have tremendous role stress, worry-

Box 7.2 Factors contributing to increased stress among relief
workers

- Greater amount of time spent within disaster zone than direct victims
- Role ambiguity
- High expectations and possible sense of failure, loss and guilt
- Duration and pace of work in an atmosphere devoid of tangible
  closure
- Removal from personal and family supports
- Need to turn off emotional life in order to keep functioning

ing at once about their own families and homes and trying to attend to their
relief role. Hurricane Hugo's devastating impact on the island of St. Croix
in 1989 saw many of the local Red Cross, community religious leaders, and
mental health providers suffer major damage and upheaval in their own
lives. The vast majority remained at their posts in the ensuing weeks of
community dependency, demoralization, and depression.[31] The care with
which national Red Cross mental health workers had to approach these
worker-victims brings up yet another way in which workers may be disadvantaged in obtaining help for their own emotional needs. With all the obvious victimization around them, worker-victims typically do not feel entitled to attend to or have others attend to their own needs.[32] Ignoring or
burying their own needs can become second nature or may even have
drawn them to relief work in the first place. In approaching a professional
caregiver, Cohen underscores the necessity of giving a clear signal that he or
she is not a patient but is reacting to extreme stressors.[33]

Role ambiguity is a particular issue when a relief operation is not working. Hartsough defines role ambiguity as "confusion and uncertainty about
the nature of one's job, its purpose, and its responsibilities."[34] He goes on to
state that "from the worker's viewpoint, role ambiguity arises when the information provided about the work role doesn't correspond to what is required for adequate performance." One can imagine that the negative feel-

ings engendered by a worker feeling off balance or unsure in his or her role might lead to significant alienation from the institution and dissatisfaction with the job.

Eight days after the start of the massacres in Rwanda in mid-April 1994, the 2,000 UN soldiers who witnessed the escalating violence were unable to intervene because they were deployed under a mandate to monitor a peace agreement that was no longer in force. The frustrated UN commander was quoted by a *New York Times* correspondent: "We have been sitting now eight or nine days in our trenches. The question is how long do you sit there or attempt to get it settled? This is not a peace enforcing mission. They haven't stopped firing so I'd say I'm not yet effective. If we don't see any light at the end of the tunnel, if we see another three weeks of being cooped up watching them pound each other then we have to seriously assess the risk of keeping these soldiers here."[35]

Expectations

There are also high expectations of rescue workers that place them at risk for a sense of failure and loss if they are not successful.[36] Disaster workers frequently become targets for victim anger as the community of disaster survivors moves through predictable phases of recovery from the event.[37] Workers unfamiliar with this common occurrence may take these negative emotions personally and feel deeply injured by this turn of events. Aid workers in humanitarian crises are likely to be perceived differently by various parties to the conflict, as a function of changing alliances, the status of resources, and events of the day. A naive worker might have difficulty handling the high likelihood that he or she will not be seen simply as an altruistic individual wishing to make a humanitarian contribution by helping those in dire need. To the extent that a staff member needs to be seen in such a light to be productive in the field, he or she might be expected to "crash" early on. Workers struggle not only with the perception of themselves by the "victim" population, but also with their professional limitations, just at the time when they must rely most strongly on their own professional identity and sense of prowess as an internal support for their disaster work. Workers often feel guilt related to their role in the spotlight, a role created by the suffering of others.[38] When the motivation and credentials of agencies and workers are questioned in the press or in the eyes of victims, does the worker have the training and sense of self not only to acknowledge these assaults but to deflect them from draining enthusiasm or from connecting with underlying guilt?

An August 1994 *New York Times* article[39] detailing the misery at the Zairean refugee camps quoted the Red Cross (ICRC) agency head in Goma, who was responding to worker stress. Asked about the psychiatric support given to two Red Cross delegates who had witnessed mass killings of Rwandans in April and May and who were in Red Cross ambulances when Tutsi patients were dragged out and killed by Hutu militia, she explained:

> The stress is immense, but part of our job is to learn to be humble and to know that you are not going to save the whole of humanity. . . . What is important is to know that it is not our fault. That if people are dying it is because of war, and we must understand that the responsibility for the problem is the war.

When asked what makes a good aid worker, she responded:

> They shouldn't have too great a heart. If you want to save the world, forget it. We don't need people who are too empathetic, we need professionals.

Duration and Pace

Burkle, a physician with a background in civilian and miliary disaster response, provides a number of insights from his experience.[40] He distinguishes between shock trauma (the type of trauma one encounters in a disaster with a single extreme event) and strain trauma (one in which there is an accumulation of difficult experiences over time). The approach of the rescue worker in the first instance includes a short-haul mindset. The affected community will at a foreseeable time be able to do without the outside relief workers and will carry on healing efforts. In contrast, in the second instance, the events fueling the cumulative strain are often human-caused and continue over a long time. Burkle sees war as the prototype example here, and humanitarian crises also clearly fit into this category. In such settings, aid workers cannot see "the light at the end of the tunnel" when there might be closure on their humanitarian interventions. With no end in sight, the worker must pace him- or herself and be able to function in an atmosphere devoid of tangible closure.

Isolation

Workers on assignment are typically removed from their own personal and family supports, so that certain key interventions one might consider for primary victims are impossible to offer workers. The disaster survivor often shares the trauma and loss with family and community. If there is a need to bridge an informational or emotional gap, such as may be the case in surviving a hostage taking or a plane crash, kin and community are well aware of that gap and are generally poised to assist in bridging it. In contrast, the emotional and geographical distance of the worker's significant others can serve to sharpen his or her distressing thoughts and feelings of isolation.

There are several other reasons why the relief worker may ultimately be more isolated. In order to be in a professional role, the worker must internally emphasize and externally project characteristics of emotional strength and technical competence. Fear and dependency needs are kept far from the surface, if at all possible.

As part of the recovery process, disaster victims typically move through a phase (which can be long-lasting) when they repeatedly tell the story of their trauma with all its attendant details. Disaster workers are invested in seeing themselves as helpers and rescuers, distinct from victims. They can be expected to resist admitting weakness and vulnerability to themselves, and are much less able to share with their community the disaster stories in which they can be seen as the victim (however truthful or helpful it might ultimately be to do so).

As traumatic stimuli escalate, a worker may need to invest increasing energy in controlling emotions or may well have developed the capacity to extinguish his or her emotional life in order to keep functioning. But learning to turn off emotions is a much simpler process than learning how to turn them back on. Relationships suffer; the sense of self narrows. If a worker has not developed a practiced mechanism for getting in touch with his or her own sense of broader personal identity and for allowing a return to normal levels of emotion, he or she may find that life outside of work and relationships back home develop chasms that are not easily bridged. Further, workers tend not to see their feelings and behaviors that occur months after participating in a disaster as related to that event. "Hazardous emotional material," as Mitchell calls it,[41] tends to get buried as soon as it arises.

Defenses and Constraints

Mitchell[41] gives a personality profile of emergency workers as detail oriented and perfectionistic; as needing to be in control of themselves (for example, flat affect) and in control of the scene; as action oriented; as easily bored and needing increasing stimulation; as cautious risk takers; and as highly dedicated. He further notes that, as a group, they have a strong need to be needed; cannot say no; need to help and save people, regardless of personal cost to themselves; and generally have a high tolerance for stress and ambiguity.

Disaster and rescue workers often share some personality characteristics and unconscious mechanisms. An exaggeration that is popularized is the stereotype of the fearless, omni-competent "cowboy" who shows no strong emotions and appears to seek out danger. This portrait points to commonly used ego defenses[42] employed by the worker to keep threat at bay. Denial, omnipotence, isolation of affect, and reaction formation (engaging in precisely that which one fears in order to manage that fear) are utilized by these "disaster cowboys." These defenses can be tremendously useful in extreme settings but can damage the self in everyday life.

The pitfalls for the aid worker in reacting to an extreme situation (Box 7.3) generally move in opposing directions: on the one hand, the worker may take a position too close to the victims to be of use and, on the other hand, the worker may employ a number of distancing measures as self-protection from pain. A worker who needs to be needed and to see victims as "all good" may become enmeshed with a group of "ideal" victims and may see only the parts of the relief drama that support his or her defensive coping. Enmeshment and "black-and-white thinking"[43] simplify complex situations for some individuals and allow them to preserve their role in a situation with clear moral boundaries. This accommodation may collide with the decision making of their institution or with a circumstance that arises and make them vulnerable to anger or fragmentation. On the other side of the defensive coin, workers may become hostile and distancing, seeing all victims as corrupt and untrustworthy and treating them with contempt. Experienced workers are at risk for the development of bitterness and cynicism, taking the "cowboy" role to a more extreme and negative position.

Another pitfall for disaster workers is a move into self-destructive behav-

Box 7.3 Pitfalls for relief workers in the crisis environment

- Employment of distancing measures as self-protection from pain
- Identification with "ideal" victims
- "Black-and-white thinking"
- Self-destructive behaviors

iors. This can range from poor self-care with regard to eating, sleeping, and the use of drugs and alcohol, to taking chances and putting oneself in harm's way. Smith et al.[44] make the incisive observation that "it is the people who maintain their own health who can look out of place and as if they do not care about all the suffering around them because they are not joining in the self-destructive behaviors."

These authors further expose a psychological mechanism, "downward comparison," that can contribute to the behaviors that place aid workers at risk. Disaster workers may feel that, compared with the suffering of the direct victims, some suffering on their part does not matter. The self-esteem of such workers is low enough that they feel better about themselves if they, too, can be vulnerable to harm. At times, dangerous behaviors arise out of alternative psychological mechanisms. A mix of grandiosity, denial, and dissociation can underlie a frequently seen sense of invulnerability to danger expressed by relief workers. Whereas in their home countries, these workers would wear seatbelts and drive carefully, they may do neither in the disaster setting. Whereas workers would be scrupulous about the use of universal blood precautions in home health-care settings, in the field, they may not use gloves to draw blood from refugees. Whereas in their home towns workers would take care to avoid dangerous neighborhoods, they may remain in an area known to be at risk for mortar attack. In each case, there is a suspension of the laws of the real world, a sense that, as one worker who spent her time in an area in Africa that was regularly shelled said, "Once I got used to the noise, I wasn't afraid anything could happen to me, just the others."[45]

Agger underscores the overwhelming powerlessness and moral conflict felt by aid workers in humanitarian crises. She suggests that by risking her life a worker might attempt to relieve moral conflict and guilt.[46]

Sense of Personal Control

Whether one is a primary or secondary victim of war, of disaster, or of over-whelming loss in everyday life, the task of the individual is to cope with the stress in adaptive ways and to process and integrate the experience into one's personhood so that productive life can go on. For all affected by extreme stressors, the critical problem for the individual appears to be the threatened or actual loss of personal control.[47] Virtually by definition, complex emergencies present for the individual and for humanitarian agencies a set of issues that combine to provide the weakest foundation for individual or institutional control. In such emergencies, there are multifaceted obstacles to the provision of aid, ongoing insecurity, and at times frank danger, chronic uncertainty, and unpredictability. Expatriate relief workers are often in an unfamiliar culture, may not speak the local language(s), are unfamiliar with the terrain, and, in situations that are constantly changing, may thus have particular difficulty in identifying or prioritizing threats. A significant portion of the suffering that fills the world of the aid worker in a humanitarian crisis is human-caused, generating more ethical conflict and anger than might a natural disaster. With such pressures, at the very least, it is difficult to focus on one's job as an aid worker, to maintain a comfortable professional role, to maintain neutrality, to remain sensitive and open to all parties in the disaster, and to function at the top of one's game. In addition to the event variables to which the victims and workers are subject within the complex emergency, additional critical variables are based in the individual: appraisal of stressors; coping techniques; defense mechanisms; and prior psychological adaptation.[48] These factors can interact to support teamwork, to build experience, and to lead to adaptive functioning. Alternatively, they can devolve into personal isolation, fragmentation, and dysfunction.

Even the most adaptable and most resilient aid workers can ultimately "crack" if the degree of stress overwhelms their ego organization. Anecdotal and word-of-mouth reports from recent humanitarian crises have provided glimpses into the severe traumatic injuries and ongoing psychological disability of a number of experienced and exemplary aid workers. At least three kinds of stresses appear to underlie their fragmentation:

1. an acute horror and helplessness (witnessing a Hutu militiaman wield a machete to sever the legs of a Rwandan youngster as he was trying to escape);
2. the killing of friends and peers (the execution of six expatriate ICRC workers in Chechnya);
3. the unwise but common practice of sending experienced aid workers from one crisis directly to the next.

Abnormal Event

The mantra of disaster psychology can be summed up in one sentence: the event is abnormal, not the individual. Teaching this concept to all persons affected by extreme events is critical. Worker training must emphasize it and agencies and institutions must be convinced of it. This is not to say that people do not become injured emotionally, rather that it is normal to be traumatized by traumatic events.

Among the factors that have been recognized in the disaster literature as contributing to such injury and prolonging what would in their absence have been a quicker recovery, the most important ones for aid workers appear to be:[49]

1. profound helplessness;
2. confrontation with death;
3. mutilation and decay of bodies;
4. emotional identification with victims;
5. death of children;
6. psychological immaturity of workers;
7. specific personal losses;
8. delayed or absent treatment;
9. secondary gain;
10. malingering;
11. impending litigation.

As experience with worker stress in humanitarian crises accumulates, this list may need to be modified. Certainly, based on anecdotal evidence, the additional issues of intense personal fear, pervasive moral uncertainty, and bureaucratic entanglements contribute greatly to the distress and emotional exhaustion of aid workers in the field.

INTERVENTIONS

Interventions to decrease worker trauma became popular in the 1980s with a variety of methods of post-event debriefing. The efforts of Mitchell and others to promote Critical Incident Stress Debriefing (CISD) within the worklife of emergency and rescue crews has worked to diminish the strong taboo against acknowledging stress and expressing emotion in that culture. Mitchell[41] details the two types of CISD debriefings, one immediately following a critical incident and the other planned 24–48 hours afterward. The initial debriefing takes place during the worker clean-up after an operation; it is informal, is often run by the rescue team leaders, and is most effective when mandatory, removing much of the stigma of seeking mental health support. The initial debriefing offers positive support, attention, and concern for the workers as well as an opportunity for them to express themselves freely. Their expressions are met with acceptance, understanding, and support. The later, more formal CISD debriefing pairs a mental health professional with a trained peer rescue worker to conduct a structured discussion with defined phases. There are six phases of a CISD formal debriefing:

1. introduction of ground rules and outline of process;
2. review of facts;
3. sharing of thoughts and feelings;
4. review of reactions and symptoms of stress;
5. teaching/cognitive phase;
6. wrap-up, follow-up.

Since 1991 the ARC has developed a Disaster Mental Health Service (DMHS) that has become an integrated function in disaster relief operations. DMHS is composed of volunteer mental health professionals who assist both ARC workers and disaster victims on site. Their activities are varied and flexible depending upon the situation and include training, crisis counseling, and debriefing.[50] DMHS has become the primary mental health responder for U.S. aviation disasters, through the National Transportation Safety Board, under a 1996 congressional mandate.

In these two mental health intervention programs, which developed with disaster workers and primary victims as their targets, the rationale behind the decision to develop and expand earlier efforts for workers was based on recognition of:

1. a direct correlation between the psychological hardiness of the relief worker and the success of the mission;
2. the psychological toll paid by workers in their line of duty;
3. the high dropout rate of rescue workers after particularly traumatic events;
4. the need for aid workers to have an awareness of their own feeling states and coping mechanisms in order to be sensitive to these issues for primary victims;
5. the importance of using the public health approach of primary prevention in reducing psychiatric disability in workers, their peer groups, families and communities;
6. a growing sense of institutional responsibility for workplace safety and support.

There is controversy about the effectiveness of debriefing for rescue workers.[51,52] Researchers are attempting to design studies that will demonstrate whether or not debriefing decreases psychological morbidity. Early studies have offered mixed results. Although there has been a tremendous growth in adherents to this intervention, a small group of detractors is also emerging. A 1995 editorial in London's *Sunday Telegraph*[53] questions this "vogue for counselling" and brings to light some of the key arguments, which highlight several central concepts in psychological support for helpers. Briefly stated, two examples are given to demonstrate: (1) the ineffectiveness of debriefing for British body handlers during the Gulf War, and (2) the effectiveness of a lack of recall or dreaming about their terrible experiences in a group of well-adjusted Holocaust survivors. The editorial author suggests that "rather than encouraging people to relive their painful memories, some method of repressing them might be more helpful."

There are several important points to be made in response to the issues raised here. First, it is vital to continue to study the outcomes of all types of psychological intervention so that the best supports can be offered. Second, it must be noted that debriefing is not the only kind of psychological support necessary to sustain disaster workers. It is, instead, one nodal point that carries the potential for positive outcomes: to increase group coherence; to help individuals feel less isolated; and to remind all involved in an extreme event that such events are upsetting and may produce symptoms in normal people. Debriefing also creates the opportunity for facilitators to identify particular disturbed individuals who stand out as having had a difficult time. Third, it is worthwhile to underscore the fact that "debriefings" can be very different from one another depending upon the model used, the expertise and experience of the facilitators, the group, the institution, and the event. Evaluators should not assume that they understand what has happened when they hear that a worker "was debriefed."

Finally, it is important to analyze the concern that counseling in disaster situations may actually exacerbate psychological injury by stirring up painful memories. A major principle of psychological debriefing includes the caveat that no one is forced to talk. It is perfectly acceptable to take part in the group and to remain silent for any or all phases of the process. Another fundamental principle is that workers are taught stress management techniques (including cognitive reframing of events) in a key phase of the debriefings discussed here. These are specific ways for individuals to contain their trauma and to wrap up their feelings. The belief that psychological support in disaster is about pulling distressing recollections out of people is fallacious. Instead, emotional supports should be timed so that workers have the opportunity to share and to mold strong feelings before they harden or become inaccessible.

The author of the editorial ends by saying, "repression can be a very good thing, and the healthiest way of dealing with unhappy events is to forget them." Although it is certainly essential to avoid a doctrinaire approach in dealing with traumatized individuals, the problem with unconscious burial of distressing material (the defense of repression) is that it can travel underground and become the stuff of nightmares and symptoms. One healthy way to deal with such things is to consciously acknowledge what happened and, then, to consciously suppress those events. The distinction is of great consequence. The ego remains in charge when suppression is employed and is beleaguered when using repression.

INSTITUTIONAL RESPONSE

As experience with humanitarian crises has proliferated, the stress incurred by aid workers has attracted increasing attention.[54] These compound disasters have drawn record numbers of aid workers and produced record numbers of traumatized staff. The responsibilities of agencies and institutions to their workers is a critical issue. A new level of attention to broad worker health needs is imperative. One aspect of this matter is sensitivity to psychological issues in the worker but another, perhaps more difficult, aspect has to do with the need for institutional change. Agency priorities must be integrated with the needs of workers. In their recent discussion of emotional responses in international aid workers, Smith et al.[55] note a disturbing gulf between what they perceive as the extra-humanitarian goals and objectives of the organization (ensuring political influence and financial support, which require visibility and high volume output from the worker) and the idealism and professionalism of the worker (which may drive quite different agendas, such as building relationships and attending to local planning and development of initiatives among local personnel). Smith et al. see this conflict as contributing to high worker recidivism rates, since a worker on short-term assignment who protests has no clout against a "huge international aid organization." It is difficult for fieldworkers to influence organizations to change. The institution must recognize its part in causing worker stress.

Insensitivity to employee needs can be disastrous to the life of the worker. The same authors detail a tragic outcome that they assert would not have occurred "if the person had experienced an average expectable work support." This account illustrates a profoundly disturbing theme in relief work:

> A United Nations field officer working for refugees in the Middle East was taken hostage and for several weeks was handled brutally, blindfolded, chained, and transported between various hiding places. More than once he had reasons to believe he would soon be executed. After he was released and had time to recover somewhat, despite his wishes to be transferred elsewhere, he was sent to a similar district. His post-traumatic stress reactions developed into a disorder when he experienced a situation similar to when he had been seized. As a part of his treatment/rehabilitation program in his native country, his agency was asked to assign him to an office job at Headquarters.

The request was turned down. He felt rejected and let down, became depressed and his condition worsened. In spite of qualified treatment, a high motivation to work through the traumatic experience, a premorbid personality without any vulnerability factors, and an unproblematic life situation, he did not recover. Unable to work, he applied for disability payments, but was turned down by his pension plan because his membership had not lasted long enough. Over time he had to sell his summer house, later on his house, and ended up poor. His depression deepened and he became suicidal. In the end, his national government had to approach the agency to negotiate a satisfactory financial settlement for him.[55]

Generic Institutional Interventions

Generic institutional interventions now developed to support the mental health of rescue workers can be expanded to provide critical supports for responders to humanitarian crises (Box 7.4). These activities fall into the following categories.

Box 7.4 Institutional supports necessary to sustain relief workers

---

- Attention to broad worker health needs
- Recognition of institutional role in causing worker stress
- Recruitment of aid workers with personality traits favorable to adaptation to stress
- Preparedness training in disaster psychology, stress managagement, and adaptive coping skills
- A plan for emotional support embedded in the institutional culture
- Operational briefings prior to complex emergency entrance
- On-site communication and emotional support; implementation of basic self-care measures
- Post-crisis psychological debriefing (on site or near site)
- Evacuation of severely impaired workers for special care
- Ongoing follow-up upon return home (professional mental health support, ongoing communication) to monitor for delayed stress response

---

Candidate selection   While aid worker recruitment remains far from a science, there is evidence that certain personality traits favor adaptation to stress. Given the multiple caveats about personal factors and stress noted throughout the literature, screeners may wish to look for the following attributes in candidates for workers in humanitarian crises: flexibility; ability to laugh at oneself; stable sense of self; developmental maturity; professionalism; demonstrated self-knowledge, particularly regarding reasons for attraction to disaster work; ability to collaborate with others; ability to utilize suppression as a defense mechanism (rather than repression); interpersonal warmth; creativity; ability to follow direction; experience in stressful/traumatic settings with insight into lessons learned.

Preparedness training   As part of the general training of an aid worker for humanitarian organizations, candidates need to learn about disaster psychology, stress managagement, and adaptive coping skills. For instance, the ICRC has developed a pamphlet for its workers on stress management.[56] Workers need to be given information about past humanitarian crisis settings, difficulties, and lessons learned. It is important that they prepare for the extreme levels of frustration and helplessness that can pervade a mission; the moral dilemmas and double binds that they might encounter; the unfair allocation of resources that they might witness or engage in; the violence that might surround them and the danger that they must recognize and manage. They must have an opportunity to anticipate their own fears, anxiety, and guilt in the setting of horror and tremendous suffering. They must work on identifying emotional strategies to cope and function technically.[57] All other variables held constant, it follows that training and experience prior to the event can change the setpoint of threat for a group or an individual.

The institution needs to develop a plan for emotional support that can be put into operation on missions through methods that use both peer interaction and chain-of-command engagement. The plan must be embedded in the institutional culture, not a last-minute add-on. A high priority should be placed on retaining only those workers and leaders who can contribute within such a system, which places added emphasis on performance assessment and exit debriefings.

Operational briefing   Before going into the site of a complex emergency, aid workers need to understand the nature of the humanitarian emergency they are about to enter, the political, cultural, and ethnic influences, the role their organization intends to play, the planned mission, its chief priorities and limits, technical capabilities expected of them, and anticipated dangers and difficulties. All this information serves to support their capacity to exercise self-control and raise their threshold for threat appraisal.

On-site monitoring, communicating, processing   On site, every effort should be made to include all workers in a communication and support network. Discussion of events by the work group should be a routine part of every difficult day. If a particularly troubling event has occurred, it will be necessary to share feelings and reactions within the group in a more deliberate manner. The aim of this group process is to "deprivatize"[45] reactions and to strengthen appropriate defenses, not to unleash deep emotions.

The work group can provide critical emotional support in the field. Peers and supervisors can encourage emotional communication, accept and understand a co-worker's stress responses, allow one another to provide support and show appreciation for that support, and in particular point out and discourage unrealistic self-expectation.[58]

In the field, it is also important to remember basic self-care and to ensure that supervisors build in simple measures for workers such as sufficient sleep, breaks in the day, days off, acknowledgment of good work, and so on.

Mission leaders need to have particular training in the assessment of threats to the operation. They must not only be qualified to fulfill all aspects of the mission, but must also be prepared to abort it for the safety of their workers.[59]

When workers are subjected to significant traumatic exposure, the behavior of their leadership can strongly influence their resilience. Wright et al. detail the positive role played by senior Air Force commanders at Fort Campbell, Kentucky, following the Gander air crash in 1985. They offer the term "grief leadership" for the way in which the commanders supported the community mourning process:

1. they publicly expressed their own grief;
2. they focused on the importance of the community's sharing its sorrow;
3. they structured a series of rituals—including having the President of the United States and the First Lady express the grief of the American people—to honor the soldiers who died in the crash.[60]

On (or Near)-site debriefing   Prior to leaving the area a worker should have an opportunity to go through a psychological debriefing. In order to have any chance of sharing observations and unloading toxic feelings, workers must be in a physically and emotionally safe setting. If the group meeting has to be held in an area of ongoing threat, the chief goal must instead be to shore up defenses and manage anxiety. It is not appropriate, in such settings, to dig for "hazardous emotional material."

A psychological debriefing is distinct from an operational review, is confidential within the bounds of worker safety, and is best conducted by a mental health professional. If a worker is highly symptomatic, an individual debriefing may be appropriate. In general, however, members of a work group or individuals who share organizational status and work responsibilities are debriefed together, with the help of one or two mental health facilitators.

Military psychiatry in war settings has demonstrated the marked increase in chronic disabling symptoms in soldiers who were evacuated away from their fighting group with the intent of providing more definitive treatment for their conditions. A rapid return to the group and ultimate pullout with the full group improves most combat stress.[61] Symptoms of psychological trauma may, perhaps, remain pliant at the scene but become entrenched at a distance. This observation may relate to the point made previously that an individual's appraisal of his or her degree of trauma is influenced by the peer group. Once apart from the group, an individual's self-assessments harden.

The concept of a "trauma membrane" may also underlie this finding. This concept, first described by Lindy in 1985, refers to the protective shield formed around a disaster survivor by concerned significant others. This membrane keeps out disturbance and intrusion into the traumatized victim's private space. It is possible for caring helpers to be allowed into that space early in the membrane formation if a strong enough bond can be formed.[62] This concept has application to the traumatized worker in a complex emergency setting. In formulating structures to support aid workers, the trauma membrane should be considered from two perspectives. First, the utility of a protected emotional space for an injured worker should be recognized, and supports should be implemented to ensure the rapid development of such a space when a critical event, such as a significant worker injury, occurs. Second, in planning the appropriate steps to help aid workers who are leaving the assignment, the possible existence of this membrane must be taken into account in designing the scope and venue of debriefing.

Assessment for off-site referral   At the time of the debriefing, individuals who are having a particularly difficult time should be identified. An individual evaluation should be done to consider the appropriate next step. In general, severely impaired international aid workers are best evacuated to a headquarters setting in order to receive care within the penumbra of the larger work group rather than being sent home to a setting unfamiliar with disaster work and the events that transpired in the particular humanitarian crisis.

Home follow-up   The aid worker returning home from a crisis will encounter difficult issues in making a transition back to his or her prior life. Family members and significant others should be educated in how to assist in the transition, what kind of stress responses to expect, what to be concerned about, and where to turn for help. Sources of professional mental health support must be available to the worker. A routine follow-up debriefing by a local professional skilled in disaster mental health a month or so after return would be an excellent structure to put in place. Institutional outreach as well as ongoing communication with members of the team is important. These networks can monitor for any new signs of stress response that may appear as a delayed reaction. Early detection, with introduction of appropriate treatment, is crucial to short- and longer-term recovery.

CONCLUSION

An understanding of the recognition of psychological trauma in the modern era is necessary in order to apprehend the levels of stress, the psychological challenges, and the kinds of emotional response that relief workers experience in humanitarian crises. During the past decade, disaster agencies and rescue workers in the United States have acquired greater understanding of the psychological vulnerability of workers in extreme settings. Many programs of support are under way.

The difficulties involved in mounting relief efforts in recent complex emergencies have thrown the spotlight on the plight of the international humanitarian aid worker. Although lessons learned from the disaster psychology literature are of great help in conceptualizing the fundamental issues, these workers face additional problems.

The event characteristics are particularly challenging. The outcomes of humanitarian crises have been frustrating to all parties, giving workers a deeply impoverished sense of positive impact or sense of closure. The absence of resolution, the inability to see any accomplishment, in itself produces stress. An appreciation of being part of something that has led to good results is an important aspect of balancing the traumatic experience.

Aid workers have also witnessed profound violence and suffering from unprecedented positions of helplessness. They have been put in harm's way as never before. Burkle draws a distinction between the protection afforded a relief worker in disaster by his or her professional stance and the absence of this protection afforded a soldier in war. In the former context, a disaster allows some objectivity on the part of the worker, a professional distance from which to organize and accomplish tasks. The situation of war is instead characterized by a loss of objectivity, as the soldier/worker is directly subject to, if not a direct target of, all the threats at hand.[40] Smith et al. review the appalling setting faced by the relief teams who responded to the crisis in Goma in the late summer and fall of 1994. They describe the psychological stress felt by all aid workers and give the following example from the experience of those with the International Rescue Committee (IRC). Along with predictable team stress, irritability, individual trouble concentrating, and serious sleep problems, "a significant number of people opted not to return to the camp after their first contact with the situation and completely avoided it." Organizing or delivering effective aid was difficult. Individuals were so affected by coming in contact with the refugee camp that "for the first time, some of the staff were instructed to limit their contact with the situation" in order to preserve some emotional equilibrium and decision-making capability.[63] In the environment that characterized Goma, one sees how quickly professional objectivity can be eroded and how much closer the aid worker can move toward the situation of a soldier in a war setting.

The broad influences governing the extent of emotional upset in a disaster setting are known. The aid community is in no position to affect the leading factor, the characteristics of the event itself.

The aid community is, however, in a position to bring influence to bear on many of the other factors. These include:

- personnel (the individual aid workers, their chain of command, the nature of the groups who work together);
- preparedness (the expressed values and mission of the institution);
- the recruitment and selection of workers;
- worker training in technical relief;
- institutional culture;
- team building and psychological support;
- the work site (worker supports within the field) and off-site settings (once out of the field).

The challenges outlined above call for a thorough reassessment of the proactive role of the relief organization in achieving new levels of resilience in workers, new tiers of support for them, and a new portfolio of realistic and achievable goals for each humanitarian crisis to which the workers commit themselves.

Relief organizations need to take on greater responsibility for the individuals they send into these very difficult settings. Unlike rescue workers and regular disaster workers who have ongoing jobs and peer groups, many international workers have loose connections with institutions and work only brief stints abroad. These are the individuals who are now under the greatest work strain. Relief organizations must develop the institutional capacity to pay attention to the world the aid worker lives in and to support the worker in his or her adjustment over time and across geographic space. Routines need to be set up within an established human resources department of each relief organization to promote more vigorous and critical screening at the staff selection phase, better preparation prior to deployment, and much more sustained and robust follow-up and interaction during and after each assignment. Assessment and follow-up support should be linked to more academic discussion of events and their implications for individuals, the team, and the mission. Aid workers should engage with people who understand their experience and can help them explore and analyze it in order to gain and secure objectivity and distance. As has been observed over the years,[64,65] psychic trauma is in great part determined not by the event alone, but by the meaning and affect it evokes in the particular individual.

The potential costs of not embarking upon institutional capacity-building strategies to support relief workers include the personal risks to individuals in these roles as well as the possibility of deploying people who are so damaged by their current or past experience that they will diminish or defeat the humanitarian intent of the helping community. Further, by failing to invest in a strategy that supports their personnel, humanitarian organizations will be repeating the past history of social response to individual trauma, which is to deny its existence, substance, relevance, and power. That repetition would in turn serve to abort our understanding of how pervasively destructive these experiences are to all those who are forced to endure them and to all those who have elected to enter them to provide help.

Developing institutional capacities to study and address the needs of the relief worker can be seen as a "win-win-win" strategy, one that will have positive effects in three directions. The individual worker and worker groups within the organization will be more resilient and more cohesive. The organization's mission will have a better chance of success. And the primary victims will gain more empathic, respectful, and focused assistance.

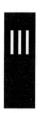

NORMATIVE AND PRACTICAL ISSUES

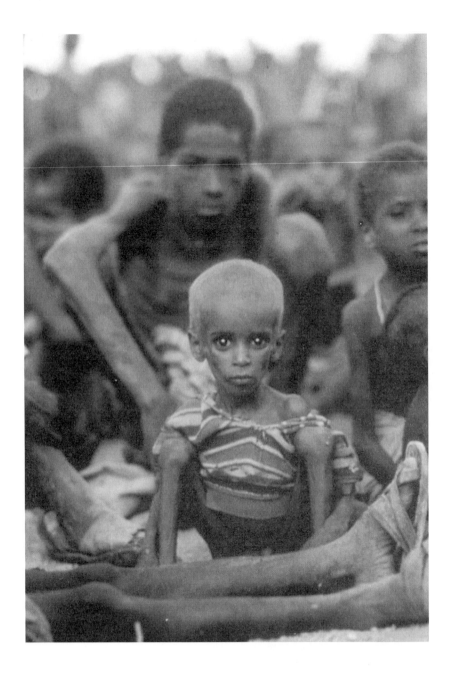

THE NEW ETHICAL BOUNDARIES

sissela bok

The expression "complex emergency," formulated in the United Nations in the early 1990s to characterize vast humanitarian crises such as those in Rwanda and Bosnia, has already passed into common parlance among NGOs and in the media. The growth in number and visibility of such crises in the post–cold war era has put unprecedented pressure on humanitarian agencies. It has also generated bewilderment among many in the international community regarding the allocation of responsibility and the costs to be borne in responding to human rights violations and desperate survival needs. Part of the bewilderment stems from a failure to sort out and examine the different factual and moral strands of expressions such as "complex emergency" and "humanitarian."

As we address the question of how to respond to the growing number of complex humanitarian emergencies worldwide, it is important, therefore, to seek greater understanding of the terms themselves. What exactly do they mean? In what sense are such collective calamities complex? How do they differ, once labeled emergencies, from equally desperate long-term human predicaments, if at all? And how is the expression "complex emergency" changed, if at all, by speaking, as is often done, of complex humanitarian emergencies? The following citations to "complex emergency" are representative of current usage:

The world's response to mass migration is most prompt and adequate when refugees cross international borders and, therefore, are protected by international legal conventions. In the case of more complex emergencies, involving civil war, famine, non-functioning governments, and mass internal displacement, the world has been slower to respond.[1]

Contemporary refugee crises tend to be complex emergencies that combine political instability, ethnic tensions, armed conflict, economic collapse, and the disintegration of civil society.[2]

Most of the latest missions have been what the UN calls "complex emergencies," in which the UN must end a war, cure a famine, resettle refugees, work with relief agencies, even rebuild whole nations.[3]

For the purposes of this document, a "complex emergency" is a humanitarian crisis that may involve armed conflict and may be exacerbated by natural disasters. It is a situation in which prevailing conditions threaten the lives of a portion of the affected population who, for a variety of reasons, are unable to obtain the minimum subsistence requirements and are dependent on external humanitarian assistance for survival.[4]

Rwanda is the latest of what United Nations and government officials call "complex emergencies," a lethal combination of starvation, economic collapse, civil strife, and disintegrating political authority.[5]

These references to "complex emergency" overlap only in part. Most, but not all, mention the plight of refugees, armed conflict, starvation, and societal collapse, whether economic or political or both. Other elements mentioned include the role of relief agencies or of humanitarian assistance, ethnic tensions, and possible natural disasters. All concern, implicitly or explicitly, vast threats to human survival.

THE NEED TO AVOID EUPHEMISM

The expression "complex emergency," used in these ways, is more than a label for such crises. It offers a starting point from which to inquire into their causes and possible remedies. And from an immediate practical point of view, the expression offers neutral, nonaccusatory language that may facilitate negotiations with obstructionist governments or warring parties for safe passage or safe havens. Like many similar abstractions, however, "complex emergency" can also function as a euphemism that makes it possible for outsiders to make dispassionate references to unspeakable forms of inhumanity and to human suffering so stark as to be almost unbearable, if truly perceived.

The constituent words "complex" and "emergency" are themselves highly abstract and multilayered, with many meanings that only partially enter into the concept of "complex emergency." When used together, the two words also take on special moral connotations that they do not otherwise possess. So long as these interlocking meanings and moral connotations are not sorted out, it is easier either to settle for the use of the concept as euphemism or to read into it unexamined moral premises and untested, undebated conclusions about responsibilities, rights, and obligations. It is worth considering each of the two constituent words in turn, therefore, along with "humanitarian," so often wedged between them, as a background to the larger debate about how moral claims should affect our responses to the crises of human survival at issue.

COMPLEXITY: PHYSICAL, POLITICAL, AND MORAL ASPECTS

Something—a fraction, a number, a musical harmony, a machine, a sentence—is complex if it consists of several parts that are connected or woven together. (The Latin "complexus" means "plaited together," and the words "plaited together," "interwoven," and "connected together" occur variously in dictionary definitions of "complex.") A heap of stones is not complex in this sense, no matter how many stones are part of it, whereas even the simplest living organism beyond the amoeba stage is. A related meaning of the word "complex" is that of something that is difficult to disentangle or analyze, as in a complex logical problem or engineering setup. In none of these circumstances does the word ordinarily carry any moral connotations, having to do with justice and injustice or good and evil.

Earthquakes, floods, and other natural disasters are often extraordinarily complex, in the sense of exhibiting a number of interacting factors and in that of being difficult to disentangle; yet such disasters are not classified as "complex emergencies" unless the complexity is also of a moral nature, in that human actions are contributing to rendering the resulting crisis more severe. The civil strife in the aftermath of the earthquake in Armenia in 1988, for example, increased the suffering of the quake's victims and rendered assistance efforts more difficult. That crisis would now count as a complex emergency, unlike the aftermath of the earthquake in the Philippines in 1990 or that in Los Angeles in 1994.

This moral aspect of complexity, in complex emergencies, attaches both to causes generating the emergency and to the effort to remedy them. Human undertakings, such as political repression, civil war, or economic pressures from the outside, contribute directly to such a state of crisis, whether or not triggered by a natural disaster. When warring factions, as in Somalia, or governments, as in Sudan or Haiti, not only heighten conditions of famine, migration, and epidemics but also interfere with the distribution of aid, confiscate supplies, and threaten the lives of relief workers, the existing emergency comes to be characterized as complex. It is an emergency, as one UN representative cautiously put it, "with complex political overtones."[6]

Such a crisis is rendered both more acute and more difficult to overcome to the extent that aid efforts become more dangerous and costly. It involves both unintended and intended causes: on the one hand, naturally occurring causes of misery such as drought, famine, epidemics, and overcrowding, and, on the other hand, the purposive interference by public officials, warring groups, or foreign powers, with the effort by victims to see to their own survival and by outsiders to come to their aid.

This is not to say that there can ever be absolute demarcations between human and nonhuman causes of emergencies. Famines typically result from mismanagement and maldistribution; earthquakes have very different effects in crowded regions than in deserts. But the difference to which the term complex speaks, in this context, is between emergencies where governments or warring factions do and do not contribute directly to societal collapse, do and do not actively threaten the survival of populations.

The moral aspects of such uses of the word "complex," then, have to do with human activities held to be rightful or wrongful, admirable or reprehensible, just or unjust. Such judgments are unavoidable when the survival of populations is at issue. But the very complexity of the causes of the emergencies makes the attribution of responsibility complex as well. As a result, moral accusations are often levied at adversaries by the contestants on each side of the related conflicts, and at outsiders.

The eighteenth-century philosopher David Hume wrote of conditions in which survival is threatened on a large scale as ones in which justice itself may be out of reach (Box 8.1).[7] He pointed to both natural and human causes of such a state of affairs. Justice can be expected, first of all, only in an intermediate range with respect to both natural scarcity and human failures. If there is such scarcity that human survival is impossible, then justice is to no avail. Conversely, if there is utter abundance of all that human beings might need, justice is unnecessary. Second, justice is only within reach and needed when human beings are neither so demoniacally evil and shortsightedly blind to future consequences that appeals to justice are to no avail, nor so uniformly generous, altruistic, kind, and foresightful that problems or disputes would never arise.

When Hume wrote, there would have been no way for him to conceive of humanly inflicted suffering on the massive scale that we now witness. The world's population had not yet reached one billion. The armaments of the time could inflict but a fraction of the casualties of contemporary wars. And reports of threats to survival in distant lands made their way slowly, if at all, to the European public. But if Hume could have foreseen a present-day complex emergency such as that in Rwanda in 1994, he might have seen it as an example of conditions in which any sort of justice is threatened because of the interweaving of human and natural forces at their most lethal: where political strife amounting to genocide, along with hunger, lack of water, epidemics, and agricultural failure, threatens millions of women, children, and men, in addition to those killed from the outset, and also poses extraordinary risks for those attempting humanitarian assistance.

As Judith Shklar points out, however, in *The Faces of Injustice,* the distinction between humanly inflicted injustices and naturally occurring misfortunes such as those from earthquakes comes more easily for outsiders than for the victims themselves: "[T]he difference between misfortune and injustice frequently involves our willingness and our capacity to act or not to act on behalf of the victims, to blame or to absolve, to help, mitigate, and compensate, or just to turn away."[8]

The concept of a complex emergency was not available as recently as 1990, when Shklar wrote. But it, too, is peculiarly a concept coined from the perspective of outsiders. To be in the midst of calamities such as those experienced by victims of such emergencies is to be beset in such ways that distinctions between human and nonhuman causes, moral and nonmoral factors, are of little or no avail.

Box 8.1 Complex humanitarian emergencies and the traditions of moral philosophy: A sampling of views

ERASMUS (16th century)	• Humans add to natural and inevitable evils through their rush to arms
HUME (18th century)	• Justice can be expected only in an intermediate range with respect to both natural scarcity and human failures. Extreme scarcity precludes justice; abundance makes justice unnecessary.
	• Justice is only within reach and needed when humans are neither so evil that appeals to justice are to no avail nor so altruistic that disputes never arise.
SIDGWICK (19th century)	• Utilitarian principle of ethics, that "another's greater good is to be preferred to one's own lesser good."
	• Commonsense view that our obligations to help others differ depending on the relationships in which we stand to them (circle of relations).
SCHWEITZER (20th century)	• In answer to question, "Am I my brother's keeper?" answered, "How could I not be?"
	• Insisted on obligation to help those in need, wherever one found them, to the best of one's ability.
KING (20th century)	• "We are all one family. We are our brothers' keepers because we are our brothers' brothers."
SHKLAR (20th century)	• Distinction between humanly inflicted injustices and naturally occurring misfortunes comes more easily for outsiders than for the victims themselves.

EMERGENCY: TO WHOM AND FOR WHOM?

An emergency is defined by the *Oxford English Dictionary* as a "juncture that arises or turns up; especially a state of things unexpectedly arising and urgently demanding immediate action"; or by the *American Heritage Dictionary* as a situation "of great danger that develops suddenly and unexpectedly." Yet the vast and many-dimensional threats to human survival labeled as "complex emergencies" do not altogether fit these dictionary definitions of emergencies. A landslide, an earthquake, a flood may come about in such a sudden and unexpected way; but the crisis in Rwanda, though it ignited with sudden force, was not unexpected; and the famine resulting from civil war in Somalia was less and less unexpected as the months wore on. Such situations are, however, emergencies in that they are "urgently demanding action." They are viewed, therefore, as emergencies in a sense that is primarily moral or valuational: namely, a situation so serious as to have priority over others. Just as emergency vehicles have priority on the road and other cars must pull to the side and let them pass, so the claim for complex emergencies is that they represent such urgent human predicaments that they must receive priority over other human needs. Funds allocated elsewhere by donor agencies and nations must be reallocated, at least for the short run.

The use of the word "emergency" to indicate priority in the distribution of resources constitutes, therefore, an implicit moral claim. Unless it is seen as such, it can serve to bypass issues of weighing and comparing responses: Why, for instance, rush to provide aid at one time rather than earlier or later? Why bring aid to one society and not to another in similar straits? How long should the aid continue, and at what costs to all involved? Merely labeling some crises and not others "emergencies" ought not to be dispositive with respect to where to rush assistance on an emergency basis.

Here again, as with the distinction between "complex" and other emergencies, the distinction between complex crises that count and do not count as emergencies is one made from the perspective of outsiders who must decide how and when to try to be of help, rather than from that of the victims themselves, for whom any threat to life is an emergency, even if no outsider learns of their predicament or comes to their help. Many instances of vast human suffering have gone largely unnoticed by those who might have come to the rescue, or, to the extent noticed and documented, have elicited little outside response. Idi Amin's reign of terror in Uganda in the 1970s, in which more than 300,000 persons were killed, would have constituted, in today's terms, a "complex emergency." But would it have been granted priority at the time by the international community? And how might such an expression have applied to the Nazi Holocaust? Or to the Chinese famine of 1959–1961, now estimated to have taken between 20 and 40 million lives? Too often, what is at stake is not so much the levels of human suffering as whether or not the outside world becomes aware of this suffering and chooses to make an issue of it.

One must distinguish, then, between collective human emergencies as experienced from within and from without. From within, they count as such whether or not aid is available—and indeed, as mentioned above, whether or not the suffering is inflicted on purpose by human forces or not. For victims, likewise, the question of whether their suffering is increased because of embargoes, sanctions, or other forms of economic warfare imposed by outside governments is also harder to assess than for outsiders. The more ruthless the regime at the receiving end of such measures, the more likely it is to expose its own people to the worst hardships resulting from them, and thus to contribute to what outsiders view as a more severe complex emergency than would otherwise have been the case.

In the age of television, attention can be thrown at one such emergency rather than another, depending, in part, on how difficult it is for reporters and photographers to gain entry into particular societies—into Somalia, say, rather than the Sudan in 1993. Here again, the more ruthlessly a regime controls entry and exit, the less likely it is that adequate documentation of the emergency by outsiders will be possible.

The question, therefore, of what constitutes a "complex emergency" has both strategic and moral aspects (Box 8.2). The strategic, or factual, aspects concern the conditions in a particular society in crisis and the magnitude of the needs to be met. The moral aspects have to do with how the determination is to be made that such an emergency exists, where responsibilities should be assigned, what kind of priority should be accorded the effort to seek remedies, and how long the state of emergency should occupy center stage if aid efforts do not bear fruit. If the moral aspects are not kept clearly in sight, it is likely that they will be blurred and thought, erroneously, to go

Box 8.2 Ethical and strategical overlaps in war and complex humanitarian emergencies

ETHICAL LANGUAGE	STRATEGIC LANGUAGE	AREAS WHERE ETHICAL AND STRATEGIC APPROACHES OVERLAP
Rooted in religion and in writings on morality	Rooted in strategic thinkers (e.g., Machiavelli, Clausewitz)	Communication, security, coordination, flexibility, transportation, deployment, supplies, interventions to bring relief and medical aid, sanitation, etc.
Stresses character, responsibility, respect, care and concern, principled conduct	Stresses competence, insight, planning	Debate about legitimate forms of intervention
Supports right relations among individuals and communities	Supports winning and survival	Focus on prevention of calamities
Raises issues of right and wrong, justice	Abandons ethical considerations in extreme versions ("All is fair in love and war")	Reconciliation of humanitarian/human rights objectives
Can provide false guidance and lead to damaging results if strategy is neglected		

without saying as long as factual answers are found to the question. This is more likely to happen whenever the third term, "humanitarian," with its seemingly self-evident moral import, is used in conjunction with the first two, as in "complex humanitarian emergencies" or when "humanitarian assistance" is rendered in the context of complex emergencies.

HUMANITARIAN: AN ALTRUIST OR A SCOUNDREL?

The word "humanitarian," unlike the first two, has inherent moral connotations from the outset. It evokes helpfulness, benevolence, and humane concern going to all who are in need, without regard to person. The *American Heritage Dictionary* in its 1993 edition defined a humanitarian as "one devoted to the promotion of human welfare and the advancement of social reforms; a philanthropist." Such a person is admired even by many who are less altruistic. So are many forms of humanitarian assistance, even by those who regard particular undertakings so described as poorly planned or executed.

This positive view of humanitarians was less prevalent in the nineteenth century, however, when the word first came into common usage in English. The adjective "humanitarian" was then used, according to the *Oxford English Dictionary,* in a manner "nearly always contemptuous, connoting one who goes to excess in humane principles." The word conveyed deep-rooted suspicion, unlike such words as "humane," "kindly," or "good." At the time, the relation of "humanitarian" to "humane" was often seen as similar to that of today's "do-gooder" to "good." Many regarded those laying claims to humanitarianism as at best wooly-headed and sentimental about humanity at large, propounding vast schemes for human improvement even as they neglected their responsibilities to their own families and communities, and at worst, as persons using the mantle of humanitarianism and the love of humankind to cover up every form of religious, commercial, or even criminal abuse and exploitation of others.

Charles Dickens's portrait of Mr. Pecksniff, in *Martin Chuzzlewit,* conveys that form of exploitative hypocrisy so perfectly that "pecksniffian" has entered the English language.[9] Pecksniff, a self-proclaimed "humanitarian philosopher," expresses unctuous concern for all of humanity, calling his own daughters (and fellow parasites until he betrays them) Mercy and Charity. He is shown up for the scoundrel he is, scheming to defraud and torment his fellow humans while intoning the language of universal love.

By the twentieth century, a great shift in the meaning of "humanitarian" was taking place, one that matters as we seek to understand current conflicts about when and how to respond to complex humanitarian emergencies. The term "humanitarian" has come to be more focused and less derogatory. It is more focused, in that it concerns specifically the effort to meet fundamental human needs and to alleviate suffering, rather than all conceivable efforts to improve the human condition. And it is less derogatory, in that suspicion is no longer part of the reaction it evokes for most people. A humanitarian, rather, is seen as someone genuinely concerned to meet urgent human needs wherever they arise, without distinction as to nationality, ethnic background, or religion.

Early in the century, Albert Schweitzer helped to dramatize the personal choice that taking such humanitarianism seriously represents. His writings on religion and music had already achieved wide recognition in Europe when he went, in 1913, to Gabon, in what was then French Equatorial Africa, to build a hospital and minister to those most need in of help. In explaining how he had come to make this choice, Schweitzer wrote that he had read about "the physical miseries of the natives in the virgin forests; . . . and the more I thought about it, the stranger it seemed to me that we Europeans trouble ourselves so little about the great humanitarian task which offers itself to us in far-off lands."[10] In answer to the question "Am I my brother's keeper?" he reputedly answered: "How could I not be? I cannot escape my responsibility." He insisted that all human beings counted as brothers, in this sense, and that his obligation was to help those in need, wherever he found them, to the best of his ability. Likewise, Martin Luther King, Jr., as quoted by Jesse Jackson in the *Los Angeles Times,* held that "We are all one family. We are our brothers' keepers because we are our brothers' brothers."

By the end of our century, however, and in no small part because of the complex emergencies now endangering the survival of so many, the term "humanitarian" has undergone yet another shift. It is a shift not yet noted, to the best of my knowledge, in any dictionaries. With the growth of UN aid agencies, of NGO assistance programs, and so many governmental and intergovernmental efforts designated as humanitarian, the word no longer denotes only persons who work to alleviate suffering and to meet human needs, nor only their attitudes, beliefs, or actions. It now connotes, also, collective assistance programs in the name of the international community, as by the United Nations, which created a Department of Humanitarian Affairs in 1992, as well as the rules of war.[11] But in the process, the term has expanded still further: it has come to concern not only the provision of aid but also the predicament of those persons and communities and populations who are in greatest need of such aid. Accordingly, when we now speak of "humanitarian crises," of "complex humanitarian emergencies," or of "international humanitarian law," we have in mind the crises for those who are afflicted as well as for those who are struggling to come to their aid.

HUMANITARIAN AID OR INVASION?

As for the concept of "humanitarian interventions," and especially military interventions on humanitarian grounds, these have long been used even by powers having nothing but conquest in mind. Throughout history, the vast majority of invasions, proxy wars, and political coups engineered from the outside have been undertaken for self-serving, often expansionist reasons quite different from any humanitarian goals invoked by their sponsors. A case in point is Hitler's claim, on September 23, 1938, that ethnic Germans and various nationalities in Czechoslovakia were being maltreated to the point that the security of more than 3 million human beings was at stake.[12]

By now, the term "humanitarian intervention" is more frequently invoked for what appear to be at least in part genuinely altruistic undertakings.[13,14] And the criteria are changing with respect to when and how it is seen as legitimate to intervene in the affairs of a state and across national frontiers to deliver humanitarian aid. But when it comes to claims that military interventions are humanitarian in nature, the original nineteenth-century suspicion of claims to humanitarianism stands as a caution against idealistic labels that risk concealing, or developing into, old-fashioned power politics.

Each of the three constituent elements of the concept of "complex humanitarian emergencies," in sum, has to be seen in the light of how it has evolved, as we consider the concept itself and the role that it now plays in debates about how best to respond to crises of human survival. Together, they point to the interlocking obstacles, and especially the human obstacles, to providing meaningful aid across national boundaries, and to the possibility that these emergencies might be not just crises in their own right, but represent, together, an unprecedented crisis for humanitarian action and intervention.

EXTENDING THE HUMAN CIRCLE

As the images of unspeakable suffering multiply, outsiders experience anguish in considering how best to allocate aid and to weigh the costs, even in human terms, of attempting to carry out such aid. There is anguish, too, at the contrast between the inestimable worth many are willing to grant to each life and their awareness—made so much more immediate and overpowering by television coverage—of the burden of suffering under which so many fellow human beings labor.[15] Most people care about the survival of at least some—at least themselves, their family and friends, often also their fellow citizens—more than about the rest of humanity. Yet many also take seriously the challenge posed by views such as those of Albert Schweitzer, and worry about the injustice in treating human beings differently on such grounds.

Henry Sidgwick, the British nineteenth-century thinker, found this contrast to be serious enough to threaten any coherent view of ethics. On the one hand, he was prepared, as a utilitarian, to hold as the fundamental principle of ethics "that another's greater good is to be preferred to one's own lesser good." According to such a principle, any sacrifice on one's own part would be called for, as long as it could achieve a greater good for others.[16] And to those who urged that we owe more to our fellow citizens than to the rest of humanity, Sidgwick responded that he had never seen, nor could even "conceive, any ethical reasoning that will provide even a plausible basis" for such a view.[17]

On the other hand, Sidgwick also took for granted what he called the commonsense view that our obligations to help others differ depending on the relationships in which we stand to them:

> We should all agree that each of us is bound to show kindness to his parents and spouse and children, and to other kinsmen in a less degree; and to those who have rendered services to him, and any others whom he may have admitted to his intimacy and called friends; and to neighbors and to fellow-countrymen more than others; and perhaps we may say to those of our own race more than to black or yellow men, and generally to human beings in proportion to their affinity to ourselves.[18]

A metaphor that has often been used, beginning in antiquity, to convey the conflict to which Sidgwick points, is that of concentric circles of human concern and allegiance, with the self in the center, surrounded by circles for family members, friends, community members, fellow citizens, and the rest of humanity.[19,20] The diagram in Figure 8.1 represents this metaphor.

The circle metaphor speaks to the necessary tensions between what is

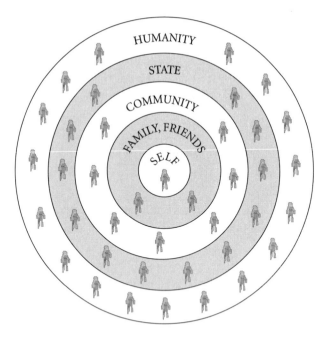

Figure 8.1   The metaphor of concentric circles, with the self at the center and progressively distant social relations in the outer circles, can be viewed in contrasting ways: as encouragement to expand one's connections with the larger world or as reinforcement of the notion that one's primary allegiances are owed to those closest to one's own station.

owed to insiders and outsiders of the many interlocking groups in which we all exist. The metaphor has long been used either to urge us to stretch our concern outward from the narrowest personal confines toward the needs of outsiders, strangers, and all of humanity (and, according to the views of some thinkers, animals);[21,22] or to stress a contrasting view: that of "my station and its duties," according to which at least some of our primary allegiances are, precisely, dependent on our situation and role in life and cannot be overridden by obligations to humanity at large.

The first view corresponds to universalist humanitarianism in many of its forms. It is expressed in statements such as those by Schweitzer and King. For them, saying that all are brothers is also saying that the boundaries of the different circles should count for little when it comes to helping those in need. The second view, which emphasizes these boundaries and stresses the priority of directly experienced allegiances over far-flung ones, is expressed in Sidgwick's "commonsense" view quoted above.

Both the universalist and the graduated view concern human survival and security, no matter how thoroughly advocates of these views suspect opponents of parochialism or hypocrisy and, in either case, blindness to genuine human need. Most proponents of both agree at least that one ought to help others when this does not mean shortchanging persons in need to whom one has preexisting obligations. Many agree, further, that certain prohibitions, such as those on killing and breaking promises and cheating, ought to hold across all the boundaries of all the circles; and that in certain acute emergencies such as that after an earthquake, the obligation to offer humanitarian aid across boundaries should supersede needs that can wait. It is when the needs of outsiders are of vast extent and prolonged duration and would constitute a considerable reallocation of scarce resources that holders of the graduated view are most likely to balk at the use of the term "emergency" to urge priority for such needs over the needs of family members or compatriots.

No matter from which of the two perspectives we intuitively view the image of the concentric circles, it is important to strive to see the importance of the other perspective and to recognize the role that both play in the conflicts over how to respond to the surge in complex humanitarian emergencies. In so doing, it matters, too, to sort out the factual and moral controversies inherent in the concept of "complex humanitarian emergencies." It is too easy, otherwise, to ignore either one: either to fail to explore the important empirical questions about how such crises arise and what forms of response are most appropriate to meet existing needs and prevent recurrences of the crises; or to ignore the genuine ambivalence many feel regarding the conflicting calls on their concern and on their sense of responsibility.

To the extent that we fail to keep such distinctions in mind, and to explore their ramifications, we risk answering too hastily the questions that today's vast humanitarian crises have raised with unprecedented starkness: Taking into account family members, friends, fellow citizens, and persons in desperate need in so many parts of the world, what loyalties should have precedence? What needs are overriding? Whose obligation is it to protect rights, such as those not to be killed or tortured, which are recognized, in principle, across all boundaries? And at what cost?

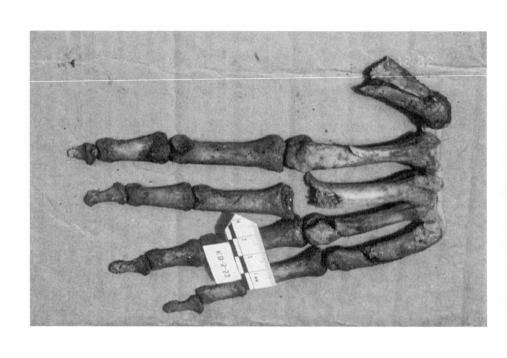

9

HUMAN RIGHTS CHALLENGES

aryeh neier

jennifer leaning

Important differences exist between the customary effort to promote human rights and the effort that must be undertaken in humanitarian crises, where human rights law is largely inapplicable and the norms of the Geneva Conventions and other agreements on international humanitarian law are those that must be invoked. A few general issues relating to these differences are discussed and then reference is made to four specific humanitarian crises. The particularities in each of these situations highlight key challenges, several of which are framed as contradictions in policy and procedure between the delivery of humanitarian assistance and the effort to promote human rights.

The modern human rights movement has a relatively brief history, dating from the immediate post–World War II period. In adopting the United Nations Charter in 1945, the governments of the world agreed to language affirming "fundamental human rights," "the dignity and worth of the human person," and "equal rights of men and women."[1] In adopting the Universal Declaration of Human Rights in 1948, the nations of the world affirmed their commitment to achieving the high standards and objectives defined in that document. The first article of the declaration asserts that "all human beings are born free and equal in dignity and rights."[2] In the intervening years, the human rights movement has focused more on individuals than on populations. It has developed its efforts less in support of civilians trapped in war, civil conflict, or complex humanitarian emergencies and more in support of individual cases in which persons around the world have been imprisoned, tortured, summarily executed, or have become victims of disappearances, usually because of their political beliefs or their political expressions. The mission of the human rights movement, to support compliance with human rights standards, has been expressed through four objectives:

1. to promulgate and create awareness of certain standards that have now been agreed to by virtually all the countries of the world that prohibit certain practices that we call human rights abuses;
2. to investigate abuses where they take place;
3. to compile information and document those abuses and disseminate information about them;
4. thereafter, to call attention to the discrepancies between the pretenses of governments in ratifying certain international agreements on human rights and their actual practices.

Essentially, these objectives have served the effort to embarrass those governments that violate the standards to which they have agreed.

In some measure, the same approach can be used and is now being used by humanitarian agencies and human rights groups in their attempts to deal with the human rights abuses spawned by humanitarian crises. Yet involvement in complex emergencies from the perspective of human rights represents a significant shift in mission and rationale for many human rights organizations and an even greater shift for humanitarian aid agencies.

LEGAL CONTEXT

Human rights organizations have thought of themselves as seeking compliance with international human rights law, as defined first by the Universal Declaration of Human Rights and then by a number of subsequent international documents (such as the Convention (1951) and Protocol (1966) Relating to the Status of Refugees, the International Covenant on Civil and Political Rights (1966), the Convention on the Elimination of All Forms of Discrimination against Women (1979), and the Convention on Torture and

Other Cruel, Inhuman or Degrading Treatment or Punishment (1984)). Various regional instruments also figure significantly in the compliance work of human rights organizations. Yet much of international human rights law is inapplicable to the situations that lead to humanitarian crises, in that these emergencies are taking place in and are in fact defined by the context of war or civil conflict. International human rights law does not apply to many of the severe abuses that take place in connection with war. An entirely separate body of international law imposes duties upon nations during wartime and constrains the way that they wage war. Within that body of law, the regulations and treaties applicable to the rights and protection of persons during war is called international humanitarian law, or IHL.[3] From this perspective, IHL can be seen as defining human rights in war.

IHL, in terms of its historical definitions and elaboration, has a much longer tradition than human rights law. Rules relating to combat are as old as the practice of war.[4,5] The robust body of rules now most frequently referred to as IHL has been built through treaty and covenant deriving since 1864 from examined experience during and after the major wars of the modern era. Most relevant to protection of persons in war and conflict are the Four Geneva Conventions (1949) and the Two Protocols (1977). Other documents of note include the Convention on Genocide (1948). To ensure compliance with the Geneva Conventions in particular and with IHL more broadly, the international community has charged the International Committee of the Red Cross with the task of assessing violations of IHL during war. Because of this assignment, ICRC delegates are accustomed to carrying out investigations within the constraints of wartime conditions. Their procedure is to make known their findings to the commanders of the camps, armies, or governments, depending upon the nature of the abuse identified. It is an explicit tenet of ICRC procedure not to publicize most of its findings.

RULES OF ENGAGEMENT

The difference between the way in which the ICRC functions and the traditional mode of operation of the international human rights movement highlights a difficult problem encountered by the human rights movement when it tries to monitor violations of international humanitarian law. That is, the ICRC obtains information about the condition of victims because the governments and the combatant forces that deal with the ICRC know that it will not publicize that information. Accordingly, they provide the ICRC with a certain degree of access to victims that would otherwise be withheld. Human rights organizations, in contrast, having the opposite approach, are not dealt with in the same way by combatant forces, because those forces know that the mission of the human rights movement is to report on abuses publicly.

The ICRC follows its mode in part because it is also an agency that delivers services. Under the terms of the Geneva Conventions, it is responsible for ensuring that relief supplies and medical care are delivered to wounded combatants on all sides, to prisoners of war, and to trapped civilians. In the more traditional wars of this century, waged by formal standing armies, the military units have organized internal medical support functions to treat their own military casualties and it has been the ICRC role to support POWs and civilians. In the more recent humanitarian crises, however, it is frequently the case that no military infrastructure exists to support the warring factions, so the ICRC is involved in providing medical care for wounded combatants and noncombatants alike, on all sides. Thus the ICRC is allowed into the war zone to deliver humanitarian assistance and is permitted to assess and attempt to support compliance with international humanitarian law only to the extent that it does so by reporting confidentially.

In the post–cold war period in which complex emergencies have been seen to erupt, some groups other than the ICRC have attempted to deliver humanitarian assistance and, simultaneously, to make public information regarding human rights abuses.[6,7] In such circumstances, the authorities who have the power to grant access are often unwilling to do so. This reluctance serves to highlight the contradiction that develops between efforts to deal with human rights and efforts to deliver humanitarian assistance. Humanitarian assistance generally requires cooperation with the authorities who are responsible in any particular area where there are victims. Human rights efforts, in contrast, by their nature are not cooperative. Human rights work attempts to rally world opinion to condemn those who engage in abuses. It attempts to generate political pressure. For example, if another government is supporting a force that is engaged in certain abuses by giving it diplomatic, political, economic, or military support, the idea is to embarrass those who are providing that support as well as those who are the actual recipients of that support.

Indeed, one of the principal ways that the human rights movement operates is by focusing on surrogate villains. Very often, the villain who is actually engaged in abuses is not susceptible to various kinds of pressure. The political sponsor, the donor, or the arms supplier may have a higher sensitivity. Accordingly, human rights organizations focus their pressure on such supporters, embarrassing them as a way of calling attention to the abuses that are being committed and also as a way of indirectly exerting pressure on those who are committing various forms of abuses.

The specific problems that arise from the differences in mandate and procedure between customary human rights work and the effort that must now be undertaken in humanitarian crises is best illustrated by reference to example.

SOMALIA

Leaders who themselves were engaged in violations of IHL, such as indiscriminate attacks or targeted attacks on civilian populations, presented the major challenge in Somalia. Their deliberate method of war was to terrorize vulnerable populations, force them to move, and thus capture territory.[8,9,10,11] Given such willful action, who is it that one can stigmatize? What political sponsors do the leaders of the different factions have who can be embarrassed as the surrogate villains? Prior to the flight of Somalia's longstanding dictator, Siad Barre, in 1991, both the United States and the former Soviet Union had long since dropped the competitive cycles of support that had helped arm the country in the 1970s and 1980s.

What about stigmatizing the Somali leaders within the country? Here issues of communication and timing intervened. There were few means of communication within the country that could have been used to point out that this or that warlord had engaged in indiscriminate attacks upon the territory controlled by the other warlord, and had thereby caused many thousands of deaths and many more thousands of injuries. Social institutions had collapsed in the setting of civil war that swept across the country, a war that helped cause and then sustain a devastating famine. How, in a time frame with any practical relevance, could one stigmatize anybody within that country, and where could one go externally to stigmatize them?

Did General Aidid care what was said about him in the *New York Times*? Did he care whether a member of Congress denounced him for the indiscriminate attacks that his forces were engaged in? Did either "President" Ali Mahdi or General Morgan care what was said about him in a column or editorial in the *Washington Post* or the *Boston Globe*? Without external support from the United States, or any other nation linked via geopolitical interests, these Somali warlords were relatively impervious to international criticism.

Thus the traditional tools of the trade of the human rights movement for stigmatizing those who are engaged in abuses were blunted by the fact that no surrogate villains could be identified and no local opposition, at that time, could be reached by outside support.

The other major problem that Somalia created for human rights workers was that the U.S. military intervention, accomplished under UN auspices, forced an accommodation with the very leaders that human rights organizations were seeking to stigmatize. The purpose of the military intervention was to protect the delivery of humanitarian assistance to a population suffering from starvation and war.[12] The paradox is that it became necessary at the very outset to establish agreements with the warlords responsible for human rights abuses in order to make sure that humanitarian assistance would not be impeded. In seeking the cooperation of the warlords, the international community went a long way toward providing them legitimacy, thus undermining all efforts to brand them as abusers of human rights and violators of IHL. Instead, the warlords were invited to various conferences; asked to negotiate peace agreements; and envoys from the United Nations were required to deal with them. Thereby their status was enhanced.

A further issue that arose in Somalia involved the alliances that humanitarian aid groups had to make with the warlords in order to secure their own protection in the delivery of relief. The warlords evinced little respect for the Geneva Conventions and exerted minimal control over their forces. In these anarchic and violent circumstances, the principle of humanitarian neutrality could not be upheld[13] and even the ICRC was forced to diverge from its usual practice. For what was probably the first time in its history, the ICRC hired armed guards.[14] Other humanitarian groups were forced to do the same. These armed guards came from the factions that were engaged in combat with one another, the combat that caused the humanitarian crisis in the first instance. Yet the ICRC and other aid groups recruited them and took advantage of their control of military equipment to protect the delivery of humanitarian assistance. The substantial payment for these armed guards developed into a significant form of financial assistance to the warlords, helping them to arm and feed their bands of men and boys and allowing them to maintain their authority and conduct the war.[15–18]

These problems identified within the context of Somalia in 1991–1993 underscore the considerable tension that arises between the human rights effort and the humanitarian assistance effort. To respond to human need in settings that force alliances with warlords undermines the effort to promote human rights.

BOSNIA

Despite the Dayton agreement, a grim quiet hangs over Bosnia, with outright war held in check but no peace in sight. During the three and a half years of the war (April 1992 to December 1995), the UN protection force saw its main mission as protecting the delivery of humanitarian assistance. Yet there are very bitter people in Bosnia who will tell you that the role of the UN was to make sure that they were fed until the time they were shot. The UN, in its peacekeeping role, has been widely criticized for its failure to protect civilian lives, whether in safe havens, besieged cities, along transport routes, or in the countryside.[19,20,21] Yet the ambiguities of the UN peacekeeping role were aggravated by conflicting and changing signals from the major powers, who as funders and determinants of overall UN policy were obliged to take ultimate responsibility for the outcome of UN actions in Bosnia.[22,23,24] The unfolding drama of humanitarian relief efforts succeeded in obscuring, for several years, the fact that a resolution of the cruelties and horrors of the conflict required decisive and coordinated political and military action. While the great powers deliberated at length on the logistic, political, and strategic obstacles in the path of concerted response, the world's NGOs provided ample diversion on the ground to distract attention from the void in policy that permitted the atrocities to continue.

A number of humanitarian organizations were keenly aware of this dilemma, yet they continued to pour in supplies and personnel. Humanitarian action, as one group sardonically noted, is a "blindfold which allows us to bask permanently in the warmth of our own generosity."[25] Human rights organizations, in general, were more outspoken regarding the need for great power intervention to put an end to the ethnic cleansings and rape. In the summer of 1995, after the shameful tragedy of Srebrenica, the human rights community took the unprecedented step of calling, in a joint statement signed by twenty-seven major human rights and humanitarian organizations, for military intervention in Bosnia to stop the war.[26] Human rights organizations are intensely aware of the violations of rights that armed intervention can entail. Yet conditions in Bosnia had so deteriorated that the balance of poor choices tilted toward the use of the military. It was not until the heavy shelling of Sarajevo later that same summer, however, that NATO took the long overdue step of sending in definitive airstrikes against the Serbian forces, an intervention that rapidly led to agreement by all sides to negotiate terms for a cease-fire.

To feed the starving population, the UN had to negotiate with and secure the cooperation of the people who were responsible for the ethnic cleansing and all the other horrors known to have occurred. The process of negotiating had the effect of dignifying the perpetrators and granting them legitimacy. In the course of acquiring that legitimacy, those who engaged in ethnic cleansing achieved a significant part of their purpose.

Since May 1993, when the UN Security Council established the International War Crimes Tribunal for the Former Yugoslavia in the Hague, the human rights community has sought to bring those persons to trial. Yet during this period the UN, as the agency trying to provide humanitarian assistance, has found it necessary to engage with a number of the perpetrators, including Radovan Karadžić and General Ratko Mladić. The United States first refused to deal with these two men after December 16, 1992, when the U.S. secretary of state, Lawrence Eagleburger, labeled them both war criminals, and then ultimately agreed to negotiate with them, beginning first with a meeting in Pale. Struck by the moral incongruity of treating these perpetrators with the respect of official recognition, Victor Jacovich, then the U.S. ambassador in Bosnia, refused to attend the Pale meeting and was subsequently removed from his post for this refusal.

From a humanitarian standpoint, it is not possible to refuse to deal with the people who control access to humanitarian assistance. Should a matter of principle cause the denial of medical care and food to others? Yet from a human rights standpoint, a different problem emerges. Members of the human rights community do not wish to grant legitimacy to the authors of ethnic cleansing. Rather, these people must be stigmatized, treated as pariahs. Only in this way is it possible for the world to demonstrate its condemnation of the crimes in which they have engaged. And by demonstrating contempt for these crimes, the world community shows its resolve to bring the perpetrators ultimately to trial.

As of mid-1998, the issue was whether the international community had the political will to bring those accused to trial and then to apply sanctions and punishments against anyone convicted. The effort to gather the evidence and construct effective prosecution requires substantial resources and expertise as well as the willingness to engage in a forceful removal of criminals from their sites of refuge. To date the requisite funds and political will have not been forthcoming. Removing Karadžić and Mladić might in the short term aggravate the security situation and place foreign personnel at further risk of attack. The rationale for this failure to pursue the perpetrators, however, is couched in humanitarian terms; in the minds of the United States and the UN, buttressed by the defending parties themselves, efforts to shore up the fragile peace and kindle development initiatives must take priority. It is argued that pursuing issues of culpability will only sow continued bitterness and revenge. The counterargument from the human rights community, that failure to punish serious crimes contributes to an erosion of the rules themselves, feeding an inevitable ongoing cycle of recurring violence and retribution within the local society and a deepening cynicism within the international community,[27] has to date acquired insufficient support from those positioned to determine the next steps.

RWANDA

The case of Rwanda poses endless challenges to the human rights movement. Genocide leads the list. How is it defined, when is it identified as occurring, at what point should military intervention be called for? Since the adoption of the 1948 Convention on Genocide, intended to respond to awful contingencies raised by Nazi attempts to exterminate the Jews during World War II, the UN Security Council has made no timely attempt to apply this term to subsequent instances of mass killings, such as those inflicted upon the residents of East Timor by the Indonesian government, the citizens of Cambodia by the Khmer Rouge, or the citizens of Ethiopia in

Mengistu's reign of Red Terror.[28] For the Convention on Genocide to apply, there has to be firm evidence that an effort exists to eliminate a population on the basis of its ethnicity, religion, or distinct communal status. Killings for political reasons, no matter how numerous these deaths may be, do not constitute genocide. If the Security Council determines that genocide does in a given instance exist, then the international community, acting through the Security Council, is obligated under international law to intervene and put a stop to the killing.

In retrospect, it can be seen that in the days just after the killings began in Rwanda on April 6, 1994, the situation crossed the definitional threshold.[29] Within a few weeks, hundreds of thousands of people of Tutsi ethnicity were killed by organized Hutu extremists and their followers. The killings, planned long in advance, began literally 30 minutes after the plane carrying Rwandan president Habyarimana and Burundian president Ntaryamira was shot down. In a matter of days it was evident to the international community that carnage, based on ethnic divisions, was under way. The only possible way to stop the killing was by military intervention; the only way to mobilize this intervention was to label the killing genocide.

At the international policy level, a protracted debate ensued over the distinctions between Tutsi and Hutu, to what extent the killings were politically motivated, and whether the killings were deliberately intended to eliminate an entire ethnic group or simply to gain a significant interim advantage.[30,31] On the ground in Kigali, the torture and massacre of a contingent of Belgian forces under UN command led the UN to pull its military force out of Rwanda, leaving the field to the Hutu militia. Had it not been for the immediate campaign of the Rwandan Patriotic Force (RPF), launched from Uganda within two days of the onset of the killings, there might well have been even greater slaughter than the estimated 500,000 to 1,000,000 killed.

The human rights community quickly assessed the killings as genocide but was far less agreed on the nature of the intervention to recommend. As the killings continued, however, the risks attendant with any military intervention appeared small compared with the atrocities it had the potential to avert. Thus, confronted with what it considered to be the first unequivocal case of genocide since the end of World War II, the human rights community found itself in the unusual position of calling for the use of international armed intervention and acknowledging the invasion of the RPF for its positive role in halting the carnage in Rwanda.[32]

A second enormously difficult challenge posed by the Rwandan situation was the question of what stance to take with regard to the refugee camps. Humanitarian aid agencies initially were divided on whether or not the masses of refugees spilling across the Rwandan border into inhospitable terrain in Zaire should be summarily turned back. The UNHCR, acting within its mandate under international law, could not force refugees to return across international borders, despite the fact that the practical arguments from the humanitarian perspective were very powerful.[33,34] Cholera broke out, and all efforts then focused on providing medical relief. As the epidemic abated and the camps became more established, it became evident that they were substantially controlled by the organizers of the genocide.[35,36,37] Provision of humanitarian aid to the camps gave political strength to the Hutu extremists, increasing the possibility that the genocide might resume from the new base they were building within Zaire. A political analysis of this situation would have dictated withholding further outside assistance; a humanitarian analysis would have led to the opposite conclusion, since hundreds of thousands, if not millions, in the camps were in need of relief and were not leaders of the genocide; and a human rights analysis would have argued for introducing a greater measure of security in the camps, extending to disarming the extremists and expelling them from the midst of the refugees. Again, as with the intervention needed to respond to the genocide, the option endorsed by the human rights community brought its members into uncomfortable proximity with a position advocating the use of external military forces, with all the collateral harm such intervention might entail.

The actual course of events brought further permutations on what was possible. As human rights abuses escalated within the camps, inflicted by Hutu extremists on other refugees, and as external aid was ever more blatantly channeled to supply these same extremists with fungible goods, a number of humanitarian aid agencies began to consider the option of pulling out from the camps altogether. Finally, in the fall of 1995, the field officers for MSF France in Goma decided to suspend operations and withdraw, signaling that this move was as much a protest against the international community for continuing to collude with Hutu murderers as it was a condemnation of the corruption in the camps.[38] Their action was noted with approval by many human rights organizations but has been interpreted by others as a "symbolic gesture," since other groups could move in to fill the niche they had vacated.[39]

CHECHNYA

In Chechnya, the international human rights movement was almost entirely ineffectual. Structurally, this case reveals the way in which human rights issues involving the former superpowers may now play out in the post–cold war period. Whereas most complex humanitarian emergencies can be seen as communal conflicts or civil wars occurring in settings where the collapse of the cold war has left an apparent superpower void, the rebellion in Chechnya uncovers the dynamics of the new alliance that now exists whenever superpower interests still pertain. Russia may be responsible for a vast number of indiscriminate killings and also a large number of targeted individual killings of noncombatants in its efforts to suppress the war in Chechnya, but as a member of the Security Council it could block any official condemnation of its acts. (The Security Council, from this perspective, is an ineffective instrument for condemning human rights abuses.) Regardless of the human rights issues, U.S. policy was determined by the fact that these brutal actions made the Yeltsin government deeply unpopular with the Russian people. Fearing that out of this weakness worse possibilities might emerge, the United States tried to support Yeltsin, to the extent that President Clinton traveled to Russia on May 9, 1995 (in the middle of the war in Chechnya), to participate in a fiftieth anniversary celebration of the end of World War II.

This kind of diplomatic support for the Russian government in what was perceived as its effort to quell an internal disturbance is precisely what the human rights movement generally tries to prevent, using all manner of information and communication to persuade other governments to take responsible action against the offending government. In this circumstance, however, the Russian government confounded the human rights movement by advertising its own instability and weakness and thereby requiring its international supporters, such as the U.S. government, to rally to its side. Human rights takes a back seat when issues of international security are invoked. Such were the prevalent dynamics in the years of the cold war. Chechnya in some ways was a structural throwback.

Consequently, in this humanitarian crisis, interlaced as it was with issues of superpower stability, the prospects for achieving a human rights agenda appeared dim from the beginning. High levels of internal insecurity also made delivery of humanitarian relief exceedingly dangerous, as evidenced by the murder of an expatriate and three Russians associated with the Open Society Institute in 1995 and of six expatriate staff of the ICRC in December 1996.[40] In strictly military terms, Chechnya again looked more like a cold war conflict than one occurring in the 1990s: there was no neutral third force, such as the UN, to provide a modicum of security for an influx of humanitarian aid agencies,[41] and there was no external party attempting to introduce peacekeeping. What existed until the cease-fire was an unmitigated state of war, conditions too inhospitable for all but the old-time, traditional providers of relief in war, the ICRC. And even that organization, as a result of the loss of its six staff members, began to reconsider its mission in war settings where adherence to the Geneva Conventions cannot be assumed.

CONCLUSION

Attempts to promote human rights in the context of humanitarian crises must deal with new bodies of law, shifting political alignments, and policy disputes with humanitarian aid agencies. The human rights community must resolve several major issues if it hopes to be effective in the future (Box 9.1).

First, the key policy instrument of human rights organizations, stigmatization, is proving useless against perpetrators who are independent of the great powers and act outside the customary network of economic and political leverage. Other instruments of persuasion are needed.

Second, negotiations undertaken by governments or aid agencies with regimes that have inflicted gross human rights violations may promote access for humanitarian aid, but they also confer international legitimacy on those regimes and vitiate the attempts of human rights groups to mount a campaign of condemnation and isolation. In some instances these two approaches may need to be pursued as mutually exclusive and thus oppo-

Box 9.1 Human rights issues in humanitarian crises

- Methods of persuasion when stigmatization proves useless
- Isolating renegade regimes or negotiating to obtain access to populations in need
- Erosion of humanitarian neutrality to promote practical arrangements
- Humanitarian aid as a cover for governmental failure to act
- Supplying refugees in need or insisting first upon disarming the militants
- Operational definition of genocide that can trigger intervention
- Focus on justice versus focus on peace and development in post-conflict setting

sitional strategies. In other situations it may be possible to work out an advance agreement between human rights and humanitarian organizations on ways to proceed in tandem.

Third, elaborate logistic and political arrangements linking aid agencies with one side of a multifaceted conflict erode the notion of humanitarian neutrality and heighten the risk that the relationship may constitute complicity in the war effort. This point of view, though perceived as critical of humanitarian aid agencies, must continue to be raised by the human rights community.

Fourth, humanitarian and human rights organizations agree that humanitarian aid in the setting of persistent wide-scale war and atrocity serves only to conceal governmental failure to act. Whenever this situation occurs, it is incumbent upon the NGO community to raise the issue in unambiguous and public ways. The crisis paradigm can be overtaken by the reality of an extremely ugly war, for which the only relief is international political and, if necessary, military action.

Fifth, the status of refugee cannot be applied to the exclusion of other considerations relating to the siting and security of massive populations. The practical and political implications of recent failures to incorporate these considerations have been great. Human rights groups and humanitarian organizations are now more poised to view each refugee situation on its own terms, weighing the legal status of refugee in the context of the larger complex emergency, the need for stability, and the potential for longer-term integration.

Sixth, events of the mid- to late 1990s have forced to the surface key ambiguities in the ways in which the international community has chosen to address the Convention on Genocide: what is the operational definition of genocide; what is the agency charged with responding; what forms of intervention are mandated? These issues must be resolved, lest the next instance further expose our collective lack of readiness to abide by a treaty of monumental import while another population faces annihilation.

Finally, the human rights community places great priority on the need to conduct swift and comprehensive trials, including war crimes trials, in order to formalize the process of truth telling and speed the path toward justice. Humanitarian agencies, in contrast, consider the establishment of peace and the launching of development initiatives much more important. Of the several areas of disagreement identified between the two groups, this one has perhaps the most serious implications for the future of the international human rights movement. To ignore the body of evidence already gathered and fail to prosecute those responsible for the savage deeds of, for example, Bosnia and Rwanda sends an intolerable message to victims, survivors, and the witnessing societies.

Human rights work has never been so difficult as it is now. If these and other issues cannot be resolved in the near term, whatever moral voice has been salvaged from this century may well be lost.

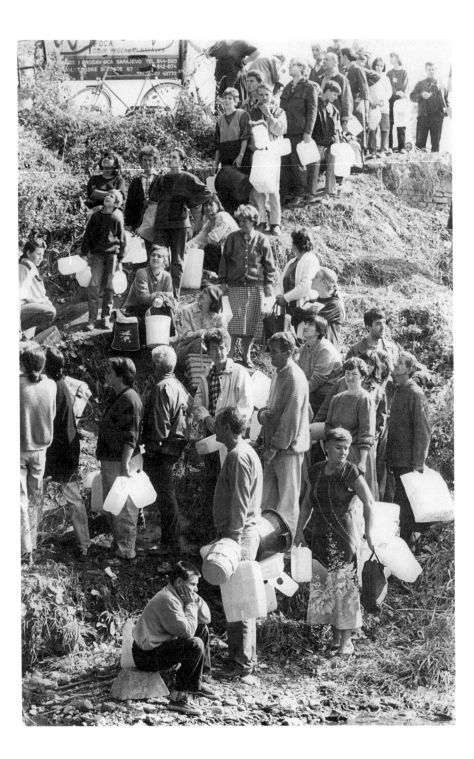

10

COMPLEX EMERGENCIES AND NGOs:
THE EXAMPLE OF CARE

marc lindenberg

Before the humanitarian crises of the late 1980s and the 1990s changed the landscape entirely, international humanitarian nonprofit organizations were thought of as highly valued, neutral providers of critical services to the innocent victims of war, famine, and national disasters. Refugee rights were well defined within the conventions of the United Nations. Safe access to civilian victims, refugees, and internally displaced people was often negotiated with belligerents. The neutral humanitarian mission of the International Committee of the Red Cross was so well known that the safety of its staff and supplies was guaranteed.

Since the collapse of the former Soviet Union, refugees have been used as pawns by warring factions in Bosnia, Chechnya, Somalia, Rwanda, Burundi, and Zaire. It has become increasingly difficult to separate civilians from insurgents. Innocent women and children are frequently the victims of intimidation. Rebel armies extort food from civilians and use them as shields. Open access to refugees must now be fought for rather than being guaranteed. NGO workers are called upon to provide medicine, food, and safe drinking water in territory where no nation will send its troops.

While the horrors of war are as old as mankind, the contemporary context of humanitarian crises has rendered the traditional roles of the UN, the international community, and NGOs obsolete. International humanitarian responses have still successfully helped large numbers of innocent people survive and begin to rebuild their lives after recent human catastrophes. But humanitarian response has taken place under the shadow of increased operational complexity and acute ethical dilemmas.

The discussion that follows provides a window into the troubling new world of complex humanitarian emergencies. It probes both the operational and the ethical dilemmas that lurk in its shadows. It describes the range of emerging NGO responses to these challenges. Finally, it focuses on ways to practice a new philosophy of "active humanitarianism," where relief and rehabilitation programs strive consciously to save lives as well as to reduce conflict rather than exacerbate it. In the wake of the tragedies of Rwanda, Zaire, and Bosnia, it is imperative to reflect about the role of NGO humanitarian response and to make important changes.

THE NEW WORLD OF COMPLEX EMERGENCIES

Before 1980, most international NGOs involved in emergency relief responded largely to natural disasters like earthquakes, cyclones, hurricanes, droughts, and floods. Since 1978 the number of natural disasters has remained relatively stable. But since 1978 the number of emergencies ignited by human conflict has grown substantially. For example, between 1978 and 1985 there were five such emergencies.[1] But between 1985 and 1995 there were twenty-six. In 1993 there were thirty-four countries with major international armed conflict (conflict with more than one thousand deaths per year) which claimed more than 68,000 deaths.[1]

The human and physical consequences of these emergencies reach far beyond the fatalities. They literally destroy the social fabric of families and communities. They put severe strains on community assets and set family well-being back years. In Angola, for example, although the hostilities are officially over, there are 20 million reported land mines, two for every inhabitant. Afghanistan has one land mine per person. The cost of making a land mine today is between US$1 and $3. The removal costs are currently between $300 and $1,000 per land mine. The economic and social costs of recent wars are astronomical, particularly for poor countries.

Today when people in the international community talk of complex humanitarian emergencies they usually think of them as "events that come up unexpectedly which demand immediate, high priority attention."[2] Such emergencies are complex because they combine a "lethal combination of starvation, economic collapse, civil strife, and disintegrating political authority."[2] They are called complex "humanitarian" emergencies because they threaten human survival and security.

While wars between two nation states are hardly a new feature of human life, several dimensions make the new complex emergencies since 1978 unique. First, the documented number of internal state conflicts (conflicts among groups within a nation-state boundary) as opposed to conflicts between nation states has risen dramatically. Second, the collapse of many nation states has been triggered by both the end of the cold war and the irrelevance of artificial national boundaries in Africa drawn during the colonial period. Third, the media is now able to bring such conflicts into people's living rooms through new communications technologies. Finally, these new emergencies present special problems to the NGO community because, with the exception of the ICRC, most NGOs responded largely to natural rather than man-made emergencies before 1978. They have been ill equipped to work in conflict situations.

These new largely internal armed conflicts have changed the world of humanitarian response in which NGOs work. Figure 10.1 highlights the critical differences between the world of traditional international armed conflict and the new world of complex emergencies.

The traditional international humanitarian response system to human-caused disasters was based on a model of struggles for territory between two belligerent sovereign states—the context for conflict. Within this context three major roles were played. First, at the level of world political action, either the United Nations or specific nation states attempted to bring warring parties to the bargaining table to end such conflicts. Second, security for refugees and humanitarian actors such as the ICRC was provided under specific UN protocols or was negotiated so that refugees' needs could be met, so that prisoners of war could be visited, and so that services could be provided. The belligerents themselves often provided the guarantees of safe access. Finally, UN organizations such as the United Nations High Commissioner for Refugees or NGOs supervised or provided direct humanitarian action through the delivery of food, medical service, water, sanitation, and refugee relocation.

The new post–cold war world of heightened intrastate ethnic, religious, and political conflict provides a radically different context for conflict and

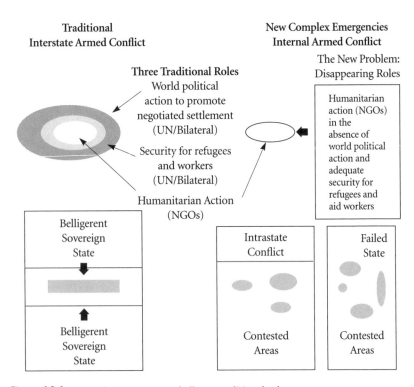

Figure 10.1 Complex emergencies challenge traditional roles.

for humanitarian action. This context is not adequately addressed in the existing international protocols that govern humanitarian response during conflict between nations. For example, in a totally failed state such as Somalia in 1993 more than five clan factions and militias were in conflict. Thus all humanitarian actors had to negotiate with a bewildering number of coalitions whose territory shifted rapidly.

Moreover, existing protocols provide few guarantees for internally displaced people who are often the main civilians at risk during conflicts within nations. Faced with collapsed states and multifaction armed struggles, new leaders and their soldiers often know little of international law or protocols and have little incentive to cooperate with humanitarian actors. As the number of child soldiers in Liberia, Somalia, Rwanda, Zaire, Sudan, and elsewhere have increased dramatically, problems of discipline have soared. Finally, in many parts of the world even regularly established armies have not honored the rights of refugees, civilians, and internally displaced people.

Post–cold war politics have also changed the nature of response by the international community in the 1990s. The UN, the international community, and individual nations such as the United States or France have been less willing to undertake diplomatic action to bring belligerents to the bargaining table in Africa. The result has been poorly defined roles for peacekeeping forces that have been extremely difficult to implement. It has been increasingly problematic to persuade UN or other actors to guarantee security for refugees or aid workers. Although troops have been assigned in Bosnia and Somalia to provide safe corridors, these have been the exceptions rather than the rule.

As a result, in the new world of complex emergencies, humanitarian action by NGOs and the ICRC has been provided without adequate security and without world pressure to bring belligerents to the bargaining table to get them to accept international human rights protocols, anti-genocide protocols, or normal guarantees to refugees and innocent civilians. Many in the NGO community now believe that humanitarian action has sometimes been used as a less expensive substitute for long-term international action to deal with causes of conflicts and to bring warring parties to the bargaining table.

DILEMMAS OF COMPLEX EMERGENCY RESPONSE

Structural Limitations

The international humanitarian community response to the new world of complex emergencies has serious structural flaws. Humanitarian action in the absence of security or broader peace-making efforts deals only with the most life-threatening symptoms of problems. Bandages and biscuits are not a substitute for negotiated political solutions or for dealing with root causes of problems. Given the unwillingness of the international community to provide security to refugees, their safety is compromised. For example, many innocent people in camps in Rwanda found themselves mixed with soldiers and officials of the Rwandan Hutu-based government in exile. Even if these civilians had wanted to return voluntarily to Rwanda, their lives were at risk. Some were killed because they publicly expressed a desire to return to Rwanda. The failure to separate civilians and belligerents in refugee camp situations became the rule rather than the exception in many places.

Another issue has been security for humanitarian workers. NGO and

Red Cross volunteers are no longer viewed as neutral helpers. Warring parties have been increasingly willing to target aid workers and to capitalize on their deaths for political purposes. In 1996 and 1997, for example, six ICRC medical personnel in Chechnya and three Doctors of the World staff and three UN human rights monitors in Rwanda were assassinated.[3,4] Since 1979 CARE has lost seventy-four workers, most recently to land mines and gunfire.[5] Even if factions want to guarantee security, such guarantees are difficult to maintain in a multifactional internal war.

There has also been the problem of access. In a world where well-institutionalized nations were at war it was often feasible to negotiate access to refugees. Although this has also been done successfully in Bosnia, and southern Sudan, warring factions today are frequently unwilling or unable to guarantee the delivery of humanitarian supplies. These structural dilemmas are often accompanied by both operational and ethical problems.

Operational Problems

NGOs have many strengths in responding to a complex emergency. They are often quick, flexible, innovative, and pragmatic. Staff are often courageous. They are capable of building useful coalitions with other organizations and building local capacity. They can draw upon a strong private resource base within their own communities. They can play roles in advocacy, operations, and conflict resolution.

NGO operational responses in places like Somalia, Rwanda, and Bosnia, however, have also revealed serious weaknesses. NGO responses to emergencies have not always been timely or orderly. NGOs have frequently duplicated services. Many organizations have arrived on a scene and have duplicated logistics chains and cost structures in "side-by-side" operations. Critics have noticed uneven levels of organizational quality.

Major problems of coordination exist among NGOs in relief operations. Since many NGOs are fiercely independent, they are reluctant to attend coordination meetings and they rationalize the use of resources. Coordination within global organizations with national chapters is also a problem. National members' desires for independence and visibility can make their work competitive. Finally, organizations that work only in emergencies often have a short-term perspective. They move in and out quickly. Their staffs frequently do not speak local languages or have sensitivity to local culture and conditions. They may work on relief without longer-term rehabilitation or development. These difficulties can be summarized as a lack of timely response, cooperation, quality, and comprehensiveness.

Ethical Dilemmas

The toughest dilemmas for NGOs working in complex emergencies revolve around whether actions that save lives help perpetuate conflict in insidious ways. "Moral calculus" is not a highly developed form of mathematics. It is difficult to know whether a hundred lives saved is worth the price of having inadvertently helped to prolong a conflict by a month. It is even harder to document the number of lives lost and saved in such situations. Furthermore, the operational choices NGOs must make to reach people create complex ethical issues. Although many of these problems are as old as war itself, the new context of complex humanitarian emergencies has brought them to even greater attention.

Supporting forced population movements   NGOs may find themselves being asked to work with people who have been forcibly moved to refugee or internally displaced persons' camps. These refugees may either be loyal supporters whom the government is trying to protect or dissidents a government is trying to control. The NGO may be able to help large numbers of innocent civilians in such camps, but may also inadvertently help one belligerent's war effort at the expense of another's by providing food, clothing, and shelter, which allows the belligerent to use its own resources for other purposes. As a result of such efforts, belligerents may maintain access to, control over, and manipulation of large numbers of civilians, internally displaced people, and refugees.

Falling victim to food diversions, looting, and war or protection taxes   When access is a problem, NGOs may find their supplies looted at gunpoint. They may find that political elements in camps extort war taxes from refugees after food distributions take place or that political groups try to control the distributions themselves. The NGOs may be asked to take on armed guards from a particular faction or to pay protection taxes to move their supplies through particular territories. Rebel factions may locate near refugee camps and divert food and supplies from NGO distribution sites to maintain their armed struggle.

Perpetuating a war economy   Warring factions may sell refugee supplies to buy guns. Relief efforts can allow factions to use their own resources for continuing the war while the international community takes care of the civilian population. In addition, importing food and other supplies may provide disincentives to the reactivation of agriculture or other key sectors.

Heightening conflict and competition   High media visibility often puts the spotlight on refugee populations at the expense of equally needy but more stable residents of communities located near such refugee camps. Favoring refugees over residents can lead to jealousy and violence. Aid providers can also inadvertently provide unbalanced assistance by favoring some ethnic, religious, or racial groups over others.

Weakening local capacity   Although there are many examples of excellent partnerships between international relief groups and local organizations, outside aid delivered by expatriates can weaken the capacity of local institutions. These include local self-help organizations, community or tribal organizations, and local NGOs.

TOUGH CHOICES FOR THE NGO COMMUNITY

The challenge of responding to humanitarian crises is daunting. Some people have argued that NGOs began their work from the perspective of "naive humanitarianism." The groups thought they could simply "do good" and "be neutral." For those who started with that perspective the last twenty years have been sobering. Many international NGOs, such as CARE, Catholic Relief Service (CRS), Médecins sans Frontières, the International Rescue Committee, Oxfam, Save the Children, and others, are reevaluating their roles and responses given the new dilemmas. Figure 10.2 provides a schematic view of the choices under consideration.

Withdrawal

Withdrawing from any form of operational response to complex humanitarian emergencies is one option for NGOs. Advocates of this viewpoint might argue as follows.[6,7,8] War is a reality and internal state conflict makes work with refugees and civilians impossibly difficult. Given the fact that NGO work is often manipulated by belligerents, it probably does more harm than good in the short term. It is better to refrain from operational response and to work instead on conflict resolution or advocacy to bring groups to the bargaining table. There is no point in putting major resources into programs that simply deal with the symptoms of problems. It makes more sense for NGOs to wait until a conflict is over and then to work on rehabili-

Withdrawal	Neutrality	Active humanitarianism

• War is a reality
• NGO work does more harm than good all or part of the time
• It is better to refrain from operational responses and to work on conflict resolution, advocacy, or long-term development
• Some principles:
  - Tough love
  - Work on the root causes of conflict only
	• War is a reality
	• Someone must try to work operationally on behalf of the victims
	• We can best help by negotiating with the belligerents on behalf of victims while maintaining a neutral position on the conflict
	  ** Three key principles
	    - Neutrality
	    - Impartiality based on need
	    - Independence
	• Role specified in Geneva Conventions + special Protocols + Mandate to monitor treatment of war prisoners
	• Separation from alliances with military humanitarian operations and human rights groups because division of labor is necessary
		• War is a reality
		• Operational NGOs can work to reduce suffering with actions that also help reduce conflict and build the conditions for peace
		• Key principles:
		  - Comprehensive long-term view
		  - Understanding social dynamics
		  - Consider how each action could contribute to conflict resolution

Clear partisanship
• War is a reality
• Operational NGOs should take sides depending on their values
  - Human rights
  - Ethnic
  - Religious
  - Political
• It is possible to mix advocacy with conflict resolution + operations
• Under appropriate conditions one can make sound alliances with military and security forces

Figure 10.2   A range of tough choices for NGOs.

tation and development efforts; or they may use resources in other places where development is possible. "Tough love" is better in the long run.

Neutrality

Those who adhere to a doctrine of neutrality might say the following: War is a reality. Regardless of the difficulties, we have a responsibility to work operationally on behalf of the victims. We can work best by negotiating access with the belligerents and simultaneously maintaining a neutral position on the conflict itself. We will not publicly judge the actions of the belligerents. Operational work should be based on three principles. First, neutrality. We take no public stands on the actions of the belligerents. We will not comment on their respect for human rights or treatment of civilians, internally displaced people, or refugees. If we did so we would never gain the access needed to permit us to save innocent lives. Second, we will respond to victims' needs impartially based on areas of greatest need. Third, we are independent. We reserve the right to respond as we see fit given our own diagnosis.

The organization that most clearly reflects much of this viewpoint is the International Committee of the Red Cross.[9] The ICRC has a proud tradition. Its role is specified by the Geneva Conventions and a series of special UN protocols. It has a special mandate to work with prisoners of war. Until recently the ICRC did not advocate the use of any form of security in its warehouses or logistics operations. It believes that to maintain neutrality a clear division of labor is necessary between advocacy groups, human rights groups, and those engaged in operational humanitarian response.

Active Humanitarianism

Many within the NGO community who initially believed that their organizations could play neutral roles in complex emergencies have begun to revise their views. After experiencing the special problems of negotiating with belligerents and of delivering services during conflicts, they have concluded that they may have exacerbated conflicts by not thinking more carefully about the implications of their work. They still believe, however, that an operational response is necessary when innocent people face death in complex emergencies. They believe that they can work positively and constructively to help reduce suffering with actions that minimize conflict and that build the conditions for peace. Their principles for action include:

1. taking a long-term comprehensive view of the conflict;
2. understanding the social dynamics and political factions in any situation;
3. considering how each program or action will either contribute to or reduce conflict;
4. acting, but choosing actions that contribute to conflict reduction.

The most articulate advocates of this view point are Anderson,[10,11] Woodrow,[12,13] and McDonald and Diamond.[14]

Clear Partisanship

Some groups believe that war is a reality and that neutrality is impossible. They believe that one group has a more just cause than another. In their view, NGOs should take sides based on human rights records, ethnic views, and religious, political, or ideological beliefs. Such groups are willing to mix advocacy activities with operational work. Under appropriate circumstances they make alliances with the military and security forces that protect the group whose side they have taken.

NGO RESPONSES TO STRUCTURAL DILEMMAS

CARE International: A Possible Framework for Active Humanitarianism

In considering the extent to which most NGOs are reorienting their views around one of the four viewpoints just described, it is helpful to examine the way in which one organization, CARE International, has been evolving its general framework. CARE staff and leadership have been involved in intense debate and reflection about the organization's future role in humanitarian response. There are few advocates of either withdrawal from humanitarian work or active partisanship. From the CARE perspective, total withdrawal from humanitarian work is a negation of the organization's origins and its belief that people "in harm's way" have a right to survive and to rebuild their lives. Withdrawal would be a rejection of the initial spirit that motivated people to send CARE packages to hungry civilians in post–World War II Europe. At the same time, CARE is a nonsectarian NGO, and few people within the organization advocate partisanship. CARE staff would find it difficult to decide definitively which ethnic, religious, or ideological group had more "right" on its side. Acknowledging hunger, malnutrition, thirst, and physical injury are clearer objectives. The CARE community is moving toward the option of active humanitarianism under some of the following general principles.

The humanitarian imperative One of CARE's key principles is that civilians in conflict situations have the right to stay alive and to survive in both natural and human-caused disasters. CARE also has an imperative to help survivors rebuild their lives once the conflict is over.

Timely operational response   When CARE staff members are convinced that a situation presents pressing humanitarian needs and a reasonable chance of having a positive impact, they will attempt to respond using the combined resources of the CARE International System.

Ensuring humanitarian access   Humanitarian response cannot take place without guaranteed, relatively safe access to people in need. CARE tries to negotiate access when and where possible. When necessary it will advocate that the UN system help provide safe access through humanitarian corridors such as the ones that existed in Bosnia and in southern Sudan through Operation Lifeline. CARE does not believe that the use of hired guards during the transport of supplies is advisable, but will ask recipient communities to guarantee safe access. Negotiations with belligerents, however, have been helpful at times in the Horn of Africa. CARE will not place its staff at risk where safe access is not guaranteed.

Refugees, internally displaced people and NGO workers have a right to safety   As a nongovernmental organization, CARE is capable of providing emergency assistance. It is not equipped, however, to provide physical security for refugees or to separate them effectively from belligerents. The UN system and the international community must hold belligerents accountable for respecting the Geneva Conventions and the protocols concerning refugees. CARE challenges the UN and the world community to find ways to provide safety to refugees in camps, and to find creative ways to separate refugees from belligerents. This is difficult, but the international community should be encouraged to experiment further with hiring local police to handle civil order in camps, with asking the government on whose soil a camp is located to ensure civil order, and with providing special camps where refugees whose lives might be at risk or who suffer from intimidation might safely live. Authorities should be urged to sort out suspected criminals, human rights violators, or perpetrators of genocide and to ensure that these individuals are treated fairly within national or international justice systems. Positive examples of such actions through UNHCR and other organizations occurred in both Zaire and Tanzania during the crisis in Rwanda.

The right to withdraw   Although CARE attempts to respond quickly to immediate humanitarian needs where reasonably safe access is ensured, the organization reserves the right to withdraw when it believes that innocent civilians have not been separated from belligerents; when it believes that refugees are being intimidated; when political groupings will not allow it to distribute resources to people in need; or when civil order cannot be maintained. In such circumstances, sometimes in coalition with other NGOs, CARE will withdraw, will encourage authorities to resolve such problems, or will publicize them if necessary.

Resisting intimidation   When CARE believes that its staff are subject to intimidation or other forms of personal threat, it will withdraw and will ask for assistance in guaranteeing the safety of its staff.

Humanitarian Response Is Not Enough

Humanitarian response is not a substitute for efforts by the international community and the UN system to promote negotiated settlements that can get at the root of conflicts rather than merely react to their symptoms. The international community has the responsibility to protect the rights of displaced and noncombatant populations and to help negotiate or provide safe access to innocent people who need assistance. Although CARE provides operational assistance, it simultaneously advocates for strong international efforts in conflict resolution and for organized ways to achieve safe access and safety for refugees and humanitarian workers.

The Goal of Active Humanitarianism

CARE builds its concept of active humanitarianism into its programs and analyzes program options to search actively for those responses that will help alleviate rather than exacerbate conflict. Emergency response programs are constructed and evaluated in the context of useful foundations that can be laid for later rehabilitation and development.

NGO RESPONSES TO OPERATIONAL DILEMMAS

The operational problems that NGOs have experienced in complex emergencies include: (1) a lack of ability to respond rapidly, (2) a lack of internal and external coordination, (3) problems with quality, and (4) problems with fielding a comprehensive response. NGOs have begun to respond to such problems in a number of ways.

FACILITATING A RAPID RESPONSE

Fast disbursal of emergency rotating funds Many NGOs have developed what they call emergency rotating funds. CARE, for example, has a $500,000 emergency response fund that it holds in reserve for emergency operations. When an emergency takes place the organization supplies initial disbursements for assessment teams, emergency setup, and full-scale operations. The fund is then replenished through private fund-raising. It may also be used as matching money for grants and contracts from UNHCR, the World Food Program (WFP), the UK Department for Internal Development, and other organizations.

New roster systems Many organizations, such as the International Rescue Committee (IRC), use roster systems in which professionals from outside the organization volunteer to be available for work of short-term duration—for example, one to three months. Other organizations, such as Save the Children and Oxfam, use a duty roster system: regular staff from headquarters and country offices are placed on the roster for several months during the year. If there is an emergency during the months when their names are on the roster, their unit or country office must release them.

Prepositioning supplies The Catholic Relief Service and the Church of the Latter Day Saints have begun to preposition standard medicines, water, food, and clothing kits around the world as well as in the United States. They can move them quickly from regional sites to particular emergencies. CARE has done this in places such as Bangladesh and in the Horn of Africa.

Special multilateral or bilateral agreements (framework agreements and indefinite quantity contracts) Some donor organizations, such as the U.S. Agency for International Development (USAID), WFP, and the European Union (EU), have looked for alternatives to slow, cumbersome contracting with NGOs at the moment of an emergency. The options they have begun to explore are framework agreements and indefinite quantity contracts. In each of these relationships the direct and indirect cost parameters, quality standards, and disbursement mechanisms are prenegotiated. During an emergency the donor can invoke the agreement and disburse funds rapidly to the NGO with whom it has the contract.

Improving Internal and External Coordination

Clear division of labor among affiliates of the same organization One of the biggest problems within global organizations such as World Vision International, Save the Children, CARE, Médecins sans Frontières, and others is the duplication of costs, support structures, and services by affiliate members of the same international organization. In the worst case five national affiliates from the same international organization may arrive on the scene and deliver the same services. They may set up costly parallel logistics operations, financial systems, and project management groups. Recently many organizations have searched for ways to cut costs and to gain economies of scale. One method has been the development of a division of labor among local affiliates. For example, one national member may specialize in primary health care or in emergency medicine, while another may take water, sanitation, or education. One affiliate may provide an umbrella for logistics, and for financial and administrative support. In the case of CARE International, a national lead or coordinating member is named who sets up the administrative infrastructure. Other members contribute to the costs of the infrastructure, and then their field programs are directly overseen by the coordinating member.

Regional plans that include other NGOs In the wake of the crises in the Horn of Africa, many NGOs have begun to plan coordinated responses for their own members and affiliates. This has resulted in the prepositioning of supplies. Donors such as USAID have sponsored multiorganizational planning through their "Horn of Africa initiative."

Joint NGO committees for coordinating operations At the field level, implementing organizations have found it useful to hold weekly meetings to identify and resolve the ongoing problems of operational response. These meetings have sometimes been prompted and chaired by representatives of UNHCR and sometimes have worked independently of UN organizations.

Joint NGO negotiations with donors, governments, and belligerents The NGO community has found it increasingly useful to form umbrella groups or ad hoc coalitions to negotiate directly with donors, governments, and belligerents. Representatives of the NGO community met with village elders in Baidoa, Somalia, in 1993, for example, and announced their combined withdrawal unless the elders could speak to their communities and control the increasing physical threat to staff. The NGO community also combined to negotiate with UNHCR in Geneva about using common costs and overhead rates for projects in 1996. Actions such as these can help minimize the problem of NGO competition.

Steps to Enhance Quality

Training, certification, and staff development   To help overcome the problem of inexperienced staff serving poorly in emergencies, many NGOs are working to provide additional training. Organizations such as CARE are considering certification processes for employees in which staff may not work in key positions in emergencies without completing training, passing an examination, and earning a formal certification. In addition, because of the high levels of stress staff experience during emergency work, many organizations are beginning to limit the length of assignments during emergencies. They also have begun to develop policies of staff rotation that move people from emergency to nonemergency assignments. Finally, some groups offer staff access to psychological counseling after particularly difficult emergency assignments (see Chapter 7).

Developing and using industrywide standards   Discussions are being held within the umbrella NGOs, such as InterAction and the International Council of Voluntary Agencies (ICVA), to develop general quality and cost standards for emergency response. Although it is difficult to mandate enforcement through umbrella organizations, such attempts at setting standards are a good beginning.

Famine early warning systems   In an effort to identify potential problems of natural and human-caused emergencies, many NGOs and government organizations in Ethiopia have developed a region-by-region food security monitoring system to identify potential crop shortages. Such systems permit better targeting of food resources to actual needs. For example, where people have food shortages for only a limited time, extra food that need not be distributed to them can be used elsewhere. At the same time, such systems allow early identification of serious droughts and potential famine conditions. The overall quality of operational response can be improved through such early assessment and can permit more appropriate responses.

Building local capacity   Some donor organizations have provided umbrella grants to NGOs to permit training and capacity building in local emergency response organizations and community groups. Such capacity building, exemplified by Save the Children's administration of umbrella grants to strengthen local NGOs in the former Soviet Union, has the potential to build stronger community infrastructure.

Promoting Comprehensive Response

Linking operations to global advocacy   Although operational groups find it difficult to engage in global advocacy for conflict resolution, organizations such as Oxfam and MSF have worked on strategies that build on the operational realities they see in emergency response to help highlight humanitarian problems and to pressure the international community to make appropriate responses.

The relief, rehabilitation, and development continuum   Organizations such as CARE, CRS, and World Vision have found it increasingly important to design emergency programs with long-term community rehabilitation and development needs in mind.

HOW NGOs ARE CONFRONTING ETHICAL DILEMMAS

There are no simple solutions to the ethical dilemmas that NGOs encounter during complex humanitarian emergencies. There have been useful pragmatic responses, however, to some of the problems outlined earlier.[8,15,16]

Countering Manipulated Access

Many NGOs have gotten around the problem of serving refugees in the territories of only one political faction by maintaining the principle of balanced service. For example, CARE works with displaced people on both sides of the conflict zones in Sudan. They have programs in both northern and southern Sudan. Insisting on negotiated humanitarian corridors in Bosnia and Sudan has allowed the NGO community more balanced access. Finally, when it is impossible to reach some groups in need through national territory, some organizations have set up cross-border operations, for example, from Rwanda into eastern Zaire (now Congo).

Reducing Diversions, Looting, and the Need for Protection

For some NGOs the solution to looting and security problems has been to hire armed guards. Other NGOs, however, have felt that there are alternative ways to minimize security problems and theft. For example, it has been possible to ask the recipient communities themselves to guarantee safe transit of goods. At times subcontracting with merchants and truckers and paying for actual quantities of commodities delivered has reduced NGO involvement in security. This approach has increased the volume of food that arrives at final distribution points. In addition, organizations have used joint negotiation of standard rates with truckers to help keep costs down. They have also used the threat of withdrawal if there is violence. More indirectly, NGOs have stayed out of food delivery entirely and relied on monetization to reduce diversion. Methods for reducing theft include using standard delivery sizes and formats that can be easily checked. Finally, there is no substitute for professional inventory management systems and qualified staff to provide supervision.

Diversion has also taken place at the level of distribution. The strategies that have worked to counter loss and to ensure that real needs are met include:

- working toward more accurate beneficiary assessments;
- getting beneficiary lists and requiring signatures upon receipt;
- using beneficiary cards;
- refusing to distribute food through paramilitary hierarchies in camps;
- distributing food and supplies to women and children directly;
- distributing food and other supplies to families;
- providing prepared meals (wet feeding) that must be eaten on the spot, instead of distributing commodities that can be sold on the black market, depress local prices, and generate hard currency for weapons purchases.

The issue of security for staff and for supplies is a difficult one. Most recently NGOs have begun to use security consultants to analyze the risks of continuing with procedures such as bringing large amounts of cash on a weekly basis into places where there is no banking system. Some organizations are hiring their own internal security staff as well as communications officers. In addition, many organizations are beginning to offer short courses and workshops on recognizing and responding to security problems in conflict situations.

Reversing the Incentives to Promote a War Economy

As NGOs have become more involved in responding to complex emergencies, they have begun to think more carefully about how to counter tendencies that might perpetuate war economies. Some of the responses have included:

- working not simply on relief but on advocacy to encourage the world community to hold belligerents accountable and to bring them to the bargaining table;
- promoting projects to reactivate the economy, such as seeds and tools programs;
- promoting barter shops to stimulate agricultural recovery.

The CARE barter shops in southern Sudan are an interesting example. In this model CARE shops provide basic goods that are currently inaccessible in return for local agricultural products. These transactions have helped to stimulate agricultural recovery. The newly produced agricultural commodities are then sold to other NGOs that need them for relief food distribution. The sales both lower the NGOs' need to bring in outside commodities and allow the barter shops to build up a cash reserve to repurchase goods. Providing food or cash for work on road and infrastructure rehabilitation also helps with economic reactivation.

Reducing the Risk of Conflict and Competition

One of the biggest concerns in the NGO community has been the intense media focus on refugees at the expense of equally needy civilian populations who may live next to refugee camps. As an alternative, some NGOs have attempted to provide balanced programs both to refugees and to the stable communities that exist side by side with them. Other alternatives have included hiring balanced numbers of returnees and individuals from stable populations for projects; developing projects that balance services among groups that have been involved in conflicts; and involving soldiers previously engaged in conflicts with one another to work on joint project implementation, such as demining teams made up of people from formerly warring factions in Angola or land titling programs for ex-combatants from both sides of the Salvadoran war. UNHCR funds CARE to establish boreholes and pumps in Sudanese refugee areas, while UNICEF funds

CARE to do the same for the Ugandans in resettlement areas adjacent to the camps.

Reinforcing Local Capacity

Although external responses to emergencies are based on the premise that local institutions have been overwhelmed by the disaster, outside groups still have opportunities to form partnerships with local organizations such as the local Red Cross or Red Crescent Society, church groups, and local NGOs. Reliance on traditional tribal or village structures for identification of people in need and for distribution of supplies and crowd control is another way to promote local engagement in disaster response.

PUTTING ACTIVE HUMANITARIANISM TO WORK IN POST-CONFLICT REHABILITATION PROGRAMS

The Case of Rwanda, 1996–97

Active humanitarianism, with an eye toward reducing rather than exacerbating conflicts, in emergency and rehabilitation programming was identified as an important principle earlier in this chapter, particularly with regard to NGO responses to ethical and operational problems. The basic tenet is to learn about community dynamics and political conflicts and then to plan each programmatic action with special attention to whether it will help reduce conflict. CARE's rehabilitation programming in Rwanda in 1996–97, in the wake of the return of more than one million refugees, illustrates both the promise and the problems in implementing this new philosophy.

The Context of a Genocide

Social relations before and after the genocide   Rwanda's social and ethnic relationships have been complex and characterized by conflict for several centuries. The literature documents the changes in the dynamics between the minority Tutsi population (estimated at 930,000, or 12 percent of the total population, in 1994) and the majority Hutu population (estimated at 6,846,000, or 88 percent) in the colonial and post-colonial period.[17,18] In the post-independence period, the Hutu population was in control of the government. There were periodic tensions and outbreaks of ethnic violence in Rwanda, with Tutsi refugee movements into Burundi, Zaire, and Uganda.

The Habyarimana regime, in power from 1973 until 1994, required its citizens to carry identity cards that identified them as either Hutu or Tutsi (though many anthropologists and social historians dispute the existence of clear ethnic or racial differences between the Hutu and Tutsi populations). The regime based its policies regarding education and jobs in government on ethnic quotas.

During the 1990s, in the wake of democratic openings in Africa, the Habyarimana regime became more supportive of the legalization of new Hutu- and Tutsi-based opposition political parties. In an attempt to diffuse its loss of political support after successful military campaigns by the Tutsi-led Rwandan Patriotic Army (RPA) in Byumba Prefecture, the Habyarimana regime became more open to participating in talks with the Tutsi opposition and to discussing multiparty government. Talks began in Arusha in 1992 and progressed slowly.

A visitor to rural areas in Gikongoro Prefecture in the southern part of Rwanda in early 1994 would have found the social structure described in Figure 10.3. In this hilly area small Tutsi extended families and communities lived close together. These communities were surrounded by more scattered Hutu houses. People of both ethnic groups walked to fields that were often interspersed among the communities. They preferred communal labor together. Each family engaged in subsistence production and sold some of its product to middlemen and traders, mostly of Tutsi origin, who traveled in the area. Those who could not provide completely for their own family's food needs and school fees worked as wage laborers on tea plantations. The government within the densely populated country had strong prefecture structures linked to the Habyarimana regime, the party in power. Each prefecture had a prefect governor, burgomeisters (mayors), counsels for smaller areas, and, finally, representatives who worked in organized communities of four hundred or fewer people. These officials were all appointed by the central party in power.

The opening of political opportunity and the success of the Tutsi-led RPF guerrilla movement operating from Uganda into northern Rwanda helped force political concessions and multiparty agreements from President Habyarimana. A growing fear and political radicalization of the right wing of the President's party, however, also resulted. The militant Hutu wing became more organized during this period, operating several radio stations and nurturing the forces of the Interahamwe, the Impuzamugambi

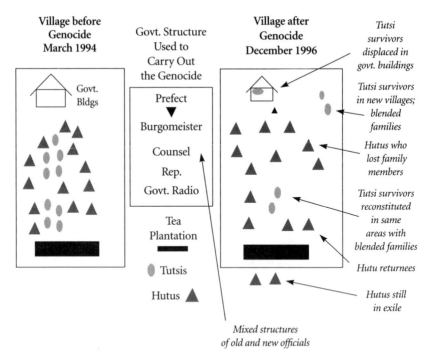

Figure 10.3 The Rwandan context: A rural area in Gikongoro prefecture.

militia, the military, the police, and the formal government structure of prefects and burgomeisters. The origins of the polarization and the eventual genocide emerged from these dynamics and from the hardening of relations that they fostered. Figures 10.4, 10.5, and 10.6 provide political maps of the key forces before, during, and after the 1994 genocide. Such maps focus on key political actors and allow a reader to visualize their alliances with or opposition to the government in power. The right side of each map is used to place Hutu groups and the left side Tutsi groups.

The word genocide is a harsh one, denoting an organized effort to systematically exterminate a population on the basis of race, religion, or ethnic origin. After careful analysis, the UN and other sources concluded that a genocide took place in Rwanda in 1994. Between 500,000 and 1 million Tutsis, along with Hutu moderates, were killed.[17,18,19] Although some sources presented this as a wave of unorganized mob killing, more detailed analysis showed that the effort was systematically organized by a

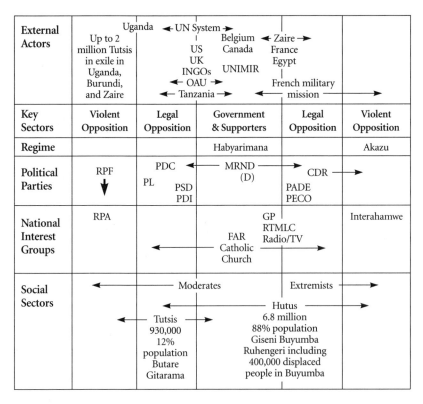

Figure 10.4 Political map of Rwanda, March 1994, before the genocide (groups are located in relation to their degree of support of the government; right side locates Hutu groups; left side locates Tutsi groups).

strong political organization. The genocide began with escalating hate messages on radio and in the media, accompanied by the preparation of lists of enemies to be killed. After the President was assassinated in April 1994, systematic implementation of the genocide was continued through the structure of prefects, burgomeisters, counsels, and representatives, who went to the villages and exhorted villagers to kill their neighbors.

In the aftermath of the genocide, the rebel RPA mounted offensives, eventually captured Kigali, the capital, and moved into the south of the country. The advances by the RPA first sent 600,000 frightened refugees fleeing into Ngara, Tanzania, and then forced several million more into Zaire and Burundi.

What ensued was a two-year period of RPF consolidation within

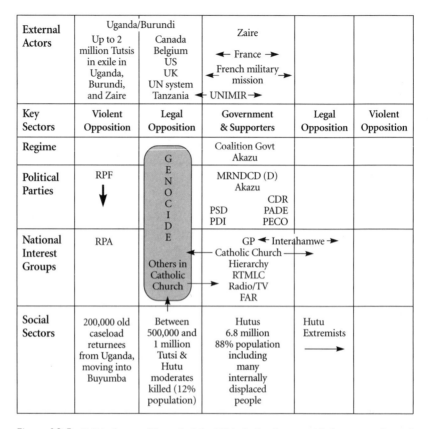

External Actors	Uganda/Burundi		Zaire		
	Up to 2 million Tutsis in exile in Uganda, Burundi, and Zaire	Canada Belgium US UK UN system Tanzania	← France → ← French military mission → ← UNIMIR →		
Key Sectors	Violent Opposition	Legal Opposition	Government & Supporters	Legal Opposition	Violent Opposition
Regime		G E N O C I D E	Coalition Govt Akazu		
Political Parties	RPF ↓		MRNDCD (D) Akazu CDR PSD PADE PDI PECO		
National Interest Groups	RPA	Others in Catholic Church	GP ← Interahamwe → — Catholic Church — Hierarchy RTMLC Radio/TV FAR		
Social Sectors	200,000 old caseload returnees from Uganda, moving into Buyumba	Between 500,000 and 1 million Tutsi & Hutu moderates killed (12% population)	Hutus 6.8 million 88% population including many internally displaced people	Hutu Extremists →	

Figure 10.5 Political map of Rwanda, May 1994, during the genocide (groups are located in relation to their degree of support of the government; right side locates Hutu groups; left side locates Tutsi groups).

Rwanda and a struggle to push the remains of the Hutu-based government and military away from the Zaire-Rwanda border. Finally, in November 1996, in the course of the civil war in Zaire, the refugee camps were broken up by the forces under the direction of Laurent Kabila and more than 800,000 refugees, largely Hutu, walked back to Rwanda. This turned out to be one of the largest movements of people since the partition of India in 1948 and the separation of North and South Vietnam in 1954.

The social fabric of rural Gikongoro prefecture broke down totally after December 1996 (Figure 10.3). A traveler returning to the same village areas at that time would have seen small clusters of Tutsi survivors, mostly widows and children, including orphans, clustered in the houses of families

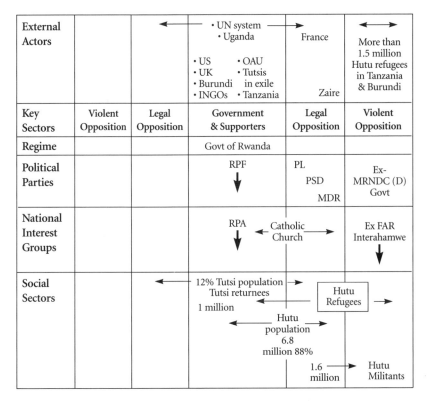

Figure 10.6   Political map of Rwanda, March 1997, after the genocide (groups are located in relation to their degree of support of the government; right side locates Hutu groups; left side locates Tutsi groups).

who had fled or living in government buildings and new housing communities. Families were often blended and were composed of several widows and their children as well as orphans. These clusters were surrounded by Hutus who had not fled, and by Hutu refugee returnees. All these groups were living together in a climate of intense distrust and a collapsed social contract.

Collapse of the social contract   It is useful to think of a society's social contract as the set of expectations that all community members have of their rights and responsibilities to one another. When the social contract is well defined, groups know what is expected of them and what they can expect from others and from institutions such as the church, the government, NGOs, cooperatives, and community associations.

In 1994, during the genocide, the social contract in Rwanda was completely destroyed. Neighbors killed neighbors, and major institutions were involved in the genocide. Today many Hutus fear the government and their neighbors. Those who survived the genocide fear those who have returned. The implications carry over into NGOs as well. Tutsi and Hutu staff members in many organizations believe that they have reason to fear each other. After what happened, people fear talking about the past. This same level of distrust exists between national and international staff. In such a climate it is difficult to use normal NGO methods of participative planning for project design or community assessment. If staff members will not talk openly about societal and community issues, it is difficult to identify problems accurately or come up with recommendations for solutions. At the same time it is hard to use participatory rural appraisal; community people do not want to talk about their neighbors or about the problems created during the genocide. Add to this the NGOs' donor pressure for three- to six-month emergency programming, and the result may be fragmented programming and short-sighted emergency responses with no connection to rehabilitation or development.

Rebuilding the Social Contract during Rehabilitation Programming

According to CARE staff in Rwanda,[20] active humanitarianism can be implemented in a number of ways. First, rehabilitation programming can do more than simply rebuild physical and economic infrastructure. Physical rehabilitation helps remove the visible signs of destruction in a devastated community, but can be slowly stretched into opportunities to rebuild the social contract among families, communities, and institutions. Where serious community trauma has taken place, however, this can only be done very slowly. The pace of these efforts depends upon the absence of major violence. One of the best ways to widen the circle of trust in post-conflict programming is to focus elsewhere. In the Rwandan context, people did not want to talk about healing, trauma, or related issues. In fact, in Rwandan circles the use of the word "reconciliation" is offensive to those who have lost family members. But by creating opportunities for people to work together on physical rehabilitation that meets family and community needs, NGO workers can help them regain mutual confidence.

CARE staff members in Rwanda and in Bosnia have identified five basic steps or stages in the approach to helping rebuild the social contract through "active humanitarianism" in post-conflict situations:

1. rebuilding the social fabric among staff;
2. rebuilding the family and community fabric;
3. widening the circle of confidence in staff;
4. widening the circle of community trust;
5. building bridges to broader society.

Each step in this lengthy process attempts to resolve a particular problem and has implications for programming.

Rebuilding the social fabric among staff   In the aftermath of the violence in Rwanda and Bosnia, many local NGO staff members have been reticent to share thoughts about one another, about their families or communities. A number of tactics have succeeded in helping to rebuild trust:

1. modeling evenhandedness in the hiring and treatment of local staff, enabling people to see that one group is not favored over the other;
2. building staff cohesion through a mixed-team approach to projects that includes staff of all backgrounds;
3. emphasizing that the NGO culture is an international culture with values that suggest an alternative to narrow identification with only one ethnic group;
4. focusing on rebuilding physical infrastructure such as water, housing, and schools without talking directly about the underlying distrust;
5. balancing project selection among potential conflict groups, which involves not favoring refugees or returnees over populations that did not flee;
6. balancing service provision among ethnic, racial, religious, and ideological groups;
7. conducting general community surveys that focus on physical rehabilitation needs and population sizes, rather than the detailed participatory rural appraisal (PRA)–type surveys that focus on past conflict.

Rebuilding the family and community fabric   In an environment of social collapse, with blended families, widows, orphans, and new communities made of people who have been uprooted from their homes and who are without real social organization, people are fearful about personal security and they distrust their neighbors. Many of these new communities are not economically viable. Some are so far from peoples' original land that they may spend four hours a day walking to and from their source of livelihood. In other cases people are too afraid to return to work their land even if they could. In such circumstances CARE staff have tried some of the following strategies with a relative degree of success:

1. insisting on community identification of needs and project selection, a participative approach that can help begin to rebuild the bonds of cooperation;
2. soliciting community involvement, labor, and organization, and, where possible, mixing groups who may have been previously involved in the conflicts;
3. promoting the reformation of community organizations such as stretcher societies, water committees, and sports teams;
4. working to get landholdings reorganized (e.g., in some cases staff have helped persuade the government of Rwanda to give farmland to new communities near their community site; this allows people to develop economically viable communities once again);
5. promoting methods to restore confidence in police and security (although this is particularly difficult, if families can see consistent evenhandedness on the part of police, confidence can slowly be restored; for NGOs that do operational work and thus find it difficult to get involved in human rights monitoring, encouraging the UN and others to do so in communities provides a channel to spot and report abuses);
6. setting limited objectives with communities and delivering what has been promised;
7. relying on physical count community surveys and needs and capacity analyses rather than on detailed surveys that have extensive questions about the past which frighten people or make them suspicious.

Widening the circle of confidence in staff   If the staff has had some success in the first two stages, cohesion may have improved to the point where people are more willing to engage in relatively open dialogue with one another. In such circumstances the following actions may become possible:

1. staff from different ethnic groups can work together on more detailed participative community survey work that looks more clearly at conflicts and how to overcome them;
2. staff can more willingly participate in joint assessment of community security issues and can evaluate the risks to life and limb of entering certain communities;
3. further staff cohesion can be promoted with group savings and credit societies.

Widening the circle of community trust   After helping with initial community physical infrastructure projects, some CARE workers report that an initial level of community trust and cohesion has been built within ethnic groups, but that people still fear relating across ethnic and ideological divides. CARE staff members have begun to work in this more positive environment in a few places in Rwanda. They are exploring the following ideas:

1. switching to truly participative community-based appraisals and household surveys;
2. developing tailored follow-on projects;
3. promoting joint community service days with all ethnic groups (as did, in fact, take place before the genocide). Genuinely voluntary community service is based on community-identified needs and priorities that support "bottom-up" decision making;
4. facilitating joint work on projects that benefit groups who were formally in conflict;
5. nurturing more open dialogue about what happened.

Building bridges to the broader society   Feasible ideas for rebuilding community organizations in Rwanda might include:

1. forming new local NGOs;
2. working to reinvolve the church, the media, and other institutions in community action.

Examples of Initial Successes and Failures in Rwanda
Some of CARE's initial rehabilitation work in Rwanda provides lessons concerning programs that proved problematic in one way or another (Figure 10.7). Other work, however, involving similar goals but differently organized projects, may hold promise for promoting conflict resolution (Figure

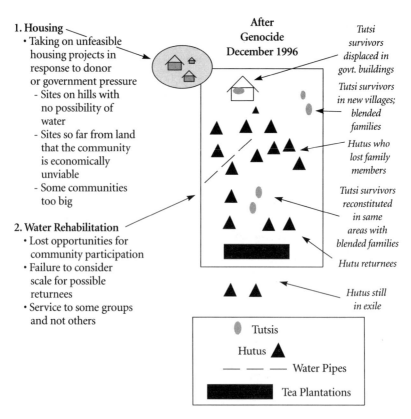

1. Housing
• Taking on unfeasible housing projects in response to donor or government pressure
 - Sites on hills with no possibility of water
 - Sites so far from land that the community is economically unviable
 - Some communities too big

2. Water Rehabilitation
• Lost opportunities for community participation
• Failure to consider scale for possible returnees
• Service to some groups and not others

After Genocide December 1996

Tutsi survivors displaced in govt. buildings

Tutsi survivors in new villages; blended families

Hutus who lost family members

Tutsi survivors reconstituted in same areas with blended families

Hutu returnees

Hutus still in exile

Tutsis ●
Hutus ▲
— — — Water Pipes
▬▬▬ Tea Plantations

Figure 10.7   Programming examples: Programs that worked less well.

10.8). Because these programs have been started only recently they need to be monitored in coming years.

Housing Rehabilitation Programs

As more than 800,000 returnees came back to their communities in Rwanda there were tremendous needs to rehabilitate damaged housing, to build new schools, and to replace vital infrastructure. This new demand for housing has also been important for those who did not leave Rwanda. Many of the Tutsi communities that were decimated by the genocide must be rebuilt away from the vicinity of destroyed villages, because the residents are afraid to return to places where their loved ones were killed. The Rwandan government has sought to locate new villages on the tops of hills in an effort to save more fertile valley agricultural land. Initially, the govern-

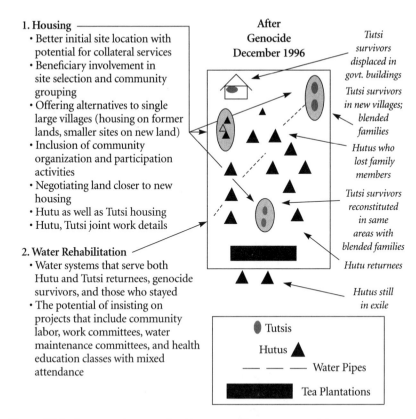

1. Housing
- Better initial site location with potential for collateral services
- Beneficiary involvement in site selection and community grouping
- Offering alternatives to single large villages (housing on former lands, smaller sites on new land)
- Inclusion of community organization and participation activities
- Negotiating land closer to new housing
- Hutu as well as Tutsi housing
- Hutu, Tutsi joint work details

2. Water Rehabilitation
- Water systems that serve both Hutu and Tutsi returnees, genocide survivors, and those who stayed
- The potential of insisting on projects that include community labor, work committees, water maintenance committees, and health education classes with mixed attendance

After Genocide December 1996

Tutsi survivors displaced in govt. buildings

Tutsi survivors in new villages; blended families

Hutus who lost family members

Tutsi survivors reconstituted in same areas with blended families

Hutu returnees

Hutus still in exile

Tutsis

Hutus

Water Pipes

Tea Plantations

Figure 10.8 Programming examples: Programs with greater potential.

ment itself selected the sites and assigned NGOs to provide particular geographic coverage.

Each housing program represents an opportunity for success or failure in reducing conflict and for rebuilding the damaged social contract. Some projects have the potential for success; others are likely to fail.

Housing projects with the potential for success As housing projects develop it will be important to monitor them to see whether those with the following features promote greater community cohesion and are more sustainable than projects that do not have these features:

1. projects with initial site locations that can accommodate collateral services (for example, housing in new villages that are close to water sites with enough capacity to meet population needs);

2. projects that give beneficiaries a chance to help select sites and also to decide in which community they want to live;
3. projects that offer alternatives to single large villages (for example, housing on former lands, or in smaller communities; poor sociopolitical management of villagization programs could lead to the creation of even more isolated Tutsi and Hutu communities);
4. projects that have strong community participation component in community rebuilding, which may help to rebuild trust;
5. projects that locate farmland near new communities so that they will be economically viable;
6. projects that offer new housing opportunities to both Hutu and Tutsi groups, in order to reduce conflict;
7. projects that have Hutu and Tutsi joint work details, which may reduce distrust.

Housing projects with less potential for success Other projects in which NGOs have been asked to participate may have poorer prospects. It will be important to monitor these projects as well.

1. In some cases NGOs have been asked to support housing rehabilitation projects that look less sustainable. Some NGOs have nevertheless taken on these projects in response to donor or government pressure. Examples are projects on hills with no possibility of water and collateral service, or sites so far from people's farmland that the community is not viable economically.
2. In other cases both the demand for housing and donor pressure have been so strong that NGOs have been forced to construct housing quickly. As a result they have not fostered community participation. Such efforts may have gotten off on the wrong foot by reinforcing an entitlement mentality.

Water Systems Rehabilitation Programs

As people began to return to Rwanda in December 1996, the government and NGO donors felt new pressure to rebuild community water systems that had been damaged during the fighting. Each new system represents an opportunity to help rebuild the social fabric in communities. As is true of housing, while it is too soon to determine which programs will help to mitigate conflict and which may exacerbate it, some programs may have more or less potential and should be monitored closely.

Programs with potential for success   Certain water programs seem to have prospects for success:

1. systems that serve Hutu and Tutsi alike, genocide survivors, returnees, and those who stayed;
2. systems that have included community labor, work committees, water maintenance committees, and health education classes with mixed community attendance as opposed to participation from only one kind of group;
3. programs that include health education based on behavioral change, which can enhance the sustainability of water projects.

Programs with less potential for success   Some programs appear to be more likely to fail:

1. water systems that were rebuilt with no community involvement;
2. systems that do not consider the increased demand generated by the large number of people returning from exile;
3. systems that clearly favor some ethnic groups as opposed to others.

CONCLUSION

The harsh world of complex emergencies has created special challenges for the international community and for NGOs that aspire to help people stay alive and rebuild their lives. This ambiguous new world has forced many NGOs to begin to redefine their roles in response to the structural, operational, and ethical dilemmas they now face. It has stimulated some within the NGO community to move away from concepts of "naive humanitarianism" and to try to overcome potentially negative aspects of their work. It also has challenged the community to become more vocal. NGOs are now more likely to say publicly that humanitarian action when people's lives are at risk is not a substitute for international action to promote peace and the resolution of the problems that lead to conflict. Food and medical relief are not a substitute for responsible international action that promotes peace settlements, that provides security to refugees as well as to aid workers, that permits refugee relief, and that provides the foundation for rehabilitation and development.

The NGO community must continue to adapt its work to the new realities of humanitarian crises. Relief organizations should pursue the further development of a philosophy of active humanitarianism, which is based upon some of the following principles:

1. Survivors of complex humanitarian emergencies have a right to rebuild their lives once the conflict is over.
2. NGOs and the international community must make a commitment to a timely operational response to pressing humanitarian needs.
3. Safe access to people in need during conflict is an important responsibility of belligerents and of the international community.
4. Refugees, internally displaced people, and NGO workers have a right to safety.
5. NGOs have a right to withdraw in conflict situations and to publicize problems where refugees are being intimidated, where political groups will not allow distribution of relief supplies to people in need, and where civil order cannot be maintained.
6. Humanitarian response is not a substitute for efforts by the international community and by the UN system to promote negotiated settlements that treat the roots of conflicts rather than their symptoms.
7. Active humanitarianism compels us to search for program responses that help alleviate rather than exacerbate conflict.
8. Emergency response should lay a foundation for subsequent rehabilitation and development for families and communities.

EPILOGUE: PUTTING ACTIVE HUMANITARIANISM INTO PRACTICE

Putting this new framework into practice presents an ongoing challenge. Initial steps at CARE have included intense discussions of the "active humanitarianism" philosophy and its implications, program training with active humanitarianism in mind, and workshops on conflict resolution in relief and rehabilitation programs. The results have begun to appear in post-genocide Rwanda and in Bosnia.

The imperative to help shape future international responses through advocacy has begun to unfold. For example, in February 1997 representatives of CARE International, Oxfam, MSF, and the ICRC had an unprecedented opportunity to share these views with the international community. They participated in the first NGO testimony to the UN Security Council, which was followed by a special meeting with the UN Secretary General, Kofi Annan.[21] A scheduled two-hour session turned into a four-hour discussion, revealing that the members of the Security Council have a high level of interest in the problem of humanitarian crises and potential solutions.

During 1997 the UN and some of its member states paid increased attention to putting a more comprehensive approach into practice. Secretary General Annan named a special representative, for the Great Lakes region in Africa, Ambassador Mohamed Sahnoun. Sahnoun's mandate has been to promote a negotiated settlement of the conflict in the Democratic Republic of the Congo (formerly Zaire), to advocate for the safety and security of refugees in the eastern part of the Democratic Republic of the Congo, to assist with rehabilitation in Rwanda, and to promote attention to refugee issues in Burundi.[22]

During this period the Secretary General, the Special Ambassador, and the head of UNHCR, Mrs. Ogata, have advocated strongly for refugee access, safety, and repatriation in the eastern Democratic Republic of the Congo. They have also denounced massacres of refugees.[23] There is every indication that this new approach to humanitarian response, which includes diplomatic action, security, and emergency relief, is beginning to work. One cannot attribute the changes to NGO adaptation and to advocacy alone. But it is fair to say that the entire international community has begun to put what it has learned from complex emergencies during recent years into practice. While there have been and will continue to be sobering setbacks, there is reason to be cautiously optimistic that these new approaches are beginning to show positive results for people whose lives are at risk.

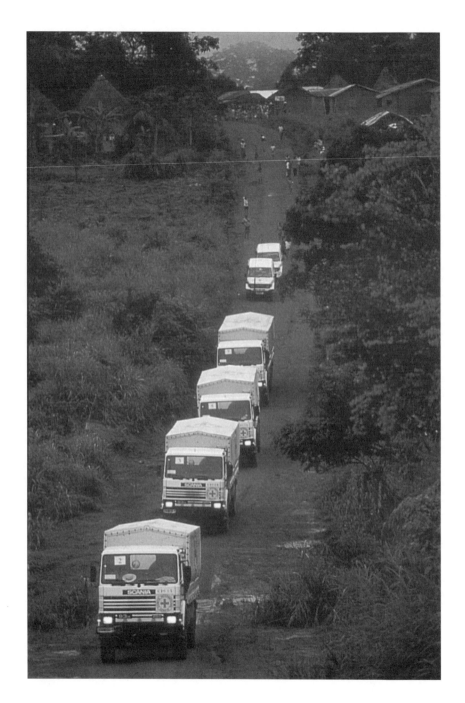

11

COORDINATION OF HEALTH RELIEF:
THE EXPERIENCE OF THE AMERICAN RED CROSS

judith b. lee

A central issue facing the international community in its response to humanitarian crises is that of mobilization and coordination of services and resources. The American Red Cross (ARC) is chartered by Congress to coordinate its work within the United States with all other nongovernmental organizations (NGOs) active in times of disasters and must continuously address aspects of structure and function in order to adapt to changing conditions.

The basic practices and theories of disaster management and coordination of relief have remained constant from the earliest days of the ARC. Advances in technology have facilitated communication and have led to efficiencies in the use of time and the movement of resources, but delivering needed services for victims of disaster remains the focal point of the Red Cross program. The lessons about relief coordination learned from previous Red Cross disaster missions, the significance of those lessons for future disasters, including complex emergencies, and the continuing problems of coordination faced by those in the field are the primary focus here.

As a member of the International Red Cross and Red Crescent movement, the American Red Cross responds to the needs of the suffering in accordance with the mandate of the Geneva Conventions of 1949 and their Additional Protocols of 1977. The ARC and its partners—the International

Committee of the Red Cross and the International Federation of Red Cross and Red Crescent Societies—provide humanitarian relief and development assistance based solely on the criterion of need (Box 11.1).

With 1,700 chapters around the United States, its territories, and its possessions, the ARC responds to approximately 55,000 disasters a year, the

---

Box 11.1 The legal basis of American Red Cross activities

In providing disaster relief, the American Red Cross has a legal and moral mandate that it has neither the authority nor the right to surrender. Red Cross has both the power and the duty to act in disaster, and prompt action is clearly expected and supported by the public.

The Red Cross's authority to perform disaster services was formalized when the organization was chartered by the Congress of the United States in 1905. Among other provisions, this charter charged Red Cross "to continue and carry on a system of national and international relief in time of peace and apply the same in mitigating the sufferings caused by pestilence, famine, fire, floods, and other great national calamities, and to devise and carry on measures for preventing the same" (U.S. Congress, act of January 5, 1905, as amended, 36 U.S.C.). The Red Cross's authority to provide disaster services was reaffirmed in U.S. federal law in the 1974 Disaster Relief Act (Public Law 93-288) and in 1988 in the Robert T. Stafford Disaster Relief Act. These laws resulted in the creation of the Federal Emergency Management Agency and made it responsible for coordinating the federal response to situations for which the President of the United States issues a disaster declaration. The Red Cross and FEMA cooperate under a statement of understanding outlining their respective roles. The Red Cross responds to all disaster events regardless of size or scope; FEMA is activated upon the request of a specific state for incident-specific federal assistance approved by the President.

In preparing for and responding to disasters, the Red Cross works with government agencies and civil authorities at all levels, other voluntary and nonprofit agencies, business and labor, and individuals and small groups. The Red Cross serves in both coordination and referral roles to match needs with resources.

Although government's role has expanded over the years, the Red Cross remains responsible for responding to disaster, but does not encroach on any action the government takes for the welfare of its citizens. The Red Cross may act as an agent for federal, state, and local agencies. For example, the Red Cross has agreed to act as the primary agency for the federal government for the coordination of mass care when the Federal Response Plan (FRP) is activated.[6]

---

majority of which affect single families. More than 250 a year are major disasters affecting large numbers of people. The initial response is made by the trained disaster workers of a local chapter. When the disaster exceeds the local chapter's capability, surrounding chapters will assist. If that response is still not sufficient, the Disaster Operations Center at ARC national headquarters will mobilize additional personnel and material support from the resources of other chapters nationwide.

THE AMERICAN RED CROSS DISASTER SERVICES PROGRAM

The Red Cross Disaster Services program is multifaceted, providing relief to victims of disaster while assisting people to plan for, prepare for, and respond to disaster. A group of documents known as the "3000 Series" provide the administrative regulations and operating procedures under which the Red Cross carries out this program. The 3000 Series enables the Red Cross to ensure that workers assist victims consistently and that the accumulated knowledge and wisdom of experienced disaster teams is captured for future responses. The program is standardized, providing services in all fifty states and the U.S. territories.

The program is organized into three areas: planning, preparedness, and response.

Planning   The planning program ensures that Red Cross chapters across the United States and its territories have written disaster plans that are tailored to their particular geographical areas, risk factors, and disaster history. Planning also includes the evaluation of responses and requisite adjustments in the written plans.

Preparedness   The preparedness program addresses disaster community education, training, and preparation for disaster response in risk areas. Preparedness activities that enable individuals and families to minimize injury, death, and loss are based on the plan written for a specific area.

Response   The response program addresses the actions required immediately following a disaster event, including the utilization of resources from outside the affected area as necessary. In essence, the Red Cross is a mutual aid society, with nonaffected chapters delivering human and material resources to those affected by a disaster. The program also works closely with other agencies active in disaster relief, to coordinate activities and to avoid duplication of services and efforts.

Disaster Services Structure

To deliver service to disaster victims quickly and effectively, the ARC has set up a function-based structure with three parts (Figure 11.1):

1. Direct Services to the individuals and families affected by disaster;
2. Internal Support Services;
3. External Support Services that interact with agencies and groups other than Red Cross Disaster Services.

When national resources are requested by local or state chapters, within hours the incoming structure sets up a multimillion-dollar organization with a goal of providing services immediately and going out of business as quickly as possible. Each function within the structure has its own procedures and practices, its own table of organization, and its own area of activity designed to ensure a quick response to serve disaster victims (Box 11.2).

Disaster Services Human Resources

A Disaster Services Human Resources (DSHR) system has been established to provide an identified, trained, and dedicated cadre of paid and volunteer staff to respond to disasters. The system permits these workers to choose three functional areas of interest and to specify a first preference. A system of reserves, maintained on a personnel roster, can be activated for a specific disaster response as paid staff. These reserves are expected to travel immediately to the site and to remain on assignment for as long as the needs of the operation require it. The DSHR system database tracks all staff, paid and volunteer, including the reserves, and contains pertinent emergency contact information, a recruitment contact point, special information such as licensure and languages spoken, job history, training record, and chosen career development path.

The ARC has developed statements of understanding with other agencies and organizations to describe areas of coordination in disaster relief such as specialized human resources. In recent years, such agreements have been made with professional associations, such as the American Psychological Association, the American Psychiatric Association, and the American Association of Critical Care Nurses. Private sector corporations also participate actively in disaster preparedness and response with personnel, goods and services, and expertise.

The Federal Response Plan designates the Red Cross as the agency that

Red Cross Disaster Response Functions

Manage-ment	Administration				
Direct Services	Disaster Health Services	Disaster Mental Health Services	Disaster Welfare Inquiry	Family Service	Mass Care
Internal Support Services	Account-ing	Building and Repair	Communi-cations	Damage Assess-ment	Disaster Computer Operations
	Local Disaster Volunteers	Logistics	Records and Reports	Staffing	Training
External Support Services	Fund Raising	Liaison, Chapter	Liaison, Govern-ment	Liaison, Human Relations	Liaison, Labor	Liaison, Volunteer Agencies	Public Affairs

This chart depicts all possible functions performed on a disaster operation. It does not illustrate lines of authority or communication.

Experienced DSHR System members in Administration, Mass Care, Disaster Health Services, Disaster Welfare Inquiry, Logistics, and the Liaison functions also will be recruited to support Emergency Support Function #6 of the Federal Response Plan in an FRP Disaster.

Figure 11.1   Red Cross disaster response functions. (ARC poster 916A, rev. 7/95)

coordinates the efforts of the voluntary agencies active in disaster and, as such, maintains close ties with those agencies, churches, and groups that are committed to responding. The Red Cross takes care to ensure that services are not duplicated and do not work at cross-purposes.

Coordination of Disaster Response

The best coordination occurs prior to a disaster, when community members allocate roles among community groups and local agencies. Virtually every area of response requires coordination for relief to be effective, efficient, rapid, and reliable. Principal areas include services (required to meet disaster-caused emergency needs), resources (personnel, material

Box 11.2 Functions within ARC Disaster Services

1. Direct Services

   - Mass Care—provides food, shelter, and bulk distribution of supplies.

   - Family Services—conducts one-on-one casework with individuals and families to ensure that disaster–caused needs, such as clothing, shoes, bed linens, and other basic household items, are met in the emergency phase; enables clients to return to their usual routines as soon as possible; assistance with long-term recovery.

   - Disaster Health Services—provides basic first aid; provides casework assistance with health-related needs caused by the disaster (for example, medication replacement, replacement of eyeglasses, hearing aids, and dentures); provides health support to disaster workers (more than 1,000 paid and/or volunteer workers may be assigned to a major relief operation).

   - Disaster Mental Health Services—supports psychological needs of assigned staff of Red Cross and their families; works cooperatively with local, state, regional, and/or federal mental health agencies to ensure that support is available to disaster clients on an individual, family, or community basis.

   - Disaster Welfare Inquiry—responds to inquiries made to chapters and sister societies around the world about the health and welfare of individuals and families within a disaster area; collects information about such persons; prepares and distributes bulletins to unaffected chapters detailing information about the disaster operation.

2. Internal Support Services

   - Accounting—administers the financial aspects of an operation; receives and expends funds to meet commitments for relief costs, travel, and maintenance of staff, salaries, and other expenditures required for a disaster relief operation.

(continued)

Box 11.2 *(continued)*

- Building and Repair—provides technical guidance in the repair and/ or reconstruction of homes; maintains liaison with contractors providing services on a disaster relief operation.

- Communications—establishes and maintains communications systems within a disaster relief operation, including telephone, cellular phone, pager, wire service, radio, satellite, and other systems; serves as liaison with voluntary groups providing such services to the operation.

- Damage Assessment—determines the size and scope of a disaster and the level of damage sustained by dwellings within the affected area; develops and distributes statistical data related to the demographics of affected populations and the effects of disaster.

- Disaster Computer Operations—provides computer hardware, software, and technical support to disaster operation staff who use the Disaster Relief Operation Management Information System (DROMIS).

- Local Disaster Volunteers (LDV)—recruits, places, retains, and recognizes local volunteers who support a disaster relief operation; collaborates with the local Red Cross Coordinator of Disaster Volunteers for recruitment of volunteers affiliated with the affected unit; works closely with the Liaisons to Voluntary Agencies and Labor for recruiting groups from other organizations; places spontaneous volunteers according to operational needs.

- Logistics—procures supplies and materials required for a disaster relief operation; stores and distributes supplies; establishes and controls the transportation system within the operation, including the acquisition, assignment, and tracking of Red Cross–owned and rental vehicles; establishes a courier system and distributes mail; acquires and releases facilities; maintains materials, equipment, and services, such as security and facilities cleaning.

(continued)

- Records and Reports—controls and processes the disbursing orders provided to victims; maintains files of the cases opened on each individual and family; compiles statistics related to a disaster relief operation.

- Staffing—recruits, places, administers, supports, and recognizes paid and volunteer staff (usually from outside the affected Red Cross chapter's jurisdiction) assigned to the operation from any of the fifty states, possessions, and territories of the United States or from sister societies such as the Canadian Red Cross and the Mexican Red Cross

Training—orients all staff assigned to a disaster relief operation; provides operational training for new staff; delivers refresher or new training in all functions.

3. External Support Services

- Fund-Raising—formulates and implements fund-raising strategy; manages and coordinates fund-raising activities required to meet the cost of a disaster relief operation; ensures gift tracking, stewardship, and recognition (the Red Cross operates solely on the donations of the American people).

- Liaison, Chapter (LC)—establishes and maintains effective working relationships with chapters in the affected area; keeps all Red Cross leadership throughout the state, as well as operational leadership and personnel, informed about the progress of an operation, problems encountered, and concerns expressed by any chapter.

- Liaison, Government—develops and maintains liaison with federal, state, and local authorities and government units.

- Liaison, Human Relations—develops and maintains community relations in an affected area, including relations with individuals and organizations representing minority, disabled, elderly, and socially and economically deprived segments of the community, to enhance service delivery to those populations and for the development of advisory committees; supports the local chapter(s) in the area of human relations.

(continued)

Box 11.2 *(continued)*

- Liaison, Labor—develops and maintains liaison with organized labor and contacts these organizations for potential recruitment of volunteer resources; secures from labor organizations and their employer companies gifts-in-kind, such as transportation of goods; serves as liaison between all levels of organized labor and the Red Cross.

- Liaison, Voluntary Agencies—develops and maintains liaison with other voluntary organizations, and contacts these organizations for potential recruitment of volunteer resources (voluntary organizations include national organizations, local components of national organizations, community organizations, and ad hoc groups involved in disaster response).

- Public Affairs—provides information about services available to people affected by disasters; provides information to the general public about disaster services; serves as liaison with all media; provides general public affairs support to the operation.

goods, and logistic supports), and information (including evaluation, in order to promote appropriate decision making, effective management, and accountability). Principal issues in coordination (Box 11.3) are discussed below.

Services

Services provided directly to the disaster victims and to the workers at a disaster site must be coordinated among agencies and groups to ensure the provision of appropriate services needed while making efficient use of manpower and resources, both material and financial. Advance community planning and preparedness, with clarification of roles and responsibilities, supports an immediate and effective response. Communities that do not prepare for disaster are unable to respond adequately when the time comes. Those communities risk additional loss of life and property as well as injury and confusion. Ultimately, the post-disaster result is a disgruntled population and a changed community that does not trust its leaders.

Box 11.3 Issues in Coordination

- Lack of preparedness planning
- No assignment of roles and responsibilities
- Spontaneous volunteers
- Unwanted or unmarked goods
- Storage bottlenecks
- Information gathering and dissemination
- Rumors
- Cultural diversity
- Tracing and identification
- Evaluation and follow-through

Innovation in Mental Health Services

As described in Chapter 5, the mental health community has slowly been learning how to address situations in which "normal" people have experienced an abnormal event. Over the years the nurses in ARC Disaster Health Services have provided counseling, compassion, and referrals for disaster workers and for disaster victims experiencing emotional reactions to the event. After good experience with the deployment of mental health professionals following Hurricane Hugo in 1989, the ARC a year later convened a task force of representative disciplines in mental health to create Disaster Mental Health Services (DMHS).

This effort has led to a busy and expanding function in disaster relief. Professional mental health associations have in turn created disaster response networks and committees at the community, state, and national levels. For certain types of disasters today, DMHS is the principal Red Cross response. Following the crash of the ValuJet aircraft in Florida in 1996, for example, the most visible and extended assistance from the Red Cross was provided by DMHS on the scene, in the area for family members of the crash victims, for the airline workers, and at the points of embarkation and destination.

Resources

Individuals who can provide specialized care, such as doctors and nurses, and those who can cook large quantities of food, drive tractor trailers, or provide child care for parents trying to reconstitute their lives are among the numerous resources needed during disaster response.

The coordination of volunteers and agency workers responding to a disaster is imperative. While the Red Cross has considerable experience in coordinating volunteers, there are also other community agencies that can fulfill this activity. The responsibility for volunteer coordination needs to be defined in the predisaster planning process. Spontaneous volunteers frequently appear at a disaster site from all over the country and, in some cases, from other countries as well. Having a clearinghouse or a designated agency to which incoming volunteers report would enable a review of credentials, assessment of skills and interests, recording of pertinent information about each volunteer, and placement of that volunteer with the appropriate agency. Specific plans must be written to guide the placement of people with varied qualifications who show up to help. Following Hurricane Andrew in Florida in 1992, 8,288 local responders worked as Red Cross volunteers—a fraction of the total number of responders to that disaster. Individuals were placed with numerous other agencies.

Once a disaster has struck there is no time to devise a plan of action. Institutions and people will react to what has happened. Spontaneous volunteers without sponsorship add to the confusion and, lacking their own shelter, food, and water, often become a part of the disaster. Not having a specific assigned role encourages these people to mingle aimlessly, without purpose or guidance, and results in unused talents and unhappy volunteers.

Material resources are a finite commodity requiring coordination. The procurement, shipping, and distribution of goods and the acceptance, shipping, and distribution of donated in-kind goods requires central warehousing, fleets of trucks, forklifts, pallet jacks, security, and all the accoutrements utilized by industry on a daily basis. Disaster logistics must be set up immediately, ready to receive and distribute equipment and supplies (Box 11.4).

Box 11.4 Logistics software

There are many "off the shelf" software programs available for managing disaster response logistics. The Supplies Management (SUMA) project, developed by the Pan American Health Organization (PAHO) Emergency Preparedness Program, is in wide use. SUMA software is user friendly and is easily put to use on a laptop computer. One of the objectives of the SUMA project is to provide support to and exchange expertise with those managing relief operations. A video provides an overview of the project and the methodology developed to quickly sort and inventory large amounts of relief supplies. Information on the video and other resources in logistics and the management of unsolicited in-kind donations is available from PAHO, 525 Twenty-third Street, NW, Washington, D.C. 20037; or on the World Wide Web at <http://www.paho.org/english/ped/pedsumaw.htm>.

Lack of preparation to handle the outpouring of donated goods will cause the diversion of personnel, transport, storage, and other resources that are badly needed elsewhere. Unless donors are informed of truly needed items, they will send what they perceive is needed or wanted.[1] The Red Cross has an In Kind Donations corporate section that closely coordinates with Disaster Services when a major relief operation is under way. Predetermined lists of goods generally used in the first ten days of any type of disaster have been prepared and are used to target donations. These lists are adjusted as needed for a specific disaster. Knowing what is available, offered, and accepted enables the logistics personnel to plan the receipt, transportation, and storage of the goods. The goods will travel consigned to the Red Cross, will be packaged appropriately with proper bills of lading, and will be marked as "disaster relief supplies." This process is particularly successful in international disasters and complex emergencies, and facilitates the entry of an approved and known consignment into the affected country.

Storage of goods in a disaster area can be a challenge. Finding warehouses with sufficient space for temporary use is often accomplished with the assistance of the local business community. In major disasters, coordination among agencies needing storage space can stretch resources to satisfy all needs. Specialized requirements for storage and resources are not always widely accessible to all agencies. For example, the ability to preserve a cold chain for certain biological supplies can determine the feasibility of an immunization program. The World Health Organization published "An Annotated Cold Chain Bibliography" in 1981 and has revised it several times since then. The bibliography refers to different aspects of the cold chain from product information sheets to descriptions of state-of-the-art solar refrigerators.[2]

Information

Background information gathered as part of a community's predisaster plan will enable the quick interpretation and comparison of post-disaster data. This information needs to be shared easily by all agencies and should include demographic data, listings of health facilities and services, locations of stores of food stocks, medicines, and key equipment and supplies, and names and points of contact for agencies active in disaster in the community.

Once a disaster has occurred, information gathered should be factual and verified to the extent possible by authorities and teams conducting assessments. The extent of damage, available local human and material resources, and potential secondary risks to the public health are the initial assessments required. Accurate information is necessary to facilitate decision making by relief agencies, to keep the public informed, and to prevent or to counteract rumors.[3]

Teams of personnel assessing and collecting information should be separate and distinct from those teams providing life-saving medical care, from search and rescue efforts, and from other services designed to protect lives and property. The Red Cross dispatches damage assessors immediately and initiates contacts at local, state, and national levels to gather as much initial data as possible. Using computer linkages with such agencies as the National Weather Service, the National Oceanic and Atmospheric Administration, and FEMA's Emergency Operations Center and having the technology to gain access to demographic data for a community within minutes provide Red Cross with considerable detailed information immediately. Information available on television can be helpful, but agencies should rely principally on verified information from authorities on or near the scene.

Red Cross operates a twenty-four-hour professionally staffed disaster operations center. Information is relayed by fax, telephone, or radio, if necessary, to the local Red Cross or to the state lead chapter. This facilitates decision making regarding the number of personnel needed, types and amounts of supplies and equipment required, and the estimated cost of the operation.

Equally important as gathering information is its dissemination. Not only is good information of critical use internally for an agency, but it must be shared with other relief entities and with the general public. The electronic media can provide guidance to the public on shelter locations, functioning health facilities, utilities, and transportation routes. It can also provide health advisories and specific relief services instructions. In 1986 the Red Cross formalized a cooperative agreement with the U.S. Centers for Disease Control and Prevention to share information related to disaster-caused deaths, injuries, and illnesses. The Red Cross has collected data for many years, and the CDC utilizes this data for scientific and educational purposes. With this agreement came increased opportunities to raise the consciousness of the health community nationwide to the epidemiological aspects of disaster events.[4]

Rumors and fears abound in the wake of disasters. An effective system for dispelling rumors and fears must include radio, television, and newspapers as well as leaflets, posters, and signs. The languages used to disseminate information must reflect the cultural diversity of the population affected. Attention should also be given to that segment of the population unable to read or unable to gain access to established media outlets.

Community disaster education has expanded in recent years to alert individuals, families, communities, and business and industry to the ways in which one can prepare for disasters, reduce death and injury, and recover from different disaster events. The Red Cross has collaborated with other agencies and private sector entities to produce multimedia informational brochures, booklets, and workshops in different languages to educate people about disasters. Those responding to the Loma Prieta earthquake relief operation quickly realized that English and Spanish versions of information were not sufficient. Large numbers of Asian-Pacific populations in the Bay Area of San Francisco also needed information in their own languages.

Because disasters can occur at any time, families can be separated within an affected area. All information related to the identification or registration of individuals should be centralized to facilitate family reunification. Lists of the positively identified dead, the hospitalized, treated and released individuals, shelter registrants, evacuees, and recipients of bulk distributed goods are examples of data that enable the Red Cross to answer health and welfare inquiries. The Federal Response Plan designates that all such information on individuals will be coordinated by the Red Cross in its Disaster Welfare Inquiry section.

EVALUATION

The determination of how well a disaster relief operation has coordinated all the necessary internal and external activities of the Red Cross is made after the conclusion of the operation. The concepts and assumptions of the disaster plan are tested during its implementation. The evaluation of an operation determines how well the integral parts of the plan—the concept of operations, management systems, procedures, and processes—addressed operational issues and requirements.

In the Red Cross, evaluation is a formal process conducted by national headquarters; the participants include those persons who provided leadership for the disaster relief operation and those who must implement the recommendations resulting from the evaluation. The methods used include questionnaires, interviews with key personnel (including local emergency management leaders), group critiques, reviews of the written narratives required of all Red Cross functional officers, and comparison and discussion of after-action reports from similar operations. With all methods, key issues are identified and recommendations are developed to ensure that future plans and relief operations build on successes and address identified problem areas. Follow-through on key issues and recommendations is fundamental to the success of the evaluation.[5]

The Impact of Improved Coordination

Even after a comprehensive evaluation and revitalization of ARC programs following Hurricane Hugo and the Loma Prieta earthquake in 1989 (Box 11.5), the effect of Hurricane Andrew in Florida in 1995 was nearly catastrophic, requiring far more coordination with federal agencies than ever before. Andrew served as a wake-up call to many organizations and to many

Box 11.5 Evaluation of the ARC response to Hurricane Hugo and subsequent follow-through

In 1989 Hurricane Hugo made landfall in Puerto Rico and the U.S. Virgin Islands and continued on to Charleston, South Carolina. Hugo's destructive path continued well inland through South Carolina and into North Carolina. The Red Cross committed personnel and equipment to all affected areas. One month later, while relief operations were still under way in the emergency phase, the Loma Prieta earthquake struck the San Francisco area in California.

As part of the response to the Loma Prieta earthquake, Red Cross was able to provide emergency relief of food, shelter, clothing, and health needs. As soon became apparent, however, coordinated efforts by governmental and nonprofit agencies were required to provide this newly homeless segment of the population with shelter and with medical assistance. Moreover, a number of social issues faced by the community before the disaster had to be addressed.

The Red Cross had not previously faced such a series of disasters so close together in time. The evaluation of those operations was intense and led to steps in subsequent years to increase ARC's capacity for multiple responses. In 1992 Hurricane Andrew struck Florida, moved on across the Gulf of Mexico, and made landfall again in Louisiana, continuing inland in a large curve to damage parts of Mississippi as well. Several days later, Typhoon Omar devastated the island of Guam and, two weeks later, Hurricane Iniki struck the Hawaiian Islands, mainly the island of Kauai. Once again the Red Cross was faced with multiple disasters.

DISASTER SERVICES REVITALIZATION
In November 1989 the ARC undertook a major response assessment to examine in detail how the Red Cross had responded to these events. The assessment sought to describe the response, to examine how services were delivered, to identify problems and points of stress in the delivery system, and to refine the evaluation tools used to assess Red Cross disaster relief services. The assessment was completed and recommendations were accepted by the Board of Governors and senior management by January 1991.

Revitalization has been a comprehensive program designed to increase the capacity of the Red Cross to deliver high-quality services. Key components of the program are:

(continued)

Box 11.5 *(continued)*

• expansion and improvement of disaster preparedness;

• immediate improvement of delivery of services to victims;

• improved communications among Red Cross units, victims and the public, and local agencies;

• improvement of the organization's capacity to meet the needs of minority and ethnic populations.

The Red Cross has placed top priority on revitalization and has taken several significant actions since 1991, including:

• centralizing Disaster Services at national headquarters to allow direct chapter/national headquarters communication;

• creating and staffing a Planning and Evaluation Unit within Disaster Services

• increasing from ten to twenty-one the number of national sector disaster specialists assigned to field sites to assist chapter preparedness activities directly;

• creating and staffing fourteen disaster planning positions to refine and enhance Red Cross disaster planning at the local and state levels

• increasing the number of trained paid and volunteer staff available for disaster assignments nationwide from 3,200 in 1989 to more than 23,000 in 1998;

• developing, testing, and implementing relief operation performance and service quality measures;

• establishing a routine casework service audit of all major disaster relief operations to determine the quality and consistency of assistance provided;

(continued)

groups of service providers who previously had felt that a disaster of any size could be managed in the United States. For the ARC, the operation demonstrated the need for a more formalized logistical response in disaster events of such magnitude. Previously, function officers had worked with a small supply team to ensure that needed supplies and equipment were available. Following Hurricane Andrew, the senior management of the or-

Box 11.5 *(continued)*

- streamlining and implementing casework procedures to enhance the pace of assistance;

- developing cultural sensitivity training, which is continually provided to both paid and volunteer staff;

- putting in place monitoring activities to increase the number of minority supervisors for disaster relief operation;

- routinely assigning human relations specialists to major disaster relief operations.

The Red Cross has also expanded its high-technology communications capabilities as part of the revitalization program. Satellite terminals capable of transmitting voice and data have been prepositioned in the Caribbean and the Pacific as well as in high-risk coastal states in the United States. The national fleet of emergency response vehicles has also been expanded, and other types of vehicles for the transportation of supplies and equipment have been added.

A review of the relationship between the Red Cross and other organizations active in disaster response has led to more positive linkages and improved client service. A commitment to avoid duplication of benefits and services has meant that all responding agencies are working more efficiently and are making more effective use of tax and donor dollars.

ganization gave its full support to the formation of a Logistics Unit in Disaster Services. This team was put in place months after Hurricane Andrew and immediately made its presence known. The implementation of a logistical approach to the needs of the direct service functions meant that materials arrived faster, more completely and reliably, and, in the long run, at lower cost. The development of a capability to make predisaster contracts, to form linkages with groups capable of providing the necessary goods, to acquire and return facilities, to make push packages (that is, prepacked supplies that can be "pushed" into the field quickly) of known equipment needs, and to implement many other logistical practices has been invaluable.

Other lessons from 1989 made a difference in the response to subsequent disasters. In 1989 the Red Cross established one relief operation in the Caribbean, requiring the assignment of key personnel at its headquarters in Puerto Rico. Other islands were staffed with supervisors and workers. The geography and interrupted communication lines made appropriate over-sight and coordination nearly impossible. When Hurricane Marilyn struck the same area in 1995, the Red Cross established three separate opera-tions—one in St. Thomas/St. John, one in Puerto Rico, and one in St. Croix. The difficulties experienced in 1989 were not repeated. Separate op-erations, instead of requiring more personnel, resulted in the more efficient assignment of fewer personnel (Table 11.1).

APPLYING DISASTER COORDINATION LESSONS TO HUMANITARIAN CRISES

Rwanda

Internationally, the Red Cross response now often centers around complex humanitarian emergencies such as that in Rwanda, which demand ex-tended assistance to affected individuals and families over a long period of time. These human-caused crises are often marked by the destruction of the local institutions and governments that would ordinarily support assis-tance and recovery. Part of the ARC input to the coordinated response to Rwanda has been to collaborate with the Peace Corps to identify and send disaster workers to Rwanda who are experienced, skilled in multiple disci-plines, and multilingual.

Table 11.1 Comparative assignment of personnel during hurricane relief

	Volunteers	Paid	Total
Hurricane Hugo (1989)			
Caribbean	5,115	685	5,800
Hurricane Marilyn (1995)			
St. Croix	1,109	104	1,213
St. Thomas/St. John	1,976	56	2,032
Puerto Rico	714	67	781
1995 totals	3,799	227	4,026

Central and South America

When the civil wars of Nicaragua and El Salvador created large numbers of refugees in Honduras, international agencies joined forces to open camps and to provide services. The UN High Commissioner for Refugees, Médecins sans Frontières, the International Committee of the Red Cross, the League (now the International Federation) of Red Cross and Red Crescent Societies, and others worked together closely to meet basic needs. An assessment made in conjunction with the international agencies demonstrated that the needs were monumental. The ARC, under a grant from the U.S. Agency for International Development, assisted in developing special programs and health services in Honduras for children from one to seventeen years of age who had been displaced from Nicaragua, with the goal of instituting programs and services that could have long-term significance and that would serve the majority of the refugees.

Following the volcanic eruption at Armero, Colombia, in 1985, the ARC provided an experienced disaster nurse to assist in the management of the emergency camps that were created. In setting up a structure, the nurse explained and demonstrated the use of the ARC 3000 Series—the regulations and procedures of the functions in a disaster operation. The Colombian Red Cross adopted this series ("La Serie Tres Mil"). Over the next seven years the ARC transferred the 3000 Series concept to eight countries in South America, to three countries in Central America, and to Mexico. The success of this information was evident during the responses to Hurricane Hugo and Hurricane Andrew, when members of the Colombia Red Cross and the Mexico Red Cross were recruited to work on the ARC relief operations. The training and experience they brought made them valuable and productive members of the teams.

Kuwait

Flexibility is a requirement for workers whether they are responding to disasters or to complex emergencies. In 1991, as U.S. forces secured Kuwait after the invasion by Iraq, the ARC, in close cooperation with the U.S. Public Health Service, deployed a team of fifty health professionals to staff a hospital whose human and material resources had been decimated while its patient load had increased. The team's role later was expanded to administer a refugee camp providing food, shelter, and medical care for three months under adverse conditions.

Tracing

Of all the aspects of suffering caused by war, the separation of families and uncertainty about the fate of a sibling, a parent, or a child must be among the most terrifying. The ICRC has understood from the time of the Franco-Prussian War the importance of providing families with lists of the wounded and of prisoners.

Tracing work is one of the responsibilities of the ARC in augmenting the ICRC's implementation of the Geneva Conventions. Although the level of activity rises and falls with levels of refugee movement, since 1975, with the admission of 2.1 million refugees into the United States, ARC tracing work has involved many U.S. communities where Vietnamese, Somali, and Iraqi refugees have settled.

Tracing work has three components:

- Location—the search for family members, which may be initiated during the conflict, but which often continues for decades (the ARC is currently conducting searches for family members separated during the Second World War and the Holocaust, the Bosnian conflict, and conflicts related to the cold war);
- Communication—the use of standardized, hand-written message forms, also known as "family messages," that contain only personal news from a prisoner of war, from a refugee, or from a displaced child and that can facilitate contact between as many people as possible in an effort to reunite families (in many conflict situations the exchange of Red Cross messages goes on for years and is the only means available for family members to keep in touch with one another);
- Family Reunification—though not so clearly defined, this may include sending documents about family relationships to the ICRC that can facilitate the repatriation of former prisoners of war or that can support their admission as refugees to the United States.

FUTURE TRENDS AND CHALLENGES

As part of its planning function, the ARC devotes resources to anticipating future trends and to weighing their implications for disaster incidence, response, and recovery. Box 11.6 includes some of the more significant trends identified.

Box 11.6 ARC planning horizon: Significant trends

- People aged eighty-five or older are the fastest-growing age group in the United States.
- Populations are shifting annually to areas at high risk for hurricanes, floods, or earthquakes.
- Immigration rates are increasing, with the world's poorest populations settling in urban areas.
- The infrastructure of large metropolitan centers is aging.
- Faster trains and increasing road traffic are using aging highways and bridges nationwide.
- Technologies are changing rapidly, with increased reliance on electrical systems.
- Issues pertaining to zoning and building permits are growing in number and complexity.
- Health care delivery will increasingly move in the direction of home health, early release from hospitals, prolongation of life, and technological advances in equipment and supplies.
- Increasingly complex home medical/nursing treatment modalities and quicker releases from hospitals are becoming the norm.
- Budgetary cuts in the public sector will continue, as will benefits cuts in health insurance packages.
- The capacity of local public health units to fulfill their responsibility to their communities in time of disaster will be tested.
- Resources, both human and material, are shrinking for disasters that are not major attention-grabbing events with casualties.
- Public expectations regarding service delivery capacities of agencies and institutions in disaster situations will increase.

(continued)

Social trends that may contribute to the lowering of hazards and risks include improved building technology, better detection and/or warning systems, and the health care sector's increased awareness of disaster implications. Environmental trends that may help mitigate disaster impact include the reduced use of some pesticides and chemicals, cleanup of toxic sites,

Box 11.6 *(continued)*

- Instant electronic media are relaying live photographs of disasters throughout in the world, of every size or type.
- Disaster relief groups unconcerned with an integrated emergency management system are mushrooming in number and size.
- The environment, including human habitat, is suffering from deforestation, wetland loss, and soil and beach erosion.
- Resources in sensitive areas continue to be overexploited.
- New areas where hazardous chemicals have been stored are being identified, and there continue to be known areas requiring long-term cleanup.
- Home and business owners and insurance companies are engaging in protracted disputes and settlement of problems following disasters.

and the growing awareness of the implications of deforestation and climate change.

Domestically and internationally, disaster relief and humanitarian organizations face an increasing challenge to learn to coordinate efforts with national governments, international institutions such as the UN, and military forces. People affected by disaster or migration may also fall under the interest or jurisdiction of an agency of the government (such as immigrants or victims of a terrorist bombing) or of industry (owners and employees affected in disasters involving transportation carriers in mass casualty incidents or with factories and chemical plants in hazardous materials accidents, fires, or floods).

Disasters will continue to occur with regularity. Preparedness can be emphasized; early warning measures can save lives; mitigation measures can be taken; and the response to emergencies can always improve in speed and efficiency. The length of time it takes for the full recovery of the community depends on the extent and quality of coordination that occurs between all individuals and agencies during each phase of disaster response. The willingness to coordinate and the flexibility of all responding agencies will be a key to successful management of disasters and humanitarian crises in the future.

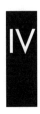

THE ROLE OF THE MILITARY

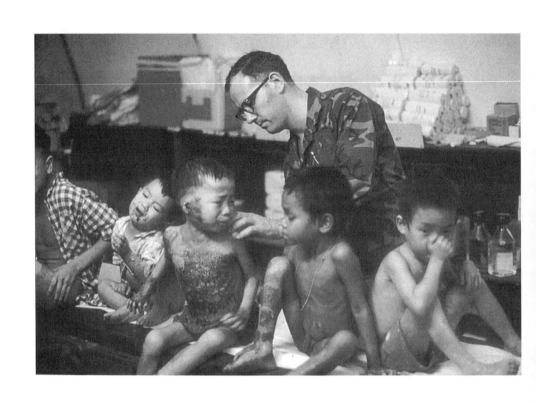

12

MILITARY SUPPORT OF RELIEF:
A CAUTIONARY REVIEW

trueman w. sharp

george a. luz

joel c. gaydos

Armed confrontation can cause tremendous devastation and destruction. War is the ultimate man-made disaster. To fight wars, military forces must be able to function in austere and devastated areas and must meet their own requirements for security, food, shelter, medical care, waste disposal, transportation, and communications. The capabilities military forces possess to provide these basic human needs to troops on the battlefield can also be used to help civilian populations cope with the adverse consequences of war and other disasters.

The use of military forces in emergency relief work has often been considered controversial. Debate has typically focused on a number of practical, political, and ethical issues.[1-10] In the post–cold war era, as the world has experienced a marked increase in armed conflict and humanitarian crises, a perceived need for external armed forces to provide security as well as emergency logistic support in highly volatile settings has led to even more controversial military assignments.[11] The following discussion undertakes a review of military capabilities for emergency disaster relief and an evaluation of critical issues and problems associated with using military forces to support this work.

HISTORICAL BACKGROUND

The expectation that military forces should provide emergency assistance to civilian populations has existed from the earliest days of organized armies.[1,12,13] The earliest recorded use of military forces for humanitarian assistance work predates Alexander the Great.[3] The commanders of many early armies viewed civilian assistance as a humane gesture to the vanquished as well as a way of winning loyalty to the conquerors.

The U.S. military and the militaries of many other nations have long traditions of providing aid to persons in distress after human-caused and natural disasters, both at home and abroad.[1] Military-civilian interactions to deal with the consequences of war for civilians first occurred in the American military during the Revolutionary War. Through the 1800s, Army physicians assigned to frontier posts were often the only medical practitioners available for great distances, and they typically addressed medical crises among Indians, hunters, lumbermen, trappers, settlers, and soldiers.[7] After the U.S. Civil War ended in 1865, the Bureau of Refugees, Freedmen, and Abandoned Lands (known as the Freedmen's Bureau) was developed to help former slaves make the transition to freedom.[7] The Freedmen's Bureau, which used Army resources extensively, provided emergency assistance, including flood and famine relief, to civilians in need throughout the South, regardless of race.

Use of the U.S. military to control and assist displaced people, refugees, and others affected by war became a critical issue in World War II.[12] The worldwide scope of this conflict and the enormous destruction caused by modern weapons created large populations of displaced people and refugees. Not only were these populations of humanitarian concern, but they also created significant obstacles to the conduct of the war. After the Korean War, an ambitious plan, Armed Forces Assistance to Korea (AFAK), used the U.S. military to assist indigenous persons with recovery efforts.[2] This experience led many politicians to believe that military forces could be used successfully in all sorts of humanitarian efforts to "win the hearts and minds" of people around the world. President John F. Kennedy declared, "The new generation of military leaders has shown an increasing awareness that armies cannot only defend their countries—they can help to build them."[2]

U.S. military forces were used extensively in the Vietnam conflict to provide emergency services to displaced persons and refugees, and in a wide variety of assistance and development programs.[6] The reasons for humanitarian assistance by military forces in Vietnam are summarized by the historian Jeffrey Greenhut:

[These programs] were reactions to U.S. domestic political pressures, they helped keep bored, underutilized medical personnel busy, and they fed the American desire to provide humanitarian assistance to peoples not as fortunate as themselves. Indeed, it is difficult to determine which reasons were paramount. . . . It must be kept in mind that the primary purpose of all the programs was to assist in winning the "hearts and minds" of the population and, in this, no reliable measure of effectiveness exists. . . . Perhaps the best that can be said is that the programs did no harm and at least some good.[6]

Humanitarian work is not unique to the U.S. military. In France, the experience of decades of military medical assistance has led to the recent development of a rapid deployment force for humanitarian assistance, the Force d'Assistance Humanitaire d'Intervention Rapide (FAHMIR).[14] The formal preparation of Swiss physicians for mass casualty management and disaster training was first started in that country's army more than fifteen years ago and continues to the present.[15] Canada has a long tradition of using its military for humanitarian missions. The militaries of many other nations have also been extensively involved in humanitarian assistance.

MILITARIES AND COMPLEX EMERGENCIES TODAY

Since the Vietnam conflict, the number of armed conflicts in the world has increased dramatically[16] and the fundamental nature of conflict has also considerably evolved.[17,18] The destructive power of weapons has increased, as has their availability. In addition to other social, political, and economic factors, armed conflict has become a predominant underlying cause of humanitarian crises today. War was a principal aspect of almost every one of the complex emergencies that affected twenty-five countries in 1994.[19]

In some crises, such as those in Kurdistan, Somalia, Rwanda, Haiti, and Bosnia, the international community, principally through the UN, has attempted to use external military forces to impose enough security and order to control the fighting and to allow relief to reach civilian victims. In recent years, peacekeeping, peacemaking, and humanitarian interventions have involved more than 750,000 soldiers, have cost more than $12 billion dollars, and have resulted in 1,200 deaths among participating soldiers. In addition to furthering humanitarian interests, militaries have been used in an effort to preserve regional peace and stability.[20]

The value of using military forces to support relief efforts, when linked to a security function, is increasingly questioned. Some challenge the preparedness of armed forces—whose main purpose is to conduct military operations—to accomplish relief activities,[3,4,5,10] whereas others have a contrary view.[9] Problems with armed soldiers projecting the "mantle of neutrality" can undermine relief or assistance efforts.[3,8] Many observers within and outside the armed forces have questioned whether it is appropriate, or even ethical, for military forces to undertake humanitarian missions, particularly as these efforts compete for increasingly limited resources such as money and training time.

MILITARY CAPABILITIES IN DISASTER RELIEF

Military forces are generally not well trained or equipped to cope with the consequences of humanitarian crises or other disasters. Military forces have many capabilities, some of them unique, that can support or strengthen a disaster relief operation. These attributes provide the basis for arguments to include the military in emergency circumstances that require response in inaccessible terrains, to large numbers of people, under insecure conditions (Box 12.1).

Security

In some complex emergencies today, effective relief is difficult or impossible because of ongoing fighting, banditry, or even anarchy. Military forces have the capability to impose sufficient security for relief efforts to proceed. Establishment of a "safe haven" during the Kurdish refugee crisis in northern Iraq enabled humanitarian relief efforts to proceed safely and encouraged the vast majority of displaced Kurds to return home.[21,22] In Somalia, the protection of relief supplies and maintenance of a credible armed presence substantially reduced the threat of violence.[8,9] One could argue that effective relief efforts were not possible in either situation without armed intervention.

TRUEMAN W. SHARP, GEORGE A. LUZ, AND JOEL C. GAYDOS

Box 12.1 Disaster capabilities of military forces

SECURITY	• Establishment of "safe havens"
	• Protection of relief supplies
	• Maintenance of a credible armed presence to reduce threat of violence
TRANSPORTATION AND LOGISTICS	• Capacity to transport personnel and supplies rapidly
	• Manage ongoing supply of equipment and materials
CONSTRUCTION AND REPAIR	• Build or repair essential infrastructure
COMMAND, CONTROL AND COMMUNICATIONS	• Sophisticated communications systems
	• Military commanders accustomed to rapid and complex contingency planning
	• Central planning and direction capabilities
	• Basic organizational and communications framework for relief organizations
DEPLOYABLE MEDICAL CARE	• Rapidly deployable medical teams, hospitals, ships, and medical evacuation systems
PREVENTIVE MEDICINE TEAMS	• Specialized teams for basic disease prevention and control
	• Sophisticated infectious disease field laboratories
	• Field water purification units

(continued)

Transportation and Logistics

Effective disaster response often hinges on being able to move people and materials rapidly into disaster-affected areas. U.S. armed forces have traditionally had a unique capacity to transport personnel and supplies rapidly to and within distant and devastated locations. Furthermore, military logistical systems, the backbone of a combat operation, can be used not only to move items but also to manage an ongoing supply of equipment and materials effectively.

In response to a typhoon in Bangladesh in 1991, military cargo planes, heavy-lift helicopters, and air-cushion landing craft rapidly transported relief workers and thousands of tons of food, medicine, and building materials into devastated areas that were otherwise inaccessible.[10,23,24] In Somalia, where few serviceable vehicles were available, the military not only provided trucks but also organized and protected convoys from the airport and seaport in Mogadishu to relief operations throughout much of the interior, enabling thousands of tons of essential relief supplies to be distributed. The U.S. military also operated the air- and seaports.[4,5,21,22]

Construction and Repair

Military engineering and construction teams, such as Navy Mobile Construction Battalions (the "Seabees"), can rapidly build or repair essential infrastructure in hostile or devastated environments. In Somalia, which had endured months of rampant destruction, military units restored the seaport, airport, main roads, and key buildings in and around the capital city. Engineering units rebuilt many of the country's main highways from Mogadishu into the interior. Military teams also repaired schools, medical clinics, water sources, and power supplies.[4,5,21,22] In Rwanda, military teams refurbished and developed key airfields and roads. In Kurdistan, Bangladesh, and Rwanda, many other critical construction and repair operations were conducted by military teams.

Command, Control, and Communications

Many observers have described the confusion and lack of coordination that often plagues disaster response efforts.[25,26] Military forces have the advantage of a clearly defined organizational structure with extensive, sophisticated communications systems. Furthermore, military commanders are accustomed to rapid and complex contingency planning. The "task organization" concept, which is familiar to the military, allows diverse units to be assembled rapidly under a unified command to work toward common goals.

Because of questions of national sovereignty and a lack of field response capability on the part of the UN, military forces became the de facto coordinating relief agency in northern Iraq during the Kurdish relief crisis.[21] This military agency facilitated central planning and direction of a medical care system, preventive medicine programs, supply distribution, and other essential relief activities. Military command and control in this situation enabled the unprecedented movement of almost half a million Kurds back to their homes over a two-week period with minimal excess morbidity and mortality (which often accompany such movements of people). In other disasters, such as in Somalia and Bangladesh, the military helped provide a basic organizational and communications framework under which many relief organizations were able to operate more cohesively and effectively.

Deployable Medical Care

In order to provide care to soldiers in combat operations, the U.S. military has a wide array of medical teams, hospitals, ships, and medical evacuation systems designed to deploy rapidly and to provide medical care in the most adverse circumstances. When used appropriately, these assets can contribute substantially to medical relief efforts.[1,4,5] For example, the U.S. Navy maintains two hospital ships that could be used for disaster relief.[27,28] High-level trauma care and medical evacuation, which are particular strengths of military medicine, can be critical after earthquakes or in situations that involve armed confrontation.

Military medical teams in northern Iraq and in Bangladesh supplemented relief agencies by treating thousands of disaster victims under field conditions. Evidence suggests that military medical care saved many lives.[22] In addition to treating the indigenous population, field and shipboard medical personnel in Somalia provided emergency care to relief workers and journalists with injuries and acute illnesses who otherwise had no access to medical services.[29,30]

Preventive Medicine Teams

Disasters may result in the loss or destruction of the public health infrastructure, which can lead to outbreaks of preventable diseases. Military medicine has specialized teams for basic disease prevention and control in austere overseas environments.

Preventive medicine teams in northern Iraq and Bangladesh performed critical rapid assessment surveys, conducted disease surveillance, provided insect control, investigated disease outbreaks, and addressed the issues of potable water and sanitation.[21,22,24] Sophisticated infectious disease field laboratories, similar to the one deployed during the Persian Gulf War,[31] were used in Bangladesh and Somalia to determine the causes of fever and diarrhea among displaced persons and to identify which antibiotics would be most effective.[29,30,32] In Goma, Zaire, the U.S. military utilized its field water purification units to produce and transport potable water to refugees.

Specialized Units

Elite units such as the U.S. Army Special Forces (USASF) have extensive training in foreign languages and intercultural interaction. Their specialized skills and diverse capabilities make them well suited in many respects to assist with emergency disaster relief. For example, special forces teams in northern Iraq quickly established important working relationships with Kurdish military and civilian leaders prior to the start of ground-based relief efforts. This work was essential for establishing security, for assessing relief requirements, and for ensuring that emergency supplies were distributed effectively in a dangerous and chaotic situation.[4,5,21]

The military field of civil affairs was developed in World War II to deal with the language, history, government, customs, and public health of occupied areas.[12] Present-day U.S. civil affairs units are almost all Army reservists and are built upon the tradition established in World War II. They provide an interface between the military and civilian populations, but they also have a wide variety of specialized skills. These units contain experts from many different areas—transportation, business, law, communications, international health, police, and many others. Civil affairs teams managed the mass relocation of Kurds out of the mountains and the construction and management of state-of-the-art resettlement camps in northern Iraq. Civil affairs units in Somalia conducted mass information campaigns for the Somali people, daily briefings for the press, and coordination with multiple relief organizations. Some argue that civil affairs units have the potential to be, and should be, the centerpiece of military disaster response.

Even infantry units and other military units with no special training can be valuable in disasters. Troops are generally an excellent source of organized and reliable manpower. Members of the National Guard are called upon routinely in U.S. domestic disasters to assist in basic tasks such as evacuation, flood control, and transportation. Active duty combat units with a few days of training have effectively relieved exhausted fire fighters in Nevada and the Pacific Northwest.[33]

Technological Disasters

The military has unique capabilities to assist in responses to chemical, biological, or nuclear incidents, which are all primary concerns in war. For example, the military has specialized units, such as the U.S. Army Institute for Chemical Defense at Aberdeen Proving Ground, Maryland, for researching and protecting against chemical warfare agents. After the sarin gas release in the Tokyo subway in 1995, the U.S. military was asked to advise local medical providers on the treatment of casualties.

Similarly, the military has a network of laboratories in the United States and overseas devoted to the study of infectious diseases of concern in military operations. These include common, naturally occurring diseases such as diarrhea and malaria, more exotic infectious diseases such as the Ebola virus, and diseases such as anthrax that are primarily of concern as biological weapons. Many of these laboratories have long, distinguished traditions of work in tropical diseases.[34] Their unique capabilities and expertise could be invaluable in disaster situations. For example, teams from the U.S. Army Medical Research Institute for Infectious Diseases in Fort Detrick, Maryland, have been extensively involved in responding to the Ebola virus outbreaks.

Disaster Preparedness

Military forces routinely conduct missions around the world to construct wells, to build medical clinics, to provide medical and dental care, to conduct immunization programs, and to supply veterinary services.[35] Sometimes these missions focus on emergency medical services and disaster preparedness. Under the MEDFLAG program, for example, U.S. military medical units based in Europe are sent for two- to three-week periods to work with civilian and military organizations in African nations. The principal focus is on training and preparedness for disasters such as plane crashes or other mass casualty situations.[1]

MAJOR ISSUES AND PROBLEMS IN DEPLOYING MILITARY FORCES FOR DISASTER RELIEF

Despite the many technical and organizational strengths the military can bring to disaster relief efforts, military forces have significant limitations in meeting many of the needs of disaster victims (Box 12.2). These limitations arise largely because the primary mission of armed forces is to fight wars, not to provide disaster assistance.[36] An institution designed and built for one objective is not well suited, in many ways outlined here, to take on another that is very different.

Box 12.2 Potential mismatches between military and
humanitarian missions

MEDICAL CARE	• Military medicine designed to stabilize young adults wounded in battle; not suited for disasters and humanitarian crises where measles, diarrhea, respiratory infections, and malaria are most common causes of death, especially among young children and women
	• Minimal quantities of medications recommended by relief agencies for disaster-affected populations
	• Little training in dealing with medical problems typical of complex emergencies (for example, epidemic diarrhea or starvation, tropical diseases)
	• Minimal quantities of vaccine taken on deployments; little experience managing large immunization campaigns among displaced persons
	• Limited transportation and communications capabilities for preventive medicine personnel
CONFLICT RESOLUTION	• Military not well suited to mobilize indigenous resources and to assist in long-term redevelopment efforts
	• Temporary imposition of security by outside militaries may impede negotiation and conflict resolution
NONMEDICAL SUPPLIES	• Supplies readily available to military forces may be inappropriate for refugees and disaster victims

(continued)

Box 12.2 *(continued)*

INTERACTIONS WITH OTHER ORGANIZATIONS	• Military commanders unfamiliar with different roles of major international organizations
	• Civilian relief personnel have minimal experience with hierarchical military structure
	• Differences in strategies, objectives, and tactics between military and civilian organizations
CONFLICT WITH HUMANITARIAN AGENDA	• Inherent tension in using military force to achieve humanitarian goals
	• Military presence can undermine appearance of neutrality of relief organizations
INADEQUATE TRAINING	• Few military officers have received training in disaster relief or humanitarian assistance
	• Military medical providers constrained by lack of training in the languages, customs, and medical practices of other populations
	• Ambiguities over role of military physicians in complex emergencies under international humanitarian law
LIMITED COMMITMENT TO DISASTER RESPONSE	• Principal mission of military is to fight and win war; no U.S. units whose primary job is disaster response
	• Little planning and few resources devoted to disaster relief

Potential Medical Care Mismatch

Disasters often present medical and public health problems that military medicine is not well prepared to handle. For example, measles, diarrhea, acute upper respiratory infections, and malaria are the most common causes of death among refugees and displaced persons.[37,38] These diseases are typically exacerbated by nutritional shortages and chronic underlying infections. Moreover, rates of illness and death in refugee situations are disproportionately high among young children and women. U.S. military medicine, however, is designed to provide emergency stabilization to young adults wounded in battle. Other acute care capabilities are limited and tend to focus on those medical problems usually found in young, healthy (and usually male) adults. Ill or injured troops who cannot be treated definitively and promptly returned to duty are evacuated.

Because of this mismatch, military medical units attempting to provide medical care after disasters have minimal quantities of the medications and supplies recommended by relief agencies for disaster-affected populations, such as oral rehydration salts, basic antibiotics, and pediatric supplies. In addition, few military health care providers have training in the unique demands of dealing with epidemic diarrhea or starvation, in diagnosing and treating tropical diseases, or in understanding the chronic medical problems and ethnic and cultural values of foreign, indigenous people.

Many of these limitations were evident in the Kurdish refugee crisis.[4,5,21,22] Early in the relief effort, children with diarrheal disease, dehydration, and malnutrition accounted for more than 75 percent of all deaths, which were occurring at greater than ten times the normal rate for this population.[21,22] Military medical personnel experienced great difficulty caring for children at the trauma-oriented field clinics and hospitals that were initially established. Critical supplies, such as oral rehydration salts, were unavailable for the first few weeks. Furthermore, medical teams were not prepared to establish the community-based oral rehydration and emergency feeding programs that could have identified and cared for many of these children. As the operation progressed past the emergency phase, medical teams became frustrated by their inability to deal with many of the endemic conditions for which survivors sought care.

Military preventive medicine teams can have substantial constraints. Preventive medicine and supply systems are geared to support a fighting force at war and have only a limited amount of flexibility to accommodate deviations from this narrow mission. Immunizations, for example, are usually administered to military personnel prior to deployment. Thus the military normally takes minimal quantities of vaccine on deployments and these are usually not for children. Few in the military have experience with managing large immunization campaigns among displaced persons or with developing the emergency sanitation and water systems needed by large disaster-affected populations. Military preventive medicine personnel typically have limited transportation and communications capabilities.

In northern Iraq, delays occurred in obtaining measles vaccine even after vaccination programs were identified as a high priority. Few trained personnel were available to improve water and sanitation despite the abysmal conditions, and those on site lacked appropriate equipment.[4,5,21,22]

Limited Focus on Redevelopment and Conflict Resolution

The critical link between emergency disaster relief and long-term redevelopment is increasingly appreciated.[39,40] For many relief organizations, restoring and developing indigenous capabilities in the affected population is an established priority in the emergency phase of relief operations. According to the UN High Commissioner for Refugees, the purpose of emergency humanitarian assistance is to "sustain dignified life, strengthen [the] local institution's efforts to relieve suffering and building self-reliance, and to assure that the first step is taken towards reconstruction, rehabilitation and development."[41]

A principle of military involvement in disaster relief, however, is to be engaged for a short time, mainly during the emergency phase, and then to transfer relief efforts to others. Most military units, with the exception of civil affairs and special forces units, are not well suited to mobilize indigenous resources and to assist in long-term redevelopment efforts. While a short-term focus is not necessarily a drawback, it can be detrimental if the mission requires a more lasting commitment or an effective transition to other relief groups who will be involved for a longer time. The importance of an early dialogue with the local community and starting sustainable development can easily be overlooked by military commanders. In addition, U.S. military medical practice is based on current standards of health care in the United States. Military health care providers may thus rely on interventions and practices that are beyond the capability of local populations.

Local physicians in northern Iraq warned that a high-technology-based medical response was undermining local physicians and was delaying the Kurds from implementing their own solutions to the crisis. With few exceptions, well-trained indigenous physicians and nurses in northern Iraq, who were familiar with their own people and their health problems, were not brought into relief efforts as an initial step in reestablishing the local health care system.[4,5]

Furthermore, the temporary imposition of security by outside militaries may not advance and, indeed, may impede progress toward negotiation and conflict resolution. In Somalia, for example, containing violence through the use of external force was not by itself enough to cause the warring factions to want to negotiate toward a peaceful settlement.

Inappropriate Nonmedical Supplies

Donated or conveniently available emergency humanitarian supplies have often been troublesome in international relief efforts.[42,43] One problem has been that these supplies are often inappropriate for the needs of the disaster victims. Similarly, the supplies that military forces have readily available may not be those most needed by refugees and disaster victims and may even cause unintended detrimental results. For example, "Meals, Ready to Eat" (MREs), the basic military field ration, may be inappropriate for nonmilitary populations. Even starving people prefer food they know and often will not eat MREs. Many MREs contain pork products, making them unacceptable to some. Most important, MREs are very high calorie meals with a high concentration of salt; providing them to dehydrated or malnourished persons, particularly children, is potentially dangerous.[44] MREs also generate an enormous volume of trash. Places where they have been used by nonmilitary populations rapidly become strewn with MRE debris.

The U.S. armed forces do not have readily available supplies of oil, flour, rice, and other basic commodities recommended by relief agencies for emergency food relief abroad. To the uniformed planner or to a politician, the use of military food rations, military medicines, and other military items such as tents may seem appropriate and expeditious. Not only may the use of these items be inappropriate, but they also may be substantially more expensive than the items recommended by relief agencies.

Interactions with Other Organizations

Emergency relief is provided most effectively when strategies and objectives are coordinated among all participating organizations.[11,25,26,45] The myriad organizations involved in almost every major relief effort—each with its own mission and agenda—makes such coordination extremely difficult. During humanitarian crises, military forces must work closely with civilian relief agencies and with the militaries of other nations, often under the umbrella of the North Atlantic Treaty Organization (NATO) or the UN. In Somalia, for example, French, Belgian, Canadian, Botswanan, and U.S. troops worked together with relief agencies under the UN to distribute posters, coloring books, and handbills advising Somalis to be aware of land-mine hazards.[46]

Military involvement adds additional levels of complexity. Few military commanders, line or medical, understand the different roles of major international organizations such as Médecins sans Frontières or the International Committee of the Red Cross. Similarly, many civilian relief personnel have minimal experience with the hierarchical and complex structure of the military. There may be major differences in strategies, objectives, and tactics between military and civilian organizations.[45] Simply learning how to interact with each other is a formidable task.[47]

In northern Iraq, poor relations between civilian and military groups contributed to confusion over command and control, to lack of direction of relief activities, to delayed implementation of high priority oral rehydration and measles vaccine campaigns, and to delayed transfer of medical care operations to relief organizations as military forces withdrew. These relations were also problematic in Somalia and Rwanda.[4,5]

Militaries from different nations—indeed sometimes the different services within the military of one country—also may have very different cultures. Under a UN or NATO coalition command there can be substantial differences in approaches toward humanitarian assistance among the different military forces. In northern Iraq, for example, while military commanders from some nations argued for a primary care orientation in their emergency medical services for displaced persons, others favored bringing in large tertiary care field hospitals. In Somalia, the militaries from some nations became much more involved in providing direct medical care and other humanitarian services than those provided by other nations, who thought such direct care was inappropriate. Within a coalition force, military commanders must still answer to commanders and civilian leaders of their own country. Coalition military forces are sometimes loosely tied together and each may pursue somewhat different strategies, goals, and objectives.

Conflicts with a Humanitarian Agenda

The provision of humanitarian relief can easily be perceived as a partisan or political act. Relief efforts can be overtly manipulated for the benefit of different warring factions.[48,49,50] Many humanitarian organizations presently struggle with the challenge of operating as impartial and neutral entities in times of conflict, particularly in situations where there are "predator" states or seemingly amoral warlords (see Chapter 14). Military intervention may serve to exacerbate or prolong the conflict by supporting some factions over others.

Whereas most international relief organizations have the mandate to be neutral and nonpartisan, U.S. military forces are directed by government policy. The military and relief organizations cooperating with them are thus easily perceived by warring factions and disaster victims as having other than solely humanitarian interests. This perception may result in adversarial relationships that interfere with both the military's and the relief organizations' ability to provide humanitarian assistance.

In the former Yugoslavia, for example, relief supplies were often viewed as aid for enemy forces, and relief organizations were often viewed as part of a highly partisan UN effort.[51,52] In Somalia, many relief workers were torn between reliance on the military for security and their mandate to be neutral parties. Assistance that appeared to favor one local armed faction over another sometimes resulted in hostilities against relief workers and, unfortunately, deaths. Even in Bangladesh, which was not a situation of conflict, some military relief teams found that local leaders did not want to be perceived as receiving aid from the U.S. military.[4,5]

It is extremely difficult for the military to intervene in a situation with force and subsequently to attempt to provide humanitarian relief. There is an inherent tension in using military force to achieve humanitarian goals. Indeed, some have argued that the use of the military, particularly the U.S. military, is fundamentally incompatible with, and may be detrimental to, humanitarian objectives.[48,53]

Inadequate Training

Few military officers have received training in disaster relief or humanitarian assistance.[54,55] Although this situation is improving somewhat, only limited guidance on appropriate principles and procedures is available in current operations orders, contingency plans, doctrinal publications, and training manuals. Military medical providers have been, and will probably continue to be, constrained by a lack of training in the languages, customs, and medical practices of other populations. In Kurdistan, for example, military-style latrines built to improve sanitary conditions were inappropriate for the culture and were not used.[4,5] In many disasters, military relief providers were not prepared to cope with a variety of ethical and medical-legal dilemmas that resulted from attempting to apply a highly developed health care system to a developing world population in extreme circumstances. Many ambiguities over the role of military physicians in complex emergencies exist under current international humanitarian law.

Limited Commitment to Disaster Response

Despite the language of the national military strategy, and the reality that the military is in fact often engaged in disaster relief today, the principal focus of the U.S. military is to be able to fight and win two nearly simultaneous major regional conflicts.[36,56,57] While some believe that the military should concentrate more on disaster relief, little planning and few resources are devoted to this area. Currently there are no units whose primary responsibility is disaster response, and there are few units that spend significant time preparing for this mission.

PROSPECTS FOR THE FUTURE

In the United States, the military may continue to handle disaster relief as an occasional assignment, as it has done in the past, or it may place greater emphasis on this mission. Which direction is taken will be determined by political decisions that dictate military priorities, size, and resources. The militaries of some other nations currently recognize humanitarian assistance as a higher priority.

The U.S. government and the military must resolve a number of fundamental issues relating to the role of the U.S. military in the post–cold war era (Box 12.3). One of the most important is whether the armed forces should embrace humanitarian assistance and disaster relief as principal roles and missions. If peacekeeping and humanitarian assistance are to become priorities, strategies to identify those crises that warrant military intervention must be elaborated.[58,59] Defining the roles of the military in preventing or intervening earlier in complex emergencies is also critical, as is a better understanding of how militaries can withdraw from situations in which they have imposed security from the outside without rekindling the original conflict. In addition, the military will need to address a number of

Box 12.3 Fundamental issues for the future role of the military in responding to disasters and humanitarian crises

- Role of U.S. and coalition militaries in post–cold war era: Should humanitarian assistance and disaster relief be a principal role and mission?
- How to identify those crises that warrant military intervention?
- What are roles of the military in early prevention or intervention; how can militaries withdraw without rekindling original conflict?

issues internally to determine how better to plan, to train, and to equip troops for these missions.

Whether or not disaster relief becomes a primary mission of the military, it remains a daunting challenge to ensure that when called upon, military forces are used appropriately. When military involvement in disasters is anticipated, the role of the military should be carefully delineated. The military is best suited for providing rapid transportation to remote locations, for restoring a functioning infrastructure in a devastated area, for providing armed intervention in unstable situations to establish and maintain security for relief operations, and for supplying certain initial medical care and evacuation for disaster victims. Not all military units can provide all services. Preventive medicine, civil affairs, and special forces units have a number of specialized and valuable capabilities.

The limitations of military medical care must be kept in mind; simply dispatching ill-prepared military clinics and hospitals is not the answer. Civilian relief organizations are better prepared to provide most relief services, particularly after the emergency phase when the focus shifts to redeveloping sustainable medical care and other human services. Furthermore, while the use of military force as an emergency measure to provide security in situations of conflict can save lives in the short run, it may delay difficult but critical efforts toward conflict resolution. In an extremely violent world that seems intent on creating increasingly more complex emergencies, determining the best roles for military forces will remain a formidable challenge.

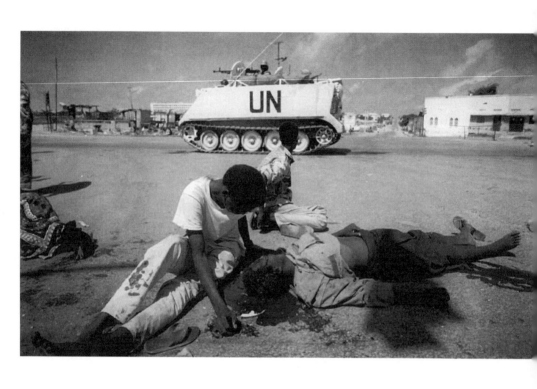

13

MILITARY SECURITY:
LESSONS FOR RELIEF

frederick m. burkle, jr.

An early humanitarian, St. Paul, questioned whether soldiers should get involved in civil affairs of any sort: "No soldier on service gets entangled in civilian pursuits, since his aim is to satisfy the one who enlisted him."[1] This
biblical passage evokes confusion in its interpretation, not unlike the current state of discomfort over the roles and responsibilities of governments
and their armies in contemporary humanitarian crises. Although armies
throughout the world have always been involved in humanitarian assistance, until recently few opportunities have existed to wage peace rather
than war. The search for meaningful responses to complex humanitarian
emergencies requires a reflection on the role of the military, especially in
peace operations where violence and security issues predominate. A brief
review of the experience of military security operations in recent crises suggests a number of problems in mandate, direction, support, and training.

SHIFTING POLITICAL VIOLENCE

Complex emergencies, in all their severity, are long-term, violence-prone
crises. Even the term "complex emergency" has drawn fire. The list of terms
used to define these events illustrates the confusion that exists over what
they actually represent. The term "complex humanitarian emergencies"

places the focus on management issues, whereas the term "complex political disaster" emphasizes that the capacity of societies to survive is primarily threatened by political factors and, in particular, by high levels of violence.

As a consequence of political violence, public infrastructure (which includes public health, transportation, communications, the judiciary, agriculture, and public safety) may be rendered inaccessible, may be made off limits to certain vulnerable populations, or may simply be damaged beyond repair. In Bosnia, 60 percent of the homes, half of the schools, and a third of the hospitals were destroyed.[2] A natural disaster, such as the Somalia drought, may create the final pathway to a complex emergency, catalyzing the migration of large populations internally or across borders. By the time the developed world becomes involved, events may have deteriorated into a catastrophic public health emergency. Cultural minorities, religions, and ethnic groups are often placed at the brink of extinction. Even if hostilities cease immediately, such events require massive international assistance. The logistical requirements for food, medicine, water, shelter, sanitation, and fuel are essential to providing a cushion of hope.

Since 1945, wars have shifted from cross-border conflicts to largely internal disputes, many of which, since the end of the cold war, have acquired the features we now ascribe to complex humanitarian emergencies. These have in recent years become more dangerous, more frequent, longer lasting, and more widespread across regions. Data from forty conflicts during the first half of 1990 enumerated 1.1 million military deaths and 5.2 million civilian deaths, the majority comprising vulnerable and repressed groups such as children, women, and ethnic minorities.[3] Complex emergencies have increasingly placed relief workers at risk from cross fire, accidents, and land mines. The ICRC suffered more than forty deaths in the mid-1990s,[4] often at the hands of warring factions who had little or no respect for either the Red Cross emblem or the sanctity of the Geneva Conventions. As requirements for humanitarian relief shift from rural areas to cities, military units are increasingly targeted in crowded marketplaces frequented by women and children. Evidence suggests that military casualty rates are statistically higher when a decisive force is absent from the scene.[5–8]

Wars within collapsing states or regions, 95 percent of all wars since 1991, are beyond the reach of intervention authorized by the UN Charter.[9,10] While the major responders to humanitarian crises are generally united by their desire to alleviate emergency conditions, they frequently differ in their motives and means to bring order out of chaos, especially where sovereignty issues exist. To categorize these events as "operations other than war," however, plays into the hands of those who have knowingly placed peacekeeping forces in environments where there is no peace to keep. Many complex emergencies can, in fact, be characterized as wars that lack only the predictable patterns known to traditional armies.

A brief overview of four recent military interventions in complex humanitarian emergencies (northern Iraq, Somalia, Bosnia, and Rwanda) demonstrates the difficulties of deploying the military in conflict situations and calling the mission one of humanitarian relief.[11] If the situation is sufficiently stable, a military-supported relief mission can remain consistently humanitarian, as in northern Iraq. In the three other situations, where hostilities were ongoing or intermittently volatile, the lack of a clear mandate and poor preparation combined to diminish or obscure the military's humanitarian contribution and highlighted the political failure to deal with the conflict.

Northern Iraq

During the 1991 intervention in northern Iraq, coalition military forces (Belgium, France, Germany, the United Kingdom, and the United States) played a major role by establishing safe havens for the Kurdish minority and by using transport aircraft and helicopters to deliver aid on behalf of UN agencies and NGOs. The coalition dealt with UN operational weakness by using a rapid-response force under a UN Security Council resolution, placing coalition forces under the command and control of a U.S. military Joint Task Force (JTF). Military forces steadfastly maintained that their role would be limited to security for humanitarian relief in the emergency phase. Approximately thirty-six NGOs required liaison and security assistance. Only resources on the scale available to the military could meet the massive logistical and security requirements of the emergency phase of this disaster.

For the first time many NGOs established mutually beneficial working relationships with the military forces. The NGOs utilized the protective transport, communication, and shelter capacities of the coalition military to carry out humanitarian assistance activities. Minear, Weiss, and Campbell claim that the success of the operation was due in part to the "basic discipline and organization injected by the military into a fluid situation, giving the NGOs a firm point of reference."[12] The humanitarian relief organizations perceived the military as an ally in their efforts to assist a persecuted minority group. With some reservations, the Kurdish refugee mission became a model of an integrated and collaborative operation.

By using coalition military forces to support the humanitarian relief operation in southern Turkey and northern Iraq, the UN Security Council set a post–cold war precedent. The Kurdish refugee crisis in many ways signified the end of the cold war, while raising expectations that the world community would be willing to share resources for a common good. A countervailing trend, however, has been the widespread proliferation and availability of weapons, which has enhanced the temptation to use violence as a strategy by disparate groups that lack conscience, discipline, or maturity. Attempts since the Kurdish mission to respond to and resolve armed violence under the umbrella of impartial international humanitarian assistance have not worked. Neither has traditional military doctrine nor deployment of force structures developed during the cold war. Predictions that the short-term emergency relief efforts employed during the Kurdish refugee crisis would become a model for future humanitarian crises soon disappeared from the discussion.

Somalia

Only a brief respite occurred before Somalia became the center of attention in 1992. Unlike the situation in northern Iraq, multiple NGOs and the ICRC had been working in Somalia for more than a decade. Their humanitarian efforts had reduced mortality rates among children under the age of five from an alarming 137 per 1,000 population down to 49 per 1,000 population in 1990.[13] With the onset of clan feuding and widespread war after the overthrow of Siad Barre in 1991, however, mortality rates from disease and starvation slipped back to an all-time high of 168 per 1,000 population in 1992.[13] The media knew this and so did the world community. The United States entered Somalia reluctantly, with a security-oriented mission statement that anticipated a rapid shift from emergency deployment to a transition phase.

Contrary to the participatory partnership and "must succeed" philosophy expressed in the Kurdish crisis, in Somalia the military proceeded with a security mission in support of a political agenda. Critics of this venture say that Somalia showed how the "traditional military doctrine . . . of overwhelming force, identifying the enemy, and secrecy, can mix badly with traditional UN peacekeeping and NGO mandates" for impartiality and dissemination of information.[14] The European Community Humanitarian Office would later comment that military humanitarian efforts were perceived as bypassing humanitarian activities already in place. This approach, the office stated, "tended to ignore entirely institution building that is critical to successful relief."[15] With improved security, however, the mortality rates for children under the age of five declined significantly, and amputee rates from war casualties and land-mine injuries dropped from 3–4 per day to 1 per month.

These results were little comfort to those who saw bad omens in military involvement that seemed merely to strengthen the resolve of the conflicting parties. The military presence blurred the distinction between civilians and military expatriates, now considered a homogeneous group at equal risk of being targeted by warring factions. Somalia exposed a widening gap between soldiers and relief workers that would persist into the future.

The UN structure was not prepared to assume responsibilities for the peacekeeping mission when it was transferred from U.S. military command to UNOSOM II. Political reconciliation in Somalia was insufficiently advanced. The transition plan was poorly defined, and the UN forces lacked command and control mechanisms. In the rush of events, UN personnel were unfamiliar with and untrained in security and operational requirements. The United States, the only power capable of projecting a force that could contain the belligerents, was accused of leaving too early. After Somalia, the United States became linked not only with UN successes but also with its failures.

Rwanda

Many indications existed in Rwanda that the 1994 slaughter would occur. Appeals from UN agencies and NGOs in Rwanda had fallen on deaf ears at public agencies and foreign governments for the preceding four years. For three years international arms sales had increased to the military regime and to the rebel Rwandan Patriotic Front (RPF).[16,17] When the genocide began the only non-UN relief organizations capable of caring for wounded in the region were the ICRC and Médecins sans Frontières. The humanitarian nightmare took place in the absence of an international military force to contain it. Despite the early entry of the RPF, 500,000 to 800,000 Rwandans, primarily Tutsi, died in the first three months of the genocide.

The Rwandan experience revealed, again, that UN forces were not operationally equipped to respond to such emergencies. At the outbreak of the killings, on April 6, 1994, the UN Security Council members had divergent views on whether to augment the small peacekeeping force that was there or to pull out. The initial decision was made to scale back just as the genocide was mounting. Under existing UN law the multilayered process leading from a request for intervention to implementation takes a minimum of three to four months.[16] On May 17, 1994, 41 days after the beginning of the massacre, the UN Security Council approved deployment of 5,500 troops for Rwanda.[16] No UN member states made firm offers of troops. On June 23, a small interim French force, sent by authorities critical of continuing delays and initially unauthorized by the UN, arrived to protect civilians and stop the killings. Reconnaissance photos from this French effort, "Operation Turquoise," warned early in July 1994 that more than one million people had fled to the Zairean border.[16,18] Near the border town of Goma that unfed population waited one week for food. Finally a UN force relieved the French on August 22, 137 days after the massacre began. Even then, no consensus existed among the Security Council members on where or how to use UN troops to protect widely scattered pockets of refugees. As a result, in this early period there were no guards to protect the refugee camps from security threats.

Just before the massacre occurred, the U.S. Presidential Decision Directive (PDD) on Reforming Multilateral Peace Operations was being circulated for approval. This directive defined intervention in terms of a clear purpose and achievable objectives, with costs and risks commensurate with the U.S. national interests at stake.[19] Clearly, the United States was not intending to provide the military presence in Rwanda that many thought necessary. Multiple forces, including some from the United States, eventually provided logistics support, medical care, and water. These forces were openly criticized by the NGOs for "not keeping the peace, policing, disarming, and isolating the militias and the exiled Rwandan Army."[20] NGOs critical of the military presence in Somalia were now critical of the lack of a large and effective force in Rwanda.

Bosnia

Critics have said that the United Nations Protection Force (UNPROFOR) did not live up to its name.[21] From the outset UN forces in Bosnia were handcuffed by an ambiguous mission statement and equally ambiguous rules of engagement. The UN Security Council granted all necessary measures for delivering aid,[22] yet did not include "force" in those measures. UNPROFOR was doomed to take a middle road between inaction and imposition. Only once were weapons actually used to real effect. Without a strong presence on the ground "the mission ended as it had lived—in confusion, ineptness, injured pride and impotence."[21] As in Somalia and Rwanda, UN peacekeeping officials bitterly opposed going into Bosnia because, as they rightly pointed out, there was no peace to keep.

The NGOs, now numbering almost two hundred, had their own dilemma. Feeling powerless, frustrated, and plagued with attacks against staff and volunteers, many relief workers found it increasingly difficult, if not impossible, to maintain a humanitarian stance of neutrality. Some NGOs came into open conflict with UNPROFOR and rejected impartiality in favor of solidarity with ethnic and vulnerable groups.[23,24]

The Intervention Force (IFOR) has had only partial success in removing indicted war criminals from the political scene. A fatal flaw in the conditions placed on military forces in Bosnia was that they could not pursue indicted war criminals; arrests could only occur if criminals were found in the normal process of daily routine. Research into post-conflict recovery supports the view that, in reality, without criminal proceedings and the enforcement of human rights and justice, prospects for a lasting peace become doubtful.

THE SEARCH FOR COMMON GROUND

The major participants in humanitarian crises are strange bedfellows indeed, and they are not immune to sectarianism. Each participant—whether a UN agency, an NGO, or the military—brings unique and critical management tools to the relief response. Cooperation and coordination among participants have recently improved. Much need for skilled leadership remains, however, primarily to offset three problems:

- distrust brought on by overlapping organizational mandates;
- lack of experience working together;
- competition for scarce resources.

Coordination is often plagued by each institution's ignorance of the other's characteristics, capabilities, and limitations.

Overlapping Mandates

Both the Kurdish crisis and the Somalia experience confirmed that a U.S.-led military coalition can rapidly field an operational force that is trained and equipped to care for itself. Such a force has extraordinary capabilities to provide relief logistics, to facilitate communications, to maintain vital infrastructure, and to deliver emergency medical services and high-priority supplies (for example, cold-chain-dependent measles vaccine). As viewed by many NGOs, the technical humanitarian roles for the military include:

- conducting airlifts;
- bringing order out of chaos;
- removing mines;
- repairing infrastructure;
- conducting intelligence briefings;
- providing transportation;
- ensuring security;
- distributing aid in active war settings.

Unfortunately, after 1992 tensions grew between NGOs and military institutions. On a cultural level NGOs were more ambivalent about accepting the military as allies or partners. The emergency phase "sledgehammer" approach of the military, effective in the Kurdish crisis, was considered "insensitive" in Somalia. Fragile but workable relationships between warring factions and NGOs often failed because of the perceived association between the NGOs and the military. A basic mismatch of cultures and political views fueled disputes over turf, image, and motives. The military was increasingly seen as the expression of uninformed political decisions that were "hierarchial, bureaucratic, cautious and uncommitted."[24] NGOs, in contrast, were acknowledged risk takers, represented the unreachables, and were present regardless of politics. In reality, military leaders seasoned in humanitarian operations shared the frustration of a disconnection in the field between what the military actually does (under the constraints of its mission statement) and what it needs to do (Figure 13.1).

The sectarian atmosphere within the NGOs can compound the dilemma. MSF founder Bernard Kouchner describes "wars [between philanthropists] as the worst of all . . . quarrelling among themselves for control of the victims of disasters and [they] fight to the death amongst themselves after having risked their lives together."[25] The military, often confused by this behavior, sees itself as an unwilling, convenient, and common scapegoat. Warring factions take advantage of any real or perceived animosities among military institutions and NGOs to provoke conflict; they build on inherent weaknesses and differences in order to take the media pressure off themselves.

Lack of Experience in Working Together

The manner in which the major participants communicate within their organizations and with one another contributes to failures in coordination. Military structure requires three levels of authority: strategic, operational, and tactical (field). The ICRC maintains similar lines of command, control, and communication. The UN and NGOs generally do not have an operational level, although the UN has since 1993 taken several steps toward establishing such a level of operational coordination for UN agencies. Some NGOs (for example, CARE and Save the Children–UK) have also developed operational sector levels (Figure 13.2).

Mutually understood levels of authority and communication are critical, especially in a hostile and fluid environment. NGO headquarters staffs, often considered the "operational" level during complex emergencies, are preoccupied with donors and recruitment and are geographically too far removed from most crisis situations. By long-standing tradition, field decisions about relief programs are left to dedicated but frequently untrained young adult relief workers, who face increased risk as a result. Because of these differences in organizational structure and communications, military decisions about security and other critical matters may not reach all relief workers in a timely manner.

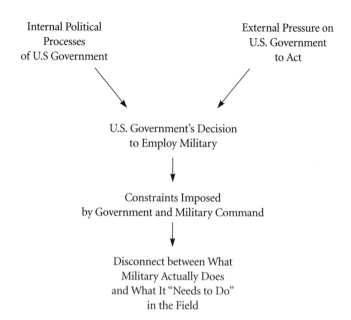

Internal Political
Processes
of U.S Government

External Pressure on
U.S. Government
to Act

U.S. Government's Decision
to Employ Military

Constraints Imposed
by Government and Military Command

Disconnect between What
Military Actually Does
and What It "Needs to Do"
in the Field

Figure 13.1 Asymmetry between mission statement and field requirements. (Adapted from work performed at Roundtable Conference on military involvement in humanitarian assistance operations, Center for Naval Analyses, Alexandria, Va., May 15, 1996)

An evolving model for linking military and civilian cooperation is the On-Site Operations Coordination Center (OSOCC) funded by Sweden and first developed by the UN Department of Humanitarian Affairs, now the Office of the Coordinator for Humanitarian Assistance, with authority to coordinate with UN and emergency management agencies in the former Yugoslavia.[26] OSOCC also provides an integrated, neutral, and ongoing forum for communications and coordination with relief agencies. OSOCC authority is derived from both the UN and the affected state. (The model for this initiative is the Civil-Military Operations Center, or CMOC, popularized in Somalia, which became both a place and a concept for daily field coordination between military forces and NGOs.)[27] A Civil-Military Operations Coordination Center (CMOCC), not a CMOC per se, was deployed by IFOR in Bosnia. The CMOCC in Bosnia has provided critical liaison with the OSOCC and further demonstrates that what began as a strict military model can now be seconded by the partners it was supposed to support. These experiences have demonstrated that some form of an opera-

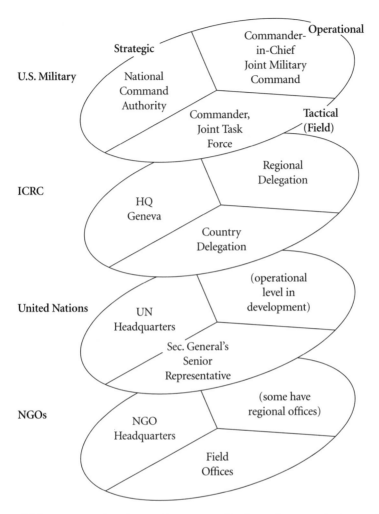

Figure 13.2 To ensure the safe, unambiguous coordination and communication required in operations to address complex emergencies, the UN and NGOs must establish clearly defined levels of authority that include the operational level.

tions center, possibly designated by the lead agency in the planning phase, is a necessity during response to a complex emergency.

Measures of Effectiveness (MOEs) were developed during a joint military and NGO humanitarian operations exercise in 1994[28] as a management tool to bring together organizations that need to support one another.

MOEs provide a common language and define priorities for humanitarian and peace operations. They help minimize confusion and risk to field workers by requiring that each organization know what the other is doing and why. By using measurable criteria to which all participants agree, trend analyses (for example, improved mortality rates), not fixed events, help determine areas of need and better define the appropriate military end states. To be effective, however, MOEs must be planned for, developed, and universally accepted by the major participants. The lack of MOEs was considered a major UNPROFOR weakness. Utilized in Haiti,[28] the concept has had little or no support in the IFOR-UNHCR organizational structure in the former Yugoslavia. When MOEs are utilized effectively, the fear of mission creep is replaced, in part, by an acceptance that "mission shifts" are expected and can often represent healthy opportunities for MOE renegotiation. (Terms such as "mission creep" have been added to an ever increasing lexicon for discussing complex emergencies. The military is compelled to work under a political agenda and a mission statement, established by the National Command Authority, and a Joint Command mission concept plan. Any escalation from this plan is interpreted as mission creep, which risks both increased cost and redeployment delays.) Presidential Decision Directive–56, dealing with the management of complex contingency operations, was signed in May 1997. It calls for the political-military or implementation plan to include measures of success that are to be updated to incorporate changes in the situation on the ground. In recognition that humanitarian crises represent catastrophic public health disasters, health, in its broadest definition, is both the implied objective and the yardstick of success.

CHALLENGES FOR THE FUTURE

Advances in early warning technologies developed during the cold war will raise alarms throughout the world community and force the Security Council to become involved in an effort to forestall complex emergencies. Crisis prevention in a potentially hostile environment will require the projection of military force. Peace enforcement (UN Charter Authority Chapter 7), not peacekeeping, is the only viable alternative to the costly post-emergency recovery and rehabilitation of a society.

Attempts to organize a rapidly deployable UN force capable of peace enforcement have met with little success for political, economic, and institutional reasons:

- the U.S. government's trust in the United Nations is at an all-time low, creating a serious political obstacle to the Secretary General's call for an international force of 50,000 active troops and an additional 50,000 reservists;[7]
- with the experience of UNOSOM II lingering in their memory, U.S. forces are wary of coalition involvement unless the U.S. President has ultimate command authority over them;
- the costs to the United States of an exclusive U.S. force, or of an international force for which the cost burdens are not shared, are prohibitive;[29]
- the command, control, intelligence, communications, and logistics expertise garnered during the cold war have become essential to effective response to a humanitarian crisis. Unfortunately peace enforcement training is either ad hoc, limited, or altogether lacking.

It may take another complex humanitarian emergency (in Burundi, Nigeria, Indonesia, or Kosovo, for example) to make an overwhelming case for a mobile, rapidly deployable international force. A U.S. military in-kind payment to the UN might come in the form of extensive multiforces training, out of which a trusted troop force and leadership might emerge. UN forces, at times inept and scandal prone, have contributed to successful peacekeeping missions in Cambodia, Cyprus, El Salvador, Haiti, and Mozambique. This record alone is a compelling argument to continue to support the UN. Emerging regional organizations such as ASEAN or OAS, though still imperfect, have the support of the United Nations and the United States alike.[30] Regional organizations, supported by UN technical staff, could conceivably become the regional alliances capable of sharing the burden of funding and fielding a protective mobile force. Whatever form they take, these forces must be rapidly deployable, their mission must be peace enforcement, and they must not be handcuffed by conflicting mandates and directives.

Responding to future humanitarian crises effectively will require interagency coordination and communication within and among relief organizations and the military, with emphasis on the following features:

- breaking down institutional barriers in the classroom and on the exercise field, where integrated training of all major participants is recognized as both cost efficient and accountable;
- providing humanitarian professionals—civilians and military alike—with core competencies in health, law, negotiation techniques, development, political science, and social anthropology;
- placing high priority on training in personal security, crisis and stress management, evacuation, mine awareness, and security of facilities and operations.

A military peace-enforcement unit would be uniquely qualified to serve the following purposes during a complex emergency—roles that are outside the capabilities of existing civilian agencies:

- to separate and contain warring factions;
- to provide civil affairs and humanitarian assistance in coordination with NGOs;
- to ensure respect for international humanitarian law.

NGOs themselves must change in response to this changing environment and will, no doubt, forge new partnerships among themselves to strengthen specialization or to become stronger full-service generalists. NGOs will have to evolve to meet the following needs growing out of future humanitarian crises.

1. New professionals in demilitarization, demining, policing, constitutional development, and rehabilitation of infrastructure will add to the ranks of NGOs, as will those with knowledge of specific countries.
2. In a peace-enforcement environment, previously trained and equipped military-NGO units will be required to provide security while distributing relief and protecting vulnerable groups. Training will be integrated, will combine both academic research and operational agendas, will be certified, and will be sought after by career-minded relief professionals.
3. NGOs, as they develop new relationships with military institutions, will have to find new ways to balance this closeness with appropriate forms of distancing, so as not to compromise organizational identities.

4. A major deficiency remains, one that must become obvious,
over time, to those who have worked in the field whether they
are NGOs or military. There is no warrant for international
intervention that guides the world in determining where, how, and
why a coalition force should intervene.

The ICRC will, by its mandate, place its personnel in harm's way. The assassinations of ICRC staff in Chechnya in 1996, however, convey a rampant disregard for the Geneva Conventions. Restoration of that respect might yet prove to be the defining benchmark of the moral integrity of governments. The UN leadership has proposed to forge a new concept, one marrying law and morality. Secretary Perez de Cuéllar concluded in 1991 that any challenge to the existing principles of sovereignty would result in international chaos.[31] At the same time, he reflected that "we have probably reached a stage in the critical and psychological evolution of western civilization in which the massive and deliberate violation of human rights will no longer be tolerated."[32]

In the last few years we have not made much progress in accepting and clarifying this observation in terms that support policy development and operational planning and implementation. Certainly as the world community continues to explore and debate the warrants for intervention and the kind of international humanitarian architecture required to support an effective response to complex emergencies, the role of the military will need to be considered carefully and integrated with the roles of other responding institutions.

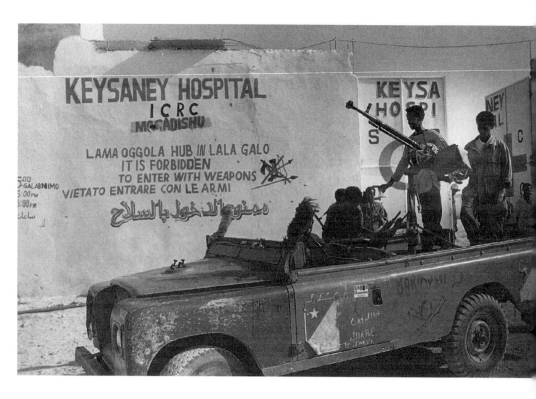

14

THE RISKS OF MILITARY PARTICIPATION

pierre perrin

Although Chapter 7, Article 42, of the United Nations Charter allows the use of armed forces under certain conditions, the Charter generally prohibits war.[1] Nevertheless, a growing number of increasingly violent armed conflicts have broken out in recent years, requiring humanitarian organizations to deal with situations of ever greater technical and political complexity. In their efforts to bring relief to the victims of war, humanitarian organizations must develop better strategies and devise more effective solutions for coping with massive and systematic violations of international humanitarian law and the increasing dangers to which relief workers are exposed in situations of armed conflict.

The international community has responded to the growing needs of war victims and the increasingly precarious conditions in which relief work is carried out by backing up a number of humanitarian operations with armed force in order to obtain access to victims and to bring them protection and assistance.

Such operations constitute a departure from the humanitarian principles of neutrality and impartiality. As a strategy for humanitarian action, moreover, the use of armed force threatens to give rise to a widening spiral of violence and tends to veil the root causes of conflicts on whose settle-

ment our human future depends. This chapter, building on the accumulated experience of the ICRC, outlines a number of issues created by linking
military action to humanitarian response.

DEFINING WAR

The strategic approach to the definition of war takes into account the
level of fighting: there are high-intensity conflicts and low-intensity conflicts. The quantitative approach defines war according to a lower limit of
1,000 deaths per year directly caused by the fighting during an armed conflict.[2] Based upon this quantitative criterion, there has been an increase in the number of wars during the last thirty years. At this writing
there are forty armed conflicts that meet the quantitative definition of
"war." This approach, however, does not take into account the indirect effects of war that, in most cases, create far more casualties than the direct
effects.

From the humanitarian point of view we may approach the problem of
wars by looking at their causes and their consequences.

CAUSES OF WAR

War can be seen as a downward spiral from a stable situation toward
conflict. Although war has many causes, those most immediately apparent
include:

- territorial disputes;
- ethnic discrimination;
- the arms race and, especially, the increasing availability of light
  weapons;
- society's growing violence.

Generally speaking, however, the basic causes of conflict are poverty and
underdevelopment. Not only does war have many causes, but their combined effect makes them all the more potent.

The factor that actually ignites a conflict may seem so inconsequential as
to be impossible to understand unless it is brought into relation with the
dispute's underlying causes. Unfortunately, the analysis of armed conflicts

often focuses exclusively on the triggering factor and thereby leads to an inadequate or unsuitable response.

THE HUMANITARIAN CONSEQUENCES OF WARS

From a pragmatic point of view, wars can be considered as conflicts between two or more parties that lead to tragic consequences: people are killed, wounded, and imprisoned; population groups are displaced; families are broken up and children made orphans.

War does not affect people only in such direct ways, however. It also cripples health services and disrupts economic activities that support the entire population, cutting people off from their traditional way of life and often depriving them of a livelihood.

In areas that are disadvantaged to begin with, life is reduced to a mere struggle for survival. Wars have changed in nature, and civilians are now the hostages and immediate victims of many armed conflicts. The indiscriminate use of antipersonnel mines produces numerous civilian casualties and also deprives farmers of their livelihood by making vast tracts of land uncultivatable.

In Mozambique, for instance:

> It is estimated that 100,000 of Mozambicans have been killed in the conflict, over 5 million have been displaced internally and up to 1.7 million have been forced to flee to neighbouring countries. Health facilities were a prime target and 2 million people had been deprived of access to health facilities. The conflict has prevented nearly 3 million people from farming land.[3]

CHALLENGES FOR HUMANITARIAN ACTION

Attitudes of Belligerents

While humanitarian organizations must respond to a growing number of tragic situations caused by war, the chaos and anarchy prevailing in such situations increasingly reduce the scope for negotiation. One should hardly be surprised, therefore, that the proliferation of conflicts is accompanied by such an increase in violence that humanitarian considerations are often swept aside.

The humanitarian strategy adopted is often conditioned by the attitude the belligerents take toward war victims. When belligerents are willing and able to take responsibility for meeting victims' needs, the role played by humanitarian organizations is confined to checking that the victims are—and continue to be—properly treated.

In some cases the parties to a conflict are not concerned about what happens to victims and rely on humanitarian organizations to cope with the consequences of war. In other cases belligerents may show concern for victims but are not equipped to protect and assist them. Whatever the situation, humanitarian organizations are faced with ethical choices regarding, for example, the attitude to be adopted toward belligerents who neglect victims, on the one hand, while denying independent and neutral humanitarian access to them, on the other.

In a growing number of situations, victims, mainly civilians, are either used for strategic ends (that is, they are taken as war hostages) or they become targets themselves (for example, as targets of systematic shelling). In keeping with the logic of such tactics, belligerents systematically block access to the victims by putting obstacles in the way of humanitarian organizations and increasing the dangers to which the staffs and volunteers of those organizations are exposed. Massive violations of international humanitarian law, insecurity, and the difficulty of reaching victims have thus become key factors in determining the strategies adopted by humanitarian organizations.

Obstacles to Defining Humanitarian Strategies in Complex Emergencies

Humanitarian operations must cope with increasingly massive violations of international humanitarian law, in particular the refusal of belligerents to grant access to victims. In such situations the standard humanitarian approach, based on negotiating with the responsible authorities, is difficult to take; it is thwarted by political leaders who have excluded humanitarian considerations from their military strategy. At other times, humanitarian action is hindered by the absence of political authorities with whom it would be possible to negotiate. Attempts have thus been made to devise new and more effective strategies.

Humanitarian organizations have adopted various approaches to cope with the difficulty of obtaining access to victims. The International Committee of the Red Cross continues to pursue its traditional strategy of negotiating with the parties to a conflict on behalf of the victims while maintaining a strictly neutral position with respect to the conflict itself.[4] In order to implement this strategy, the ICRC relies on the instruments of international humanitarian law and on its own institutional resources, which enable it to respond rapidly to the many types of humanitarian needs that must be met in armed conflicts: protecting detainees, reuniting families separated by events, restoring access to a safe water supply, and providing food and medical care.

Whereas the ICRC handles violations of international humanitarian law by dealing directly and confidentially with the authorities, other organizations denounce such violations and stigmatize those who commit them. The two strategies are complementary, but they cannot be used by the same organization. How can any organization obtain access to victims if those who are responsible for violations believe that it is going to denounce them? After a conflict, the punishment of offenders helps to reduce tension, and it is important that justice be achieved. Cooperation between those who investigate human rights violations and those whose task it is to mete out justice, however, has certain limits. Since the ICRC's role is to protect victims, it chooses not to testify in the International Court of Justice about the violations it learns of in the course of its activities. Knowing that the information gathered by the ICRC will remain confidential, those who are guilty of violations will be less tempted to eliminate their victims in order to avoid having to answer for their acts.

Seeking complementarity between strategies meant to address different problems, where none exists, is pointless. For example, people assume that humanitarian action can alleviate the suffering caused when economic sanctions are imposed on a given state. Since such sanctions affect the victims of a war rather than those responsible for the war, the notion that sanctions are complementary with humanitarian action is illusory. An organization attempting to respond to a complex emergency will find it difficult to combine humanitarian activities with coercive action.

The complementary effect sought by the UN in combining humanitarian action with peacekeeping operations (the carrot and the stick) has limits that make it necessary to draw a clear distinction between the various UN agencies and to define the role played by those specifically involved in humanitarian operations.

Military-Backed Humanitarian Operations
as a Substitute for Political Action

Adopting a strategy that uses armed force to gain forcible access to victims entails a certain number of risks, not only for the organizations involved but especially for those who pursue a traditional approach based on negotiations.

Backing humanitarian operations with military force enables states to avoid taking the types of political action needed to deal with belligerents who engage in massive violations of international humanitarian law. Such operations minimize the importance of taking more drastic action and dealing with the problem of war at its source.

The purpose of militarily backed humanitarian operations is to obtain access to victims so that they can receive assistance either from humanitarian organizations or from the peacekeeping forces themselves. Such operations can also be seen as a response to the deterioration of security conditions in recent years. While it is true that, at the risk of betraying the principles of neutrality and impartiality, military forces sometimes facilitate access to victims, there is also the concern that their presence may cause the level of violence to increase.[5] Such operations may lead to direct clashes with the parties to a conflict. Alternatively, by attempting to reach victims without taking appropriate action against those who violate international humanitarian law, these operations may convince the leaders of the warring parties that the international community is willing to adjust the military backing it gives to humanitarian operations to account for ever higher levels of insecurity. As can be seen in the former Yugoslavia, allowing humanitarian operations to be carried out under worsening security conditions may simply lead to mounting violence.

The ICRC remains convinced that humanitarian strategies should be founded on the principles of neutrality and impartiality and bases it own approach on the belief that negotiations with belligerents will eventually produce results. The fundamental role of ICRC delegates, therefore, is to keep on negotiating with the leaders of the parties to a conflict, come what may, in order to persuade them that it is both necessary and in their own interest to ensure scope for humanitarian action.

The steadfast pursuit of this strategy has eventually paid off in a number of situations. After months of negotiations the ICRC obtained permission to visit the victims of the Afghan conflict in Kabul and, eventually, to work in the rest of the country. While a great number of lives were lost during these negotiations, once the ICRC had gained acceptance it was able to develop its activities and can still pursue them today. Would a military operation have been more effective? The examples of Somalia and the former Yugoslavia show how fragile such operations can be. Although not perfect, a strategy based on negotiation makes it possible to protect and assist victims by securing agreement to an initial number of humanitarian activities and by gradually increasing their scope.

In extreme cases, of course, belligerents' total lack of concern for the suffering caused by a conflict has tragic consequences about which humanitarian organizations can do very little. Militarily backed humanitarian action, however, is not a suitable response in such situations, where a clear distinction must be drawn between exclusively humanitarian operations carried out in a neutral, impartial, and independent fashion and political action taken to restore law and order. While humanitarian work certainly benefits from operations that seek to keep or restore peace, it must be kept completely separate from such operations if it is to preserve its neutral and impartial status.

The choice of means and the way in which they are used are of no small importance. In practice, organizations that are backed up by armed force— even within the framework of a UN operation—forfeit their neutral status. Humanitarian operations will have to adopt ever greater means of protection in response to the increasingly dangerous conditions that belligerents will impose on them. By using armed force to provide humanitarian aid instead of making conditions appropriate for the application of international humanitarian law, these organizations run the risk of fueling a spiral of violence that will contribute, in the medium term, to the causes of conflict.

PRINCIPLES OF HUMANITARIAN STRATEGY: THE ICRC APPROACH

International Humanitarian Law

The consequences of war can be mitigated by applying the rules of international humanitarian law (IHL). This is achieved by regulating the conduct of hostilities and protecting persons who take no part in hostilities. The regulation of the conduct of hostilities is based on a body of law that aims to alleviate the effects of armed conflicts by regulating and limiting the methods and means of warfare used by the parties to the conflict.[6,7] Application of these rules does not imply an acceptance of war, but constitutes an ultimate means to reduce its impact.

The two major areas of regulation are the choice of targets and the use of weapons. Box 14.1 provides some examples of regulation regarding the use of weapons.

International humanitarian law is constantly being developed, and health personnel have a role to play in this development. For instance, the epidemiological study of mine injuries in ICRC hospitals[8] led the ICRC to call for a complete ban on antipersonnel mines at the 1996 review of the 1980 Conventional Weapons Convention. Although the review conferences were not immediately successful in banning mines (a treaty banning antipersonnel mines was finally signed in Ottawa in December 1997), the first conference in Vienna successfully prohibited the use of blinding laser weapons. Article 1 of the Protocol on Blinding Weapons stipulates:

> It is prohibited to employ laser weapons specifically designed, as their sole combat function or as one of their combat functions, to cause permanent blindness to enhanced vision, that is to naked eye or to the eye with corrective eyesight devices. The High Contracting Parties shall not transfer such weapons to any State or non-State entity.[9]

Box 14.1 Examples of rules in the conduct of hostilities

- Declaration of St. Petersburg Concerning Explosive Projectiles (1868)
- Geneva Protocol Prohibiting the Use of Asphyxiating, Poisonous, or Other Gases, and Bacteriological Methods of Warfare (1925)
- Convention on the Prohibition of Military or Other Hostile Use of Environmental Modification Techniques (1977)
- Convention Relating to the Use of Certain Conventional Weapons (1980)
- Convention on the Prohibition of the Use, Stockpiling, Production, and Transfer of Anti-Personnel Mines and on Their Destruction (1997)

International humanitarian law provides protection for the victims of war. Such protection is guaranteed in situations of international armed conflict (the four 1949 Geneva Conventions and their Additional Protocol I) and of noninternational armed conflict (Article 3 common to the four Geneva Conventions and their Additional Protocol II). IHL protects the fundamental rights of victims, whether they are wounded, prisoners, detainees, or civilians: the right to life, the right to be humanely treated, and the right to receive medical care. Box 14.2 lists the Conventions and their Protocols.

There are specific ways in which IHL protects the health system: Protocol I, Article 54, requires the protection of objects indispensable to the survival of the civilian population; Geneva Convention IV, Article 18, sets the rules for the protection of hospitals.

The consequences of war depend greatly on the degree of respect

---

Box 14.2 The Geneva Conventions and their Additional Protocols

- First Convention: Geneva Convention for the Amelioration of the Condition of the Wounded and Sick in Armed Forces in the Field (1864)
- Second Convention: Geneva Convention for the Amelioration of the Condition of the Wounded, Sick and Shipwrecked Members of Armed Forces at Sea (1899)
- Third Convention: Geneva Convention Relative to the Treatment of Prisoners of War (1929)
- Fourth Convention: Geneva Convention Relative to the Protection of Civilian Persons in Time of War (1949)
- The 1977 Diplomatic Conference adopted two Protocols Additional to the Geneva Conventions:
- Protocol Additional to the Geneva Conventions of 12 August 1949, and Relating to the Protection of Victims of International Armed Conflicts (Protocol I)
- Protocol Additional to the Geneva Conventions of 12 August 1949, and Relating to the Protection of Victims of Non-International Armed Conflicts (Protocol II)

belligerents show for international humanitarian law. The ICRC, which is responsible for the development and promotion of that law, conducts large-scale campaigns to acquaint the armed forces of all countries with its rules. Cooperation between various groups of professionals, legal experts, and health-care personnel must be reinforced.

Principles of Action

Humanitarian action is based on the principles of:

- neutrality (refraining from taking a position on a conflict or its causes);
- impartiality (all victims must be protected and assisted without discrimination and according to their needs);
- independence (freedom to choose objectives and strategies).

The neutrality of a humanitarian operation must be considered from two points of view, that of the organizations taking part in the operation and that of the belligerents. The daily task of ICRC delegates is to explain— and often to justify—the underlying reasons for their neutrality. If they are to be able to defend their position and hold up the principle of neutrality, they must have an unambiguous attitude toward the parties to a conflict, especially in pursuing their own strategies and goals. Belligerents are reluctant to recognize the neutral status of humanitarian organizations that report and publicly denounce human rights violations about which they have learned in the course of their activities. Furthermore, when organizations rely on military means—whether to ensure their own protection or, more especially, when used to exert pressure on those responsible for blocking a particular operation—those organizations find it difficult to provide belligerents with a credible explanation of the concept of neutrality. This is a challenge faced by the UN High Commissioner for Refugees, which, in certain situations, as in the former Yugoslavia, has found itself submerged by the military forces deployed by the UN.

The concept of impartiality is embodied in the set of specific circumstances in which everyone is to be afforded protection according to his or her assessed needs and without discrimination regarding his or her race, religion, ethnic origin, or other characteristics. Some humanitarian organizations have been pressed to distribute assistance not in proportion to need but according to demands made by belligerents who make the organizations pay for access to the victims. To give in to such demands is not simply a concession, it is a moral compromise that seriously jeopardizes the reputation for impartiality that all humanitarian operations must strive to maintain.

The principle of independence allows the ICRC to choose those objectives and strategies that, in its judgment, will best protect the victims of armed conflicts.

Defining Areas of Responsibility

In defining areas of responsibility, clear distinctions must be made regarding:

- the aims pursued, which must be strictly humanitarian when the object is to act on behalf of victims and strictly political when the object is to restore peace and punish those guilty of violating international humanitarian law;
- the means adopted, which, when they are military, must be exclusively reserved for political aims such as peacekeeping operations and not used for humanitarian aims as well;
- all the players present in the field who, to prevent confusion, must be clearly identified with respect to their aims and means of action, which, in the case of humanitarian operations, must not include armed forces.

Levels of Action

Wars have been considered historical accidents and peace the general rule. Various destabilizing factors arise and lead to war, after which peace is restored on the basis of a new equilibrium. Given this general framework, it is possible to distinguish five levels of action:

1. Fostering peace by promoting development in the broadest sense: harmonious socioeconomic development accompanied by respect for human rights.
2. Identifying potential sources of conflict and putting a rapid end to fighting in its early stages (this level includes preventive diplomacy and the deployment of peacekeeping forces).
3. Handling the political crisis by acting to stop the conflict

(setting up peace-enforcement operations, imposing economic sanctions and arms embargoes, and so on).

4. Taking steps to attenuate the consequences of war and to protect and assist war victims.
5. Beginning the process of rehabilitation, reconstruction, and all steps conducive to stabilizing the situation and fostering peace.

Figure 14.1 provides a conceptual framework of the various areas of responsibilities.

Conflict Prevention

Individual states, the United Nations, intergovernmental agencies, and specialized nongovernmental organizations all play leading roles in promoting development in the broadest sense. Such development is based on respect for human rights (evidenced at the national level by fair social and economic policies, ethnic tolerance, and democracy) and on equity (the harmonious social and economic development of nations, respect for democratic principles, and coherent policies dealing with global problems such as demography, climate, and natural resources). This is the field of primary conflict prevention, since action taken at the developmental level helps to prevent potential causes of armed conflict from arising within and among nations.

One would be naive to think that the causes of conflict will ever be totally eliminated through international cooperation, economic and social development, and respect for human rights. Both the UN and individual states have crucial roles to play in identifying problems that could lead to war. An early warning system based on an epidemiological approach to human rights violations could facilitate the steps needed to put an end to those violations and thus eliminate a direct cause of conflict. Such steps belong to the field of preventive diplomacy and may require the deployment of peacekeeping forces as a precautionary measure.

Mitigation

When secondary prevention fails, conflicts must be dealt with at two levels, with a clear division of responsibilities:

- political entities, including states, the UN, and intergovernmental organizations, have a critical part to play in defusing political cri-

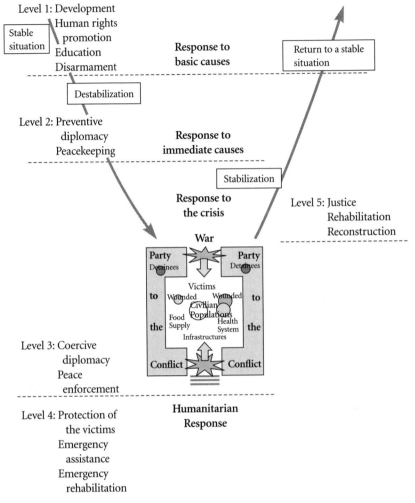

Figure 14.1   Levels of responsibility for intervention prior to, during, and after complex humanitarian emergencies. (ICRC)

ses and in prosecuting those guilty of violating international humanitarian law;

• humanitarian organizations, including the ICRC and specialized nongovernmental organizations, have the task of coping with the suffering caused by conflicts.

Reconstruction

Reconstruction is carried out by the same institutions that take part in primary prevention: states, the United Nations, intergovernmental organizations, and nongovernmental organizations specialized in development work.

This clear division of responsibilities is meant not only to protect institutional interests, but above all to defend a certain philosophy of humanitarian action and to ensure the most effective strategy for reaching the goals pursued. Humanitarian organizations must make clear where they stand in relation to these areas of responsibility. When a humanitarian organization relies on armed force to obtain access to victims it adopts a strategy that affects the way in which all humanitarian organizations are perceived. The result is a loss of humanitarian identity, with all the disadvantages such a loss entails.

GLOBAL SECURITY AS A RESPONSE TO CONFLICT MANAGEMENT

The world is in the throes of a major crisis caused by emerging problems:

- an increasingly violent society
- inequitable development;
- ethnic intolerance;
- climate changes that threaten to modify the geostrategic world map;
- the transfer of arms;
- the development of new weapons;
- the rise of new forms of terrorism;
- struggles over depleted natural resources such as topsoil and water.

Such challenges are likely to result in new conflicts in the years ahead.

The United Nations and individual states must give high priority to addressing the basic causes of future conflicts if the world is to remain committed to peace and development and if war is to remain an episodic occurrence (Figure 14.2). Otherwise the diversion of assets and energy to the sole end of managing conflicts threatens to create a world in which peace is the exception and war the rule. The UN must resist the temptation to engage

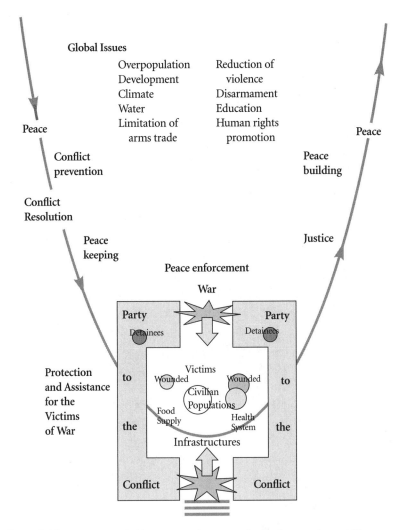

Figure 14.2 Wars and global human security: Humanitarian interventions within an overall view of the world's problems.

most of its resources in humanitarian action—thereby shirking its duty to provide the world with political guidance. As for humanitarian organizations, in particular the ICRC, they must coordinate their strategies and operations so as to be able to respond more effectively to the increasingly tragic situations caused by war.

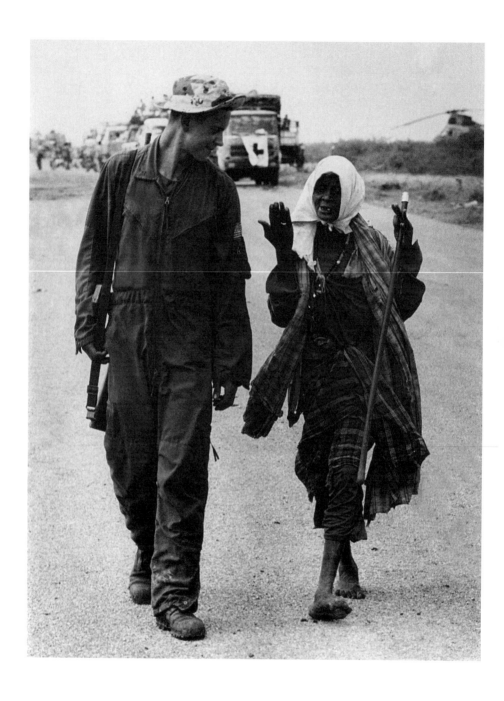

CONCLUSION

jennifer leaning

Humanitarian crises create great waste and suffering. They divert attention and resources from efforts to promote social and economic development over the long term. As shown in the preceding chapters, current attempts to respond to the morbidity and mortality of these events have had mixed results. The international community is in the midst of active efforts to improve substantially upon its short-term response strategies. Many of these areas for improvement lie in the realm of medical and public health practice and are identified and discussed in this book.

IMPROVEMENTS IN SHORT-TERM RESPONSE

To improve short-term response, relief agencies need to strengthen their internal capacity for the deployment of seasoned and expert personnel. This improvement will require establishing a professional career track for their responder cadre, including all aspects of recruitment, training and education, psychological support, retention, advancement and progression, and, as needed, outplacement.

International agencies and governments must also improve their coordination of response activities. The surge in humanitarian work since 1990 has caused a proliferation of different actors with different capacities and traditions, leading to confusion in the field regarding mission, mandate, and expertise.[1,2]

Aid agencies and governments must also expand substantially upon the skills and resources they bring to the functions of logistics and operations. In this regard, the military may play a potentially important role in support of humanitarian aid, provided the chain of command is clear and a security role is not also envisioned or indicated. Considerable controversy and uncertainty continues to attend all discussion about coordination between military and humanitarian roles in hostile situations where the military is needed for security or defense.

The extent to which the human rights dimension of these emergencies contributes as an inciting event or as an ugly accompaniment is not uniformly appreciated by the humanitarian community in general and by medical and public health workers in particular. Among these relief workers there is also an incomplete practical understanding of the body of IHL, which through its precepts of impartiality and medical neutrality provides protection but also imposes obligations. Serious and ongoing education in human rights and IHL is needed for all levels of staff in humanitarian NGOs.[3] Medical and public health workers must be helped to understand the significance of their potential to provide clinical testimony and data for the compilation of testimony to be used in trials and other judicial proceedings.

Populations affected by armed conflict experience severe direct and secondary public health consequences, usually mediated by population displacement, food scarcity, and the collapse of basic health services. Refugees and internally displaced persons have experienced high mortality rates during the period immediately following their migration. Rapid health assessments using established methodologies and the setting of priorities for health intervention are often key to ensuring civilian protection and to reducing the morbidity and mortality of affected populations.

A number of important research issues have surfaced out of recent relief experience.[4] In terms of sheer numbers, complex humanitarian emergencies have strained if not overwhelmed the technical assessment and response methods of the medical and public health participants in the humanitarian response. At a basic level, we lack innovative and proven ways to count vast populations and identify their demographic characteristics, especially when they are on the move or have rapidly accumulated in camps holding hundreds of thousands of people. Plant management, population security, health assessment, and distribution procedures for camps of this size have not been developed or tested. Field experience must be sifted and evaluated with regard to how to attend to the health and social needs of population subgroups; how to best allocate resources to optimize the mix among preventive, curative, or supportive treatment of a wide range of conditions endemic in these populations (such as malnutrition, undernutrition, diarrheal disease, upper respiratory infections, sexually transmitted diseases, land-mine and other war injuries, sexual violence, and psychological distress and trauma); and how to evaluate interventions undertaken on this scale.

This long hard look at methods and capacities must also recognize that these crises are extremely costly, long-lasting, and chronically disruptive to local and regional societies and governments. The implications of this recognition for the humanitarian community are that (1) the classic division of NGO responsibility into relief and development roles may no longer be relevant; (2) funding resources and commitments may need to be reexamined in terms of potential for staying power; and (3) individual NGO missions and mandates may need in the future to be framed in more collaborative and coordinated contexts with local actors and stakeholders.[5]

THE LONGER-TERM AGENDA

As with all catastrophes that bring large-scale human and ecological distress, the application of the public health paradigm to an examination of underlying political, economic, and social causes provides conceptual strength. Where there is no cure and no simple remedy, the strategy must shift to anticipatory action launched in the service of mitigation and prevention. Here, however, the scope of action for medicine and public health is relatively limited and the responsibilities shift to significant political players and stakeholders such as the UN agencies, the European Union, and major national governments such as the United States.

In support of the analytic power of the public health paradigm, and to place the suggestions for improvements in short-term response within a larger framework, the following points briefly outline what is at stake in this longer-term agenda.[6,7]

Mitigation

Mitigation, defined as intervention aimed to reduce the impact of a crisis and block its routes toward escalation, invokes three sequential steps: early warning, intervention based upon that warning, and stabilization in the immediate post-intervention phase.

Early warning indicators must be defined, assessed, validated, and followed by the introduction of measures to permit anticipatory action based upon the information flowing in. A number of candidate indicators can be discerned from a retrospective analysis of the circumstances preceding the eruption of acute crisis in recent emergencies in Somalia, Bosnia, and Rwanda.[8,9] These include human rights violations; arms trade and the proliferation of weapons; failure to punish lawlessness and murder; growing economic distress or outbreak of famine; suppression of the press; hate-filled propaganda; intensifying ethnic segregation; and growing internal migration and a surge in cross-border refugees.

Agreement on what constitutes intervention, when to engage in it, who must go first, and what methods to use are all tasks that lie ahead. Resolution of these issues, by individual NGOs and by the international community, is pivotal to the success or failure of the concept and strategy of early warning. Evaluation of recent experience in Somalia, Bosnia, and Rwanda is critical in providing guidance for future policy design.

An extended period after intervention awaits acknowledgment and definition by the international community. This period, referred to as the "gray period of chronic insecurity" by USAID officials[10] may persist for months or years. The challenge of stabilization during this period includes deciding among a number of economic and security options:[11,12] peace enhancement or crisis resolution; whether or not to disarm the population; policy regarding demobilization and reentry of soldiers and militia from border areas; maintenance of an ongoing external security presence or helping to establish an internal one; and whether or not to support, with expertise and finances, a process of trials or truth commissions. Time is frequently of the essence, in that the stakes of not succeeding in reinstituting some acceptable semblance of the rule of law can be very high.[13]

Currently, no government or institution wishes to accept the fact that these issues are pervasive and unavoidable. A major and legitimate concern is national sovereignty. Another is the financial burden these mitigation efforts impose upon those who assume responsibility. A third is how the inevitable loss of life among forces involved in peace enhancement or crisis resolution will be perceived back home. Maintenance of law and order in areas that have not seen such for decades is a long and perilous effort. The world community has had very few recent successful examples of this work.

Prevention: Search for Root Causes

The categories of root causes listed here have been developed by seasoned observers[14,15,16] over the last decades and are familiar to those working in this field: political instability or outright collapse of the state; long-standing violations of human rights; festering ethnic or communal hostilities; widespread economic hardship; gross income inequities; demographic pressure on resources; and environmental degradation or destruction.

What has not been defined for these factors is the metric to use in each category, or the mix of factors that leads to conflagration. These factors, singly or together, can certainly be found in many more places on earth than those where complex emergencies have currently been identified. The issues of causation constitute an agenda for a large number of professions and institutions, national and international.

Prevention: Initiatives

Long before we complete the search for and definitive measurement of root causes, we must accelerate the work we already know need to be taking place.[17,18,19] In societies where the struggle for resources is not desperate, where civil and political liberties are established and not threatened, and where opportunities for individual and group well-being are widely available, these emergencies will not develop or ignite. International institutions, governments, NGOs, and the academy must together engage in the design, implementation, and assessment of prevention strategies such as the ones outlined here: civic education (literacy, human rights, role of women); political and legal reform; resolution of gross economic inequities (land redistribution); integration into the regional and world economy; health sector improvements; and environmental restoration and reclamation. These initiatives, if undertaken early in the chain of causation, would be linked to empowerment of the local community, economic development, education in and promotion of human rights, and the development of civic institutions, such as schools, the press, and administrative and judicial systems.

These initiatives are expensive, but not costly when weighed against the price humanitarian crises are now exacting from us. These initiatives are fundamentally political, a feature they share with all influential group ventures. The public health paradigm positions us to accept, even embrace, the expense and political nature of these initiatives. Medicine and public health advance within the advances created and secured by world society. As we in this book endeavor to understand and improve our practice in this new and terrible arena of humanitarian crises, we also welcome the opportunity to participate in the larger effort to establish the conditions for a more just and peaceful world.

NOTES / ACKNOWLEDGMENTS / CREDITS / INDEX

NOTES

INTRODUCTION

1. Duffield, M. "The political economy of complex emergencies." Report for UNICEF. New York: United Nations, 1997.

2. Leaning, J. "The bell tolls." Editorial. *Medicine and Global Survival* 1994; 1: 122–123.

3. Toole, M. J., and R. J. Waldman. "Refugees and displaced persons: War, hunger, and public health." *JAMA* 1993; 270: 600–605.

4. Burkholder, B. T., and M. J. Toole. "Evolution of complex disasters." *Lancet* 1995; 346: 1012–1015.

5. Rhodes, R. "Man-made death: A neglected mortality." *JAMA* 1988; 260: 686–687.

6. De Lupis, I. D. "The law of war." LSE Monographs in International Studies. New York: Cambridge University Press, 1987: 167–168.

7. Prendergast, J. *Crisis Response: Humanitarian Band-aids in Sudan and Somalia.* Chicago: Pluto Press and Center of Concern, 1997: 11–13.

8. Weiss, T. G. Seminar presentation to Fall Migration Series. Cambridge, Mass.: Massachusetts Institute of Technology, November 24, 1997.

9. Jean, F., ed. *Populations in Danger 1995.* London: Médecins sans Frontières, 1995: 130–131.

10. Beaumont, R. "Small wars: Definitions and dimensions." *Annals of the American Academy of Political and Social Science* 1995; 541: 20–35.

11. Hansch, S. "An explosion of complex humanitarian emergencies." In: *Hunger 1996: Countries in Crisis.* Silver Spring, Md.: Bread for the World Institute, 1995.

12. Macrae, J., and A. Zwi. "Famine, complex emergencies, and international policy in Africa: An overview." In: J. Macrae and A. Zwi, eds. *War and Hunger: Rethinking International Responses to Complex Emergencies.* London: Zed Press, 1994: 6–36.

13. Nafziger, E. W. "The political economy of humanitarian emergencies: From Bosnia to Rwanda." UNU/WIDER, Sweden, March 1997.

14. Rieff, D. "Charity on the rampage." *Foreign Affairs* 1997; 76: 132–138.

15. International Federation of Red Cross and Red Crescent Societies. *World Disasters Report 1997*. Geneva: IFRC, 1997: 11.

16. Girardet, E. R. *Somalia, Rwanda, and Beyond: The Role of International Media in Wars and Humanitarian Crises*. Dublin: Crosslines Communications, 1995.

17. Benthall, J. *Disasters, Relief, and the Media*. London: I. B. Tauris, 1993.

18. Rotberg, R. I., and T. G. Weiss, eds. *From Massacres to Genocide: The Media, Public Policy, and Humanitarian Crises*. Cambridge, Mass.: World Peace Foundation, 1996.

19. U.S. Mission to the UN. *Global Humanitarian Emergencies, 1998*. New York: United Nations, September 1998: 26–29.

20. Baskett, P., and R. Weller (eds). *Medicine for Disasters*. Boston: John Wright, 1988.

21. Noji, E., ed. *The Public Health Consequences of Disasters*. New York: Oxford University Press, 1997.

22. Noji, E. K., and M. J. Toole. "The historical development of public health responses to disasters." *Disasters* 1996; 21: 366–376.

23. Beauchamp, T., and J. F. Childress. *Principles of Biomedical Ethics*. New York: Oxford University Press, 1979.

24. Veatch, R. M. *A Theory of Medical Ethics*. New York: Basic Books, 1981.

25. United Nations High Commissioner for Refugees. World Wide Website: http://www.unhcr.ch. February 28, 1998.

26. Proudfoot, M. J. *European Refugees, 1939–1952: A Study in Forced Population Movement*. Chicago: Northwestern University Press, 1956.

27. Human Rights Watch and Physicians for Human Rights. *Landmines: A Deadly Legacy*. New York: Human Rights Watch, 1993.

28. International Physicians for the Prevention of Nuclear War. *Landmines: A Global Health Crisis*. Cambridge, Mass.: IPPNW, 1997.

29. Hansch, S., and K. Jacobsen. "Environmentally induced population displacements and environmental impacts resulting from mass migrations." Symposium at Geneva, Switzerland, April 1996. Washington, D.C.: Refugee Policy Group, 1996.

30. Kibreab, G. "Environmental causes and impact of refugee movements: A critique of the current debate." *Disasters* 1997; 21: 20–38.

31. Russbach, R., and D. Fink. "Humanitarian action in current armed conflicts: Opportunities and obstacles." *Medicine and Global Survival* 1994; 1: 188–199.

32. Kaldor, M., and Basker Vashee, eds. *Restructuring the Global Military Sector. Vol. I: New Wars.* London: Pinter, 1997.

33. UN Commission of Experts. "Final report pursuant to Security Council resolution 780 (1992) to provide evidence of grave breaches of the Geneva Conventions and other violations of international humanitarian law committed in the territory of the former Yugoslavia." S/1994/674. New York: United Nations, May 27, 1994.

34. Destexhe, A. "The third genocide." *Foreign Policy* 1994; 97: 3–17.

35. Physicians for Human Rights. "Report on Congo Investigation." Boston: PHR, 1997.

36. Human Rights Watch. "Report on Democratic Republic of the Congo: What Kabila is hiding." Washington, D.C.: Human Rights Watch, October 1997.

37. European Community Humanitarian Office. Ethics of Humanitarian Action. Conference report. Geneva: ECHO, 1996.

38. Rigal, J. "Crisis medicine." In J. François, ed. *Populations in Danger.* London: Médecins sans Frontières, John Libbey, 1992: 139–143.

39. Conflict Management Group. "Peacekeeping, peacemaking, and humanitarian assistance in areas of conflict." Working Paper. Cambridge, Mass.: Conflict Management Group, 1994.

40. Gaydos, J. C., and G. A. Luz. "Military participation in emergency humanitarian assistance." *Disasters* 1994; 18: 48–57.

41. Jean, F., ed. "The former Yugoslavia." In: J. François, ed. *Populations in Danger.* London: Médecins sans Frontières, John Libbey, 1992: 15–19.

42. de Waal, A., and R. Omaar. "Humanitarianism unbound? Current dilemmas facing multi-mandate relief operations in political emergencies." Discussion Paper no. 5. London: African Rights, November 1994.

43. Leavitt, L. A., and N. A. Fox, eds. *The Psychological Effects of War and Violence on Children.* Hillsdale, N.J.: Lawrence Erlbaum Associates, 1993.

44. Desjarlais, R., et al., eds. *World Mental Health: Problems and Priorities in Low Income Countries.* New York: Oxford University Press, 1995: 116–135.

45. Weaver, J. D. *Disasters: Mental Health Interventions.* Crisis Management Series. Sarasota, Fla.: Professional Resource Press, 1995.

1 THE ROLE OF RAPID ASSESSMENT

1. Cobey, J., A. Flanigin, and W. Foege. "Effective humanitarian aid: Our only hope for intervention in civil war." *JAMA* 1993; 270: 632–634.

2. Carballo, M., S. Simic, and D. Zeric. "Health in countries torn by conflict: Lessons from Sarajevo." *Lancet* 1996; 348: 872–874.

3. Sivard, R. L. *World Military and Social Expenditures 1996*. Washington, D.C.: World Priorities, 1996.

4. U.S. Committee for Refugees. *World Refugee Survey, 1995*. Washington, D.C.: 1995.

5. United Nations High Commissioner for Refugees. World Wide Website: http//www.unhcr.ch, February 28, 1998.

6. Toole, M. J., and R. J. Waldman. "Refugees and displaced persons: War, hunger, and public health." *JAMA* 1993; 270: 600–605.

7. Goma Epidemiology Group. "Public health impact of the Rwandan refugee crisis: What happened in Goma, Zaire, in July 1994?" *Lancet* 1995; 345: 339–344.

8. Yip, R., and T. W. Sharp. "Acute malnutrition and high childhood mortality related to diarrhea." *JAMA* 1993; 270: 587–590.

9. Toole, M. J., and R. J. Waldman. "The prevention of excess mortality in displaced populations in the developing world." *JAMA* 1990; 263: 3296–3302.

10. Toole, M. J., and R. J. Waldman. "The public health aspects of complex emergencies and refugee situations." *Annual Review of Public Health* 1996; 18.

11. Moore, P. S., et al. "Mortality rates in displaced and resident populations of central Somalia during 1992 famine disaster." *Lancet* 1993; 41: 913–917.

12. Centers for Disease Control and Prevention. "Nutrition and mortality assessment—Southern Sudan, March 1993." *Morbidity and Mortality Weekly Report* 1993; 42: 304–308.

13. Centers for Disease Control and Prevention. "Status of public health—Bosnia and Herzegovina, August–September, 1993." *Morbidity and Mortality Weekly Report* 1993; 42: 973, 979–982.

14. Centers for Disease Control and Prevention. "Emergency public health surveillance in response to food and energy sources—Armenia, 1992." *Morbidity and Mortality Weekly Report* 1993; 42: 69–71.

15. Médecins sans Frontières. *Evaluation Rapide de l'État de Santé d'une Population Déplacée ou Réfugié* (available in French only). Paris: Médecins sans Frontières, 1996.

16. Centers for Disease Control and Prevention. "Famine-affected, refugee, and displaced populations: Recommendations for public health issues." *Morbidity and Mortality Weekly Report* 1992; 41 (no. RR-13): 1–76.

17. Toole, M. J., and R. Bhatia. "A case study of Somali refugees in Hartisheik A camp, eastern Ethiopia: health and nutrition profile, July 1988–June 1989." *Journal of Refugee Studies* 1992; 5: 313–326.

18. Davis, A. P. "Targeting the vulnerable in emergency situations: Who is vulnerable?" *Lancet* 1996; 348: 868–871.

19. Boss, L. P., M. J. Toole, and R. Yip. "Assessments of mortality, morbidity, and nutritional status in Somalia during the 1991–1992 famine: Recommendations for standardization of methods." *JAMA* 1994; 272: 371–376.

20. Hurwitz, E. S. "Malaria among newly arrived refugees in Thailand, 1979–80." In: D. T. Allegra, P. Nieburg, and M. Grabe, eds. *Emergency Refugee Health Care—A Chronicle of the Khmer Refugee Assistance Operation 1979–80*. Atlanta: Centers for Disease Control and Prevention, 1980: 43–47.

21. Centers for Disease Control and Prevention. "Health status of displaced persons following civil war—Burundi, December 1993–January 1994." *Morbidity and Mortality Weekly Report* 1994; 43: 701–703.

22. Mast, E. E., et al. "Hepatitis E among refugees in Kenya: Minimal apparent person-to-person transmission, evidence for age-dependent disease expression, and new serological assays." In: K. Kishioka et al., eds. *Viral Hepatitis and Liver Disease*. Tokyo: Springer-Verlag, 1994: 375–378.

23. Desenclos, J. C., et al. "Epidemiologic patterns of scurvy among Ethiopian refugees." *Bulletin of the World Health Organization* 1989; 67: 309–316.

24. Centers for Disease Control and Prevention. "Outbreak of pellagra among Mozambican refugees—Malawi, 1990." *Morbidity and Mortality Weekly Report* 1991; 40: 209–213.

25. World Health Organization Working Group. "Use and interpretation of anthropometric indicators of nutritional status." *Bulletin of the World Health Organization* 1986; 64: 929–941.

26. United Nations High Commissioner for Refugees. *Water Manual for Refugee Situations*. Geneva: UNHCR, 1992.

27. Report of a workshop on the improvement of the nutrition of refugees and displaced people in Africa. Machakos, Kenya. 5–7 December 1994. Geneva: United Nations Administrative Committee on Coordination, Sub-Committee on Nutrition, November 1995.

2 PUBLIC HEALTH INTERVENTIONS

1. Toole, M. J., and R. J. Waldman. "Refugees and displaced persons: War, hunger and public health." *JAMA* 1993; 270: 600–605.

2. Centers for Disease Control and Prevention. "Status of public health—Bosnia and Herzegovina, August–September 1993." *Morbidity and Mortality Weekly Report* 1993; 42: 973, 979–982.

3. Gessner, B. D. "Mortality rates, causes of death, and health status among displaced and resident populations of Kabul, Afghanistan." *JAMA* 1994; 272: 382–385.

4. Russbach, R. "Health problems in conflict situations." In: M. Ohta, T. Ukai, and Y. Yamamoto, eds. *New Aspects of Disaster Medicine.* Tokyo: Herusu Publishing Co., 1989: 169–172.

5. Toole, M. J. "The rapid assessment of health problems in refugee and displaced populations." *Medicine and Global Survival* 1994; 1: 200–207.

6. Centers for Disease Control and Prevention. "Famine-affected, refugee, and displaced populations: Recommendations for public health issues." *Morbidity and Mortality Weekly Report* 1992; 41 (no. RR-13): 1–76.

7. Burkholder, B. T., and M. J. Toole. "Evolution of a complex emergency." *Lancet* 1995; 346: 1012–1015.

8. Allegra, D. R., et al. *Emergency Refugee Healthcare—A Chronicle of Experience in the Khmer Assistance Operation, 1979–1980.* Atlanta: Centers for Disease Control, 1984.

9. Centers for Disease Control. "Health status of Kampuchean refugees, Sakaeo, Thailand." *Morbidity and Mortality Weekly Report* 1979; 28: 545–546.

10. Glass, R. I., et al. "Rapid assessment of health status and preventive medicine needs of newly arrived Kampuchean refugees, Sa Kaeo, Thailand." *Lancet* 1980; 1 (8173): 868–872.

11. Cuny, F. *Situational Awareness: Improving Emergency Decision-Making in Refugee Emergencies.* Dallas: Intertect, 1990.

12. de Waal, A. "Dangerous precedents? Famine relief in Somalia, 1991–1993." In: J. Macrae and A. Zwi, eds. *War and Hunger: Rethinking International Responses to Complex Emergencies.* London: Zed Books, 1994.

13. Leaning, J. "When the system doesn't work: Somalia 1992." In: K. Cahill, ed. *A Framework for Survival: Health, Human Rights, and Humanitarian Assistance in Conflicts and Disasters.* New York: Basic Books and the Council on Foreign Relations, 1993.

14. Toole, M. J., and R. J. Waldman. "An analysis of mortality trends among refugee populations in Somalia, Sudan and Thailand." *Bulletin of the World Health Organization* 1988; 66: 237–247.

15. Centers for Disease Control and Prevention. "Mortality among newly arrived Mozambican refugees, Zimbabwe and Malawi, 1992." *Morbidity and Mortality Weekly Report* 1993; 42: 468–469,475–477.

16. Telford, J. "Lessons learned from the Sudan and Gulf emergencies." *Refugees* 1992; 91: 16–18.

17. Centers for Disease Control and Prevention. "Public health consequences of acute displacement of Iraqi citizens—March–May, 1991." *Morbidity and Mortality Weekly Report* 1991; 40: 443–446.

18. UNICEF. *State of the World's Children, 1990*. New York: Oxford University Press, 1990.

19. Sayegh, J. *Child Survival in Wartime: A Case Study from Iraq, 1983–1989*. Baltimore: Johns Hopkins University Press, 1992.

20. Yip, R., and T. W. Sharp. "Acute malnutrition and high childhood mortality related to diarrhea." *JAMA* 1993; 270: 587–590.

21. Intertect. *Assessing Emergencies Involving Civilians Displaced by Conflict*. Training module prepared for the UNDP/DHA Disaster Management Training Programme. Dallas: Intertect, 1993.

22. UNICEF. *Assisting in Emergencies: A Resource Handbook for UNICEF and Field Staff*. New York: UNICEF, 1986.

23. UN High Commissioner for Refugees. *Handbook for Emergencies*. Geneva: UNHCR, 1982.

24. Goethert, R., and N. Hamdi. *Refugee Camps: A Primer for Rapid Site Planning, Land, Shelter, Infrastructure, Services*. Geneva: UN High Commissioner for Refugees, Technical Services Section, 1988.

25. Manancourt, S., et al. "Public health consequences of the civil war in Somalia, April 1992." *Lancet* 1992; 340: 176–177.

26. Moore, P. S., et al. "Mortality rates in displaced and resident populations of central Somalia during the famine of 1992." *Lancet* 1993; 341: 935–938.

27. Centers for Disease Control and Prevention. "Health status of displaced persons following civil war—Burundi, December 1993–January 1994." *Morbidity and Mortality Weekly Report* 1994; 43: 701–703.

28. Goma Epidemiology Group. "Public health impact of the Rwandan refugee crisis: What happened in Goma, Zaire, in July, 1994?" *Lancet* 1995; 345: 339–344.

29. Hansch, S., et al. *Lives Lost, Lives Saved: Excess Mortality and the Impact of Health Interventions in the Somalia Emergency*. Washington, D.C.: Refugee Policy Group, November 1994.

30. Zetter, R., and C. J. K. Henry. "The nutrition crisis among refugees." *Journal of Refugee Studies* 1992; 5: 201–380.

31. Toole, M. J., and R. Bhatia. "A case study of Somali refugees in Hartisheik A camp, eastern Ethiopia: Health and nutrition profile, July 1988–June 1990." *Journal of Refugee Studies* 1992; 5: 313–326.

32. Toole, M. J. "Micronutrient deficiencies in refugees." *Lancet* 1992; 339: 1214–1216.

33. Toole, M. J., and R. J. Waldman. "Prevention of excess mortality in refugee and displaced populations in developing countries." *JAMA* 1990; 263: 3296–3302.

34. Centers for Disease Control and Prevention. "Outbreak of pellagra among Mozambican refugees—Malawi, 1990." *Morbidity and Mortality Weekly Report* 1991; 40: 209–213.

35. Harrell-Bond, B. E. "Pitch the tents: An alternative to refugee camps." *New Republic* 1994; 15–19.

36. "The health of refugees." Editorial. *Lancet* 1985; 1 (8430): 673–674.

37. Van Damme, W. "Do refugees belong in camps? Experiences from Goma and Guinea." *Lancet* 1995; 346: 360–362.

38. Baker, R., ed. *The Psychosocial Problems of Refugees.* London: British Refugee Council, 1983.

39. Toole, M. J., and R. J. Waldman. "Nowhere a promised land: The plight of the world's refugees." *Encyclopedia Britannica* 1995.

40. Centers for Disease Control and Prevention. "Nutritional needs surveys among the elderly—Russia and Armenia, 1992." *Morbidity and Mortality Weekly Report* 1992; 41: 809–810.

41. Cuny, F. "Cities under siege: Problems, priorities, and programs." *Disasters* 1994; 18: 152–159.

42. Médecins sans Frontières. "Report of a household survey in Sarajevo, Bosnia Herzergovina." Paris: MSF, April 1993.

43. World Health Organization Nutrition Unit, Zagreb. "Summary report of nutritional health surveys carried out in Bosnia-Herzegovina during June/July 1993." Zagreb, Croatia: World Health Organization, 1993.

44. Weinberg, J., and S. Simmonds. "Public health, epidemiology, and war." *Social Science and Medicine* 1995; 40: 1663–1669.

45. Watson, F., and J. Vespa. "The impact of a reduced and uncertain food supply in three besieged cities of Bosnia-Herzegovina." *Disasters* 1995; 19: 216–234.

46. Pan American Health Organization. "Environmental health management after natural disasters." Scientific Publication no. 432. Washington, D.C.: PAHO, 1982.

47. Chalinder, A. "Good practice review no. 1—Water and sanitation in emergencies." London: Relief and Rehabilitation Network, Overseas Development Institute, 1994.

48. Shook, G., and A. J. Englande. "Environmental health criteria for disaster relief and refugee camps." *International Journal of Environmental Health Research* 1992; 2: 212–220.

49. United Nations High Commissioner for Refugees. *Water Manual for Refugee Situations.* Geneva: UNHCR, 1992.

50. Chartier, Y., G. Malenga, and L. Roberts. "UNHCR improved water container study final report." Geneva: UNHCR, 1993.

51. Noji, E. K. "Public health recommendations for the Greystone Compound, Monrovia, Liberia, April 26, 1996." Atlanta: Centers for Disease Control and Prevention, 1996.

52. Franceys, R., F. Pickford, and R. Reed. *A Guide to the Development of On-site Sanitation.* Geneva: World Health Organization, 1992.

53. Pan American Health Organization. "Emergency vector control after natural disasters." Scientific Publication no. 419. Washington, D.C.: PAHO, 1982.

54. World Health Organization (WHO). *Health Principles of Housing.* Geneva: WHO, 1989.

55. Office of U.S. Foreign Disaster Assistance (OFDA). *Field Operations Guide (FOG) for Disaster Assessment and Response, version 2.0.* Washington, D.C.: USAID, 1994.

56. University of Wisconsin Disaster Management Center. First International Emergency Settlement Conference: New Approaches to New Realities. April 15–19, 1996. Madison, Wisc.: University of Wisconsin Disaster Management Center, 1996.

57. World Health Organization. *Treatment and Prevention of Acute Diarrhea: Practical Guidelines.* 2nd ed. Geneva: WHO, 1989.

58. World Health Organization. *Guidelines for Cholera Control.* Geneva: WHO, 1992.

59. Toole, M. J., et al. "Measles prevention and control in emergency settings." *Bulletin of the World Health Organization* 1989; 67: 381–388.

60. Toole, M. J., P. Nieburg, and R. J. Waldman. "Association between inadequate rations, undernutrition prevalence, and mortality in refugee camps." *Journal of Tropical Pediatrics* 1990; 34: 218–224.

61. UN Administrative Committee on Coordination, Sub-Committee on Nutrition. Proceedings of the African Refugee Nutrition Conference, Machakos, Kenya, December 1994. Geneva: UN Administrative Committee on Coordination, Sub-Committee on Nutrition, 1995.

62. Yip, R. "Famine." In: E. K. Noji, ed. *The Public Health Consequences of Disasters.* Oxford: Oxford University Press, 1997.

63. Toole, M. J. "Guidelines for the organization of health services in Rwandan refugee camps in North Kivu region, Zaire." Goma, Zaire: UN High Commissioner for Refugees, 1994.

64. Centers for Disease Control. "Morbidity and mortality surveillance in Rwandan refugees Burundi and Zaire, 1994." *Morbidity and Mortality Weekly Report* 1996; 45: 104–107.

65. Sandler, R. H., and T. C. Jones, eds. *Medical Care of Refugees.* New York: Oxford University Press, 1987.

66. World Health Organization. "Clinical management of acute respiratory infections in children." *Bulletin of the World Health Organization* 1981; 59: 707–716.

67. Desenclos, J. C., ed. *Clinical Guidelines: Diagnostic and Treatment Manual,* 2nd ed. Paris: Médecins sans Frontières, 1992.

68. World Health Organization. *The New Emergency Health Kit.* Geneva: WHO, 1990.

69. Glass, R. I., and E. K. Noji. "Epidemiologic surveillance following disasters." In: W. E. Halperin, E. L. Baker, and R. R. Monson, eds. *Public Health Surveillance.* New York: Van Nostrand Reinhold, 1992: 195–205.

70. Aall, C. "Disastrous international relief failure: A report on Burmese refugees in Bangladesh from May to December 1978." *Disasters* 1979; 3: 429–434.

71. Moren, A. "Health and nutrition information systems among refugees and displaced persons." In: UN Administrative Committee on Coordination, Sub-Committee on Nutrition: Proceedings of the African Refugee Nutrition Conference, Machakos, Kenya, December 1994. Geneva: UN Administrative Committee on Coordination, Sub-Committee on Nutrition, 1995.

72. Nieburg, P., et al. "Limitations of anthropometry during acute food shortages: High mortality can mask refugees' deteriorating nutritional status." *Disasters* 1988; 12: 253–258.

73. Burkle, F. M., et al. "Complex humanitarian emergencies III: Measures of effectiveness." *Prehospital and Disaster Medicine* 1995; 10: 68–76.

74. Hakewill, P. A., and A. Moren. "Monitoring and evaluation of relief programmes." *Tropical Doctor* 1991(suppl. 1): 24–28.

75. Hallam, A. "Cost-effectiveness analysis: A useful tool for the assessment and evaluation of relief operations." Network Paper 15. London: Relief and Rehabilitation Network, Overseas Development Institute, 1996.

76. Overseas Development Institute. "Joint evaluation of emergency assistance to Rwanda." London: Overseas Development Institute, 1996.

3 CLASSIC CONCEPTS IN DISASTER MEDICAL RESPONSE

1. Toole, M. J., and R. J. Waldman. "The prevention of mass mortality in displaced populations in the developing world." *JAMA* 1990; 263: 3296–3302.

2. Noji, E. K., ed. *The Public Health Consequences of Disasters.* New York: Oxford University Press, 1997.

3. Waeckerle, J. M. "Disaster planning and response." *New England Journal of Medicine* 1991; 324: 815–821.

4. Burkle, F. M., et al. "Complex humanitarian emergencies: Measures of effectiveness." *Prehospital and Disaster Medicine* 1995; 10: 68–78.

5. Briggs, S. M., et al. Proceedings of the First Harvard Symposium on Complex Humanitarian Disasters. Boston, 1995.

6. Federal Emergency Management Agency. Mass Fatalities—Incident Response Course. (Instructor Guide 403.) Emmitsburg, Md.: Emergency Management Institute, 1992.

7. Barrier, G. "Emergency medical services for treatment of mass casualties." *Critical Care Medicine* 1989; 17: 1062–1067.

8. Treaster, J. B. "A lagging effort: Workers cite heat and a shortage of personnel—U.S. offers aid." *New York Times,* November 16, 1985: A-1.

9. Noji, E. K., et al. "Issues of rescue and medical care following the 1988 Armenian earthquake." *International Journal of Epidemiology* 1993, 22: 1070–1076.

10. Dressler, D. P., and J. L. Hozid. "Austere military medical care: A graded response." *Military Medicine* 1994; 159: 196–200.

11. Kumar, P., et al. "A review of triage and mangement of burn victims following a nuclear disaster." *Burns* 1994; 20: 397–402.

12. Pepe, P. E., and V. Kvetan. "Field management and critical care in mass disasters." *Critical Care Clinics* 1991; 7: 401–420.

13. Schultz, C. H., et al. "A medical disaster response to reduce immediate mortality after an earthquake." *New England Journal of Medicine* 1996; 334: 438–444.

14. Champion, H. R. "Triage." In: R. H. Cales and R. W. Heilig, Jr., eds. *Trauma Care Systems.* Rockville, Md.: Aspen, 1986: 79–109.

15. Gerace, R. V. "Role of medical teams in a community disaster plan." *Canadian Medical Association Journal* 1979; 120: 923–928.

16. van Amerogen, R. H., et al. "The Avianca plan crash: An emergency medical system's response to pediatric survivors of the disaster." *Pediatrics* 1993; 92: 105–110.

17. Vayer, J. S., et al. "New concepts in triage." *Annals of Emergency Medicine* 1986; 15: 927–930.

18. Walsh, D. P., et al. "The emergency medicine specialist in combat triage: A new and untapped resource." *Military Medicine* 1990; 155: 187–189.

19. Gray, R. "Surgery of war and disaster." *Tropical Doctor* 1991; 21(suppl.): 56–60.

20. Neel, S. "Medical support of the U.S. Army in Vietnam, 1965–1970." Washington, D.C.: Department of the Army, 1973.

21. Kennedy, K., et al. "Triage: Techniques and applications in decision-making." *Annals of Emergency Medicine* 1996; 28: 136–144.

22. MacMahon, A. G. "Sorting out triage in urban disasters." *South African Medical Journal* 1985; 67: 555–556.

23. Sklar, D. "Disaster planning and organization: Casualty patterns in disasters." *Journal of the World Association of Emergency and Disaster Medicine* 1987; 3:49–51.

24. Seletz, J. M. "Flugtag-88 (Ramstein air show disaster): An army response to a MASCAL." *Military Medicine* 1990; 155: 153–155.

25. Laurent, C. L. "Disaster triage of massive casualties from thermonuclear detonation." *Journal of Emergency Nursing* 1990; 16: 248–251.

26. Summons, G. M. "Mental health issues related to the development of a national disaster response system." *Military Medicine* 1991; 155: 187–189.

27. Southall, D. P., et al. "Medical evacuation from Mostar." *Lancet* 1996; 347: 244–245.

28. Pan American Health Organization. *Establishing a Mass Casualty Management System.* Washington, D.C.: PAHO, 1995.

29. Fykeberg, E. R., et al. "Disaster medicine: Advances in local catastrophic response." *Academy of Emergency Medicine* 1994; I: 133–136.

30. Duffy, J., ed. *Health and Medical Aspects of Disaster Preparedness.* New York: NATO, Plenum Press, 1990.

31. Lillibridge, S. R. "Disaster medicine: Current assessment and blueprint for the future." *Academy of Emergency Medicine* 1995; 22: 1068.

32. Kent, R. *Anatomy of Disaster Relief: The International Network in Action.* New York: Pinter Publishers, 1987.

4 EMERGENCY CARE

1. Cutting, P. A., and R. Agha. "Surgery in a Palestinian refugee camp." *Injury* 1992, 23: 405–409.

2. Bharnagar, M. K., and G. S. Smith. "Trauma in the Afghan guerrilla war: Effects of lack of access to care." *Surgery* 1989; 105: 699–705.

3. Labeeu, F., et al. "External fixation in war traumatology: Report from the Rwandese war." *Journal of Trauma* 1996; 40(3 suppl.) S223–S227.

4. Bowyer, G. W. "Afghan war wounded: Application of the Red Cross wound classification." *Journal of Trauma: Injury, Infection, and Critical Care* 1995; 38: 64–67.

5. Morris, D. S, and W. J. Sugrue. "Abdominal injuries in the war-wounded of Afghanistan: A report from the International Committee of the Red Cross." *British Journal of Surgery* 1991; 78: 1301–1304.

6. Gray, R. "Surgery of war and disaster." *Tropical Doctor* 1991 (suppl.); 21: 56–60.

7. Schnitzer, J. "Gunshot injuries with plastic bullets treated in a small community hospital in the Gaza strip." *PSR Quarterly* 1992; 2: 25–32.

8. Chernack, R. S., and L. Dressner. "A letter from Osijek." *Medicine and Global Survival* 1994; 1: 87–91.

9. Korver, A. J. H. "Outcome of war-injured patients treated at first aid posts of the International Committee of the Red Cross." *Injury* 1994; 25: 25–30.

10. Meddings, D. R. "Weapons injuries during and after periods of conflict: Retrospective analysis." *British Medical Journal* 1997; 315: 1417–1420.

11. Al-Harby, S. W. "The evolving pattern of war-related injuries from the Afghanistan conflict." *Military Medicine* 1996; 161: 163–164.

12. Coupland, R. M., and P. R. Howell. "An experience of war surgery and wounds presenting after three days on the border of Afghanistan." *Injury* 1988; 19: 259–962.

13. Russbach, R., R. C. Gray, and R. M. Coupland. "Short bibliography on war surgery." *International Review of the Red Cross* 1991; 284: 488–490.

14. Perrin, P. *War and Public Health*. Geneva: International Committee of the Red Cross, 1996.

15. Dufour, D., et al. *Surgery for the victims of war*. Geneva: International Committee of the Red Cross, 1990.

16. International Federation of Red Cross and Red Crescent Societies. *The Delegates' Handbook*. Geneva: IFRC.

17. World Health Organization. *The New Emergency Health Kit*. Geneva: WHO, 1990.

18. Office of Foreign Disaster Assistance. *Field Operations Guide for Disaster Assessment and Response*. F.O.G. Version 2.0. OFDA. Washington, D.C.: U.S. Agency for International Development, 1994.

19. International Committee of the Red Cross. Health Emergencies in Large Populations (H.E.L.P.) Courses. Offered several times a year worldwide by ICRC, Geneva.

20. Coupland, R. "Epidemiological approach to surgical management of the casualties of war." *British Medical Journal* 1994; 308: 1693–1697.

21. Dressler, D., and J. L. Hozid. "Austere military medical care: A graded response." *Military Medicine* 1994; 159: 196–200.

22. Russbach, R. "Health protection in armed conflict." *International Review of the Red Cross* 1991; 284: 460–468.

23. Pretto, E. A., M. Begovic, and M. Begovic. "Emergency medical services during the siege of Sarajevo, Bosnia and Herzegovina: A preliminary report." *Prehospital and Disaster Medicine* 1994; 9(suppl.): S39–S45.

24. Russbach, R., and D. Fink. "Humanitarian action in current armed conflicts: Opportunities and obstacles." *Medicine and Global Survival* 1994; 1: 188–199.

25. Ignatieff, M. *The Warrior's Honor: Ethnic War and the Modern Conscience.* New York: Henry Holt and Co., 1997.

26. de Waal, A., and J. Leaning. *No Mercy in Mogadishu: The Human Cost of the Conflict and the Struggle for Relief.* Boston: Physicians for Human Rights and Africa Watch, July 1992.

27. Rozin, R., and H. Klausner. "New concepts of forward combat surgery." *Injury* 1988; 19: 193–197.

28. Houdelette, P. "Triage of the injured in military surgery and in exceptional situations." *Journal of Chirurgie* 1996; 133: 363–371.

29. Llewellyn, C. H. "Triage: In austere environments and echeloned medical systems." *World Journal of Surgery* 1992; 16: 904–909.

30. Russbach, R., R. C. Gray, and R. M. Coupland. "ICRC surgical activities." *International Review of the Red Cross* 1991; 284: 483–491.

31. Coupland, R. M., P. J. Parker, and R. C. Gray. "Triage of war wounded: The experience of the International Committee of the Red Cross." *Injury* 1992; 23: 507–510.

32. Coupland, R. Presentation delivered at the Twelfth Annual Conference on Military Medicine. "Surgery for Victims of Conflict." R. Adams Cowley Shock Trauma Center and Uniformed Services University of the Health Sciences. Baltimore, April 17, 1998.

33. Rund, D. A., and T. S. Rausch. *Triage.* St. Louis, MO: C. V. Mosby, 1981.

34. Kennedy, K., et al. "Triage: Techniques and applications in decision making." *Annals of Emergency Medicine* 1996; 28: 136–144.

35. Coupland, R. "Abdominal wounds in war." *British Journal of Surgery* 1996; 83: 1505–1511.

36. Coupland, R. M., and A. Korver. "Injuries from antipersonnel mines: The experience of the International Committee of the Red Cross." *British Medical Journal* 1991; 303: 1509–1512.

37. Coupland, R. M. *War Wounds of Limbs: Surgical Management.* Oxford: Butterworth Heinemann, 1993.

38. Médecins sans Frontières. *Refugee Health: An approach to emergency situations.* London: Macmillan, 1997.

39. Kleinman, A. *The Illness Narratives: Suffering, Healing, and the Human Condition.* New York: Basic Books, 1988.

40. Slim, H. "Doing the right thing: Relief agencies, moral dilemmas and moral responsibility in political emergencies and war." *Disasters* 1997; 21: 244–257.

41. Southall, D. P., et al. "Medical evacuation from Mostar." *Lancet* 1996; 347: 244–245.

42. Quaglio, G. L., and P. Mezzelani. "Medical evacuation in war-torn countries." Letter. *Lancet* 1996; 347: 270–271.

43. Richter, D., et al. "Sending Croatian and Bosnian children for treatment abroad." Letter. *JAMA* 1993; 270: 574.

44. Council on Medical Education. "Principles for graduate medical education, American Medical Association." *JAMA* 1990; 263: 2927–2930.

45. WHO Consultation on Applied Health Research Priorities in Complex Emergencies, October 1997; Multi-donor Evaluation of Emergency Assistance to Rwanda; InterAction/OFDA Training: Health in Complex Humanitarian Emergencies; UNDP/UNDRO Disaster Management Training Programme; Sphere Project on Minimum Standards in Humanitarian Response.

5 DISASTER MENTAL HEALTH

1. Kinston, W., and R. Rosser. "Disaster: Effects on mental and physical state." *Journal of Psychosomatic Research,* 1974; 18: 437–456.

2. Thompson, J. "Psychological consequences of disaster: Analogies for the nuclear case." In: F. Solomon, and R. Q. Marston, eds. *The Medical Implications of Nuclear War.* Washington, D.C.: National Academy Press, 1986.

3. Lifton, R. J., E. Markusen, and D. Austin. "The second death: Psychological survival after nuclear war." In: J. Leaning, and L. Keyes, eds. *The Counterfeit Ark: Crisis Relocation for Nuclear War.* Cambridge, Mass.: Ballinger, 1984.

4. Green, B. L. "Psychosocial research in traumatic stress: An update." *Journal of Traumatic Stress* 1994; 7(3): 341–362.

5. Smith, E. M., et al. "Psychosocial consequences of disaster." In: J. Shore, ed. *Disaster Stress Studies: New Methods and Findings.* Washington, D.C.: American Psychiatric Press, 1986.

6. Baum, A., and I. Flemming. "Implications of psychological research on stress and technological accidents." *American Psychologist* 1993; 48(6): 665–672.

7. Meichenbaum, D. "Disasters, stress, and cognition." Paper presented for the NATO Workshop on Stress and Communities. Château de Bonas, France, June 14–18, 1994.

8. Solomon, S., and B. L. Green. "Mental health effects of natural and man-made disasters." *Post Traumatic Stress Disorder Research Quarterly* 1992; 3: 1–7.

9. Solomon, S. "Research issues in assessing disaster's effects." In: R. Gist and B. Lubin, eds. *Psychosocial Aspects of Disaster.* New York: John Wiley & Sons, 1989.

10. Ursano, R. J. "The Vietnam era prisoner of war: Perceptivity, personality, and

development of psychiatric illness." *American Journal of Psychiatry* 1981; 138: 315–318.

11. Sledge, W. H., J. A. Boydstun, and A. J. Rahe. "Self-concept changes related to war captivity." *Archives of General Psychiatry* 1980; 37: 430–443.

12. Taylor, V. "Good news about disaster." *Psychology Today* 1977; 11: 93–94, 124–126.

13. Quarentelli, E. L. "An assessment of conflicting views on mental health: the consequences of traumatic events." In: C. R. Figley, ed. *Trauma and Its Wake.* New York: Brunner/Mazel, 1985.

14. Green, B. L., and S. D. Solomon. "The mental health impact of natural and technological disasters." In: J. R. Freedy and S. E. Hofoll, eds. *Traumatic Stress: From Theory to Practice.* New York: Plenum Press, 1995.

15. Bromet, E. J. "The nature and effects of technological failures." In: R. Gist and B. Lubin, eds. *Psychosocial Aspects of Disaster.* New York: John Wiley & Sons, 1989.

16. Butcher, J. N., and L. A. Dunn. "Human response and treatment needs in airline disasters." In: R. Gist and B. Lubin, eds. *Psychosocial Aspects of Disaster.* New York: John Wiley & Sons, 1989.

17. Erikson, K. "Further thoughts on Chernobyl." *PSR Quarterly* 1992; 2: 98–103.

18. Green, B. L., et al. "Buffalo Creek survivors in the second decade: Comparison with unexposed and nonlitigant groups." *Journal of Applied Social Psychology* 1990; 20: 1033–1050.

19. Lifton, R. J., and E. Olson. "The human meaning of total disaster: The Buffalo Creek experience." *Psychiatry* 1976; 39: 1–18.

20. Krug, E. G., et al. "Suicide after natural disasters." *New England Journal of Medicine* 1998; 338: 373–378.

21. Cook, J., and L. Bickman. "Social support and psychological symptomatology following a natural disaster." *Journal of Traumatic Stress* 1990; 3: 541–556.

22. Steinglass, P., and E. Gerrity. "Natural disasters and post traumatic stress disorder: Short-term versus long-term recovery in two disaster-affected communities." *Journal of Applied Social Psychology* 1990; 20: 1746–1765.

23. Green, B. L. "Defining trauma: Terminology and generic dimension." *Journal of Applied Social Psychology* 1990; 20: 1632–1642.

24. Bolin, R. "Natural disasters." In: R. Gist, and B. Lubin, eds. *Psychosocial Aspects of Disaster.* New York: John Wiley & Sons, 1989.

25. Myers D. Mental health and disaster. In: Gist, R., and B. Lubin (eds). *Psychosocial Aspects of Disaster.* New York: John Wiley & Sons, 1989.

26. Logue, J., H. Hansen, and E. Struening. "Some indications of the long term health effects of a natural disaster." *Public Health Reports* 1981; 96: 67–79.

27. Huerta, F., and R. Horton. "Coping behavior of elderly flood victims." *Gerontologist* 1978; 18: 541–546.

28. Freedy, J., et al. "Towards an understanding of the psychological impact of natural disasters: An application of the conservation resources stress model." *Journal of Traumatic Stress* 1992; 5: 441–454.

29. Hansson, R., D. Noulles, and S. Bellovich. "Knowledge, warning, and stress: A study of comparative roles in an urban floodplain." *Environment and Behavior* 1982; 14: 171–185.

30. Phifer, J. "Psychological symptoms in older adults following natural disaster: Differential vulnerability among older adults." *Psychology and Aging* 1990; 5: 412–420.

31. Emergency Services and Disaster Relief Branch. "Responding to the needs of people with serious and persistent mental illness in times of major disasters." DHHS Publication no. (SMA) 96–3077. Washington, D.C.: Department of Health and Human Services, 1996.

32. Gerrity, E., and B. Flynn. "Mental health consequences of disasters." In: E. K. Noji, ed. *The Public Health Consequences of Disasters.* New York: Oxford University Press, 1997.

33. American Red Cross. *Disaster Mental Health Services, I.* American Red Cross Publication 3077. Washington, D.C.: American Red Cross, 1993.

34. Cohen, R. E., and F. L. Ahearn. *Handbook for Mental Health Care of Disaster Victims.* Baltimore, Md.: Johns Hopkins University Press, 1980.

35. Farberow, N. L., and C. J. Fredrick. *Training Manual for Human Service Workers in Major Disasters.* Publication no. (ADM) 90–538. Rockville, Md.: Substance Abuse and Mental Health Services Administration, 1978.

36. Myers, D., and L. Zunin. Unpublished training material. 1996. Used with permission. Available from Diane Myers, 1701 Andraes Estates Place, Watsonville, CA 95076.

37. American Psychiatric Association. *Diagnostic and Statistical Manual of Mental Disorders,* 4th ed. Washington, D.C.: American Psychiatric Association, 1994.

38. Myers, D. *Disaster Response and Recovery: A Handbook for Mental Health Professionals.* Publication no. (SMA) 94–3010. Washington, D.C.: Department of Health and Human Services, 1994.

39. Wilkinson, C. B., and E. Vera. "Clinical responses to disaster: Assessment, management, and treatment." In: R. Gist and B. Lubin, eds. *Psychosocial Aspects of Disaster.* New York: John Wiley & Sons, 1989.

40. Hartsough, D. M., and D. G. Myers. *Disaster Work in Mental Health: Prevention and Control of Stress among Workers.* Publication no. (ADM) 87–1422. Washington, D.C.: Department of Health and Human Services, 1985.

41. Hiegel, J. P. "Use of indigenous concepts and healers in the care of refugees: Some experiences from the Thai border camps." In: A. J. Marcella et al., eds. *Amidst Peril and Pain: The Mental Health and Well Being of the World's Refugees.* Washington, DC: American Psychological Association, 1994.

42. Emergency Services and Disaster Relief Branch. "Psychosocial issues for children and families in disaster: A guide for the primary care physician." Publication no. (SMA) 95–3022. Washington, D.C.: Department of Health and Human Services, 1995.

43. Ursano, R. J., C. S. Fullerton, and A. E. Norwood. "Psychiatric dimensions of disaster: Patient care, community consultation, and preventive medicine." *Harvard Review of Psychiatry* 1995; 3(4): 196–209.

44. Martin, S. F. "A policy perspective on the mental health and psychosocial needs of refugees." In: A. J. Marcella et al., eds. *Amidst Peril and Pain: The Mental Health and Well Being of the World's Refugees.* Washington, D.C.: American Psychological Association, 1994.

6 MENTAL HEALTH AND PSYCHOSOCIAL EFFECTS OF MASS VIOLENCE

1. UN High Commissioner for Refugees. *The State of the World's Refugees: The Challenge of Protection.* New York: Penguin Books, 1993.

2. U.S. Committee for Refugees. *World Refugee Survey 1997.* Washington, D.C.: USCR, 1997.

3. Desjarlais, R., et al. *World Mental Health: Problems and Priorities in Low Income Countries.* New York: Oxford University Press, 1995.

4. Murray, C. J., and A. D. Lopez. *The Global Burden of Disease,* vol. 1. Cambridge, Mass.: Harvard University Press, 1996.

5. Lifton, R. J. *Death in Life: Survivors of Hiroshima.* New York: Basic Books, 1968.

6. United Nations Economic and Social Council. *Peace: Refugee and Displaced Women.* Document E/CN.61991/4. New York: United Nations Economic and Social Council, November 9, 1990.

7. Muscat, R. J. "Conflict and reconstruction: Roles for the World Bank." Unpublished manuscript. Washington, D.C.: OED, World Bank, 1995.

8. Foucault, M. *The Order of Things: An Archaeology of the Human Sciences.* New York: Pantheon Books, 1970.

9. Mollica, R. F., and R. R. Jalbert. *Community of Confinement: The Mental Health Crisis in Site Two (Displaced Persons Camps on the Thai-Kampuchean Border).* Alexandria, Va.: World Federation for Mental Health, 1989.

10. Henderson, D. C., et al. "The Crisis in Rwanda: Mental health in the service of

justice and healing." Report. Cambridge, Mass.: Harvard Program in Refugee Trauma, 1996.

11. Levav, I. "Individuals under conditions of maximum adversity: The Holocaust." In: B. P. Dohrenwend, ed. *Adversity, Stress, and Psychopathology.* Washington, D.C.: American Psychiatric Press, 1998.

12. Basoglu, M. ed. *Torture and Its Consequences: Current Treatment Approaches.* Cambridge: Cambridge University Press, 1992.

13. Marsella, A. J., et al. *Amidst Peril and Pain: The Mental Health and Well Being of the World's Refugees.* Washington, D.C.: American Psychiatric Press, 1994.

14. Wolfe, J., and T. M. Keane. "Diagnostic validity of post-traumatic stress disorder." In: M. Wolf, et al., eds. *Post-Traumatic Stress Disorder: Etiology, Phenomenology, and Treatment.* Washington, D.C.: American Psychiatric Press, 1990: 48–63.

15. Mollica, R. F., and Y. Caspi-Yavin. "Measuring torture and torture-related symptoms." *Psychological Assessment* 1991; 3: 1–7.

16. Mollica, R. F. "The trauma story: The psychiatric care of refugee survivors of violence and torture." In: F. M. Ochberg. *Post-Traumatic Therapy and Victims of Violence.* New York: Brunner/Mazel, 1988.

17. Mollica, R. F., and L. Son. "Cultural dimensions in the evolution and treatment of sexual trauma: An overview." *Psychiatric Clinics of North America* 1989; 12: 363–379.

18. Mollica, R. F., C. Poole, and S. Tor. "Symptoms, functioning, and health problems in a massively traumatized population: The legacy of the Cambodian tragedy." In: B. P. Dohrenwend, ed. *Adversity, Stress, and Psychopathology.* Washington, D.C.: American Psychiatric Press, 1998.

19. Eitinger, L., and A. Strom. *Mortality and Morbidity after Excessive Stress.* Oslo: Oslo University Press; New York: Humanities Press, 1973.

20. Eitinger, L. *Concentration Camp Survivors in Norway and Israel.* Oslo: Oslo University Press; London: Allen & Unwin, 1964.

21. Strom, A., ed. *Norwegian Concentration Camp Survivors.* Oslo: Oslo University Press; New York: Humanities Press, 1968.

22. Wilson, J. P., and B. Raphael. *International Handbook of Traumatic Stress Syndromes.* New York: Plenum Press, 1993.

23. Mollica, R. F., et al. "The effect of trauma and confinement on functional health and mental health status of Cambodians living in Thailand-Cambodia border camps." *JAMA* 1993; 270: 581–586.

24. Flaherty, J. A., et al. "Developing instruments for cross-cultural psychiatric research." *Journal of Nervous and Mental Disease* 1988; 176: 257–263.

25. Mollica, R. F., et al. "Indochinese versions of the Hopkins Symptom Checklist-25: A screening instrument for the psychiatric care of refugees." *American Journal of Psychiatry* 1987; 144: 497–500.

26. Mollica, R. F., et al. "The Harvard Trauma Questionnaire (HTQ) Manual; Cambodian, Laotian, and Vietnamese versions." *Torture Quarterly* 1996; Supp. 1: 19–42.

27. Eisenbruch, M. "Commentary: Toward a culturally sensitive DSM: cultural bereavement in Cambodian refugees and the traditional healer as taxonomist." *Journal of Nervous and Mental Disease* 1992; 180: 8–10.

28. Weine, S. M., et al. "Psychiatric consequences of 'Ethnic Cleansing': Clinical assessments and trauma testimonies of newly resettled Bosnian refugees." *American Journal of Psychiatry* 1995; 152: 536–542.

29. Mollica, R. F., G. Wyshak, and J. Lavelle. "The psychosocial impact of war trauma and torture on Southeast Asian refugees." *American Journal of Psychiatry* 1987; 144: 1567–1572.

30. Kinzie, D. J., et al. "The prevalence of posttraumatic stress disorder and its clinical significance among Southeast Asian refugees." *American Journal of Psychiatry* 1990; 147: 913–917.

31. Green, B. L. "Psychosocial research in traumatic stress: An update." *Journal of Traumatic Stress* 1994; 341–357.

32. Ormel, J., et al. "Common mental disorders and disability across cultures." *JAMA* 1994; 272: 1741–1748.

33. March, J. S. "What constitutes a stressor? The 'Criterion A' Issue." In: J. R. T. Davidson, and E. B. Foa. *Posttraumatic Stress Disorder; DSM-IV and Beyond.* Washington, D.C.: American Psychiatric Press, 1993.

34. Stewart, A. L., and J. E. Ware, Jr., eds. *Measuring Functioning and Well-Being: The Medical Outcomes Study Approach.* Durham, N.C.: Duke University Press, 1992.

35. Wilson, I. B., and P. D. Cleary. "Linking clinical variables with health-related quality of life: A conceptual model of patient outcomes." *JAMA* 1995; 273: 59–64.

36. Wilson, I. B., and S. Kaplan. "Clinical practice and patients' health status: How are the two related?" *Medical Care* 1995; 33: AS209–AS214.

37. Lyons, J. "Strategies for assessing the potential for positive adjustment following trauma." *Journal of Traumatic Stress* 1991; 4: 93–111.

38. Watts, F. N., and D. H. Bennett, eds. *Theory and Practice of Psychiatric Rehabilitation.* Chichester: John Wiley & Sons, 1983.

39. Bowling, A. *Measuring Health: A Review of Quality of Life Measurement Scales.* Philadelphia: Open University Press, 1991.

40. Cienfuegos, A. J., and C. Monelli. "The testimony of political repression as a therapeutic instrument." *American Journal of Orthopsychiatry* 1983; 53: 43–51.

41. Goldfeld, A. E., et al. "The physical and psychological sequelae of torture: Symptomatology and diagnosis." *JAMA* 1988; 259: 2725–2729.

42. Sack, W. H., et al. "The Khmer adolescent project: Epidemiologic findings in two generations of Cambodian refugees." *Journal of Nervous and Mental Disease* 1994; 182: 387–395.

7 PSYCHOLOGICAL TRAUMA AND RELIEF WORKERS

1. Wilkinson, C. B., and E. Vera. "Clinical responses to disaster: Assessment, management, and treatment." In: R. Gist and B. Lubin, eds. *Psychosocial Aspects of Disaster.* New York: John Wiley & Sons, 1989: 230.

2. Herman, J. L. *Trauma and Recovery.* New York: Basic Books, 1992: 9.

3. Herman, J. L., 1992: 12.

4. Herman, J. L., 1992: 18.

5. Herman, J. L., 1992: 28.

6. Lerner, M. J. *The Belief in a Just World: A Fundamental Decision.* New York: Plenum, 1980.

7. Cobb, S., and E. Lindemann. "Neuropsychiatric observations." *Annals of Surgery* 1943; 117: 814–824.

8. *Diagnostic and Statistical Manual of Mental Disorders (DSM-III).* Washington, D.C.: American Psychiatric Association, 1980.

9. Cobb, S., and E. Lindemann, 1943: 816.

10. Lindemann, E. "Symptomatology and management of acute grief." *American Journal of Psychiatry* 1944; 101: 141–148.

11. Lifton, R. J. *Death in Life: Survivors of Hiroshima.* New York: Random House, 1967.

12. Lifton, R. J. *The Broken Connection.* New York: Simon & Schuster, 1979.

13. *Diagnostic and Statistical Manual of Mental Disorders (DSM-IV).* Washington, D.C.: American Psychiatric Association, 1994: 427–429.

14. Ibid., pp. 429–432.

15. McCann, I. L., and L. A. Pearlman. "Vicarious traumatization: A framework for understanding the psychological effects of working with victims." *Journal of Traumatic Stress* 1990; 3: 139–149.

16. Mitchell, J. S. "Crisis worker stress and burn out." In: J. S. Mitchell and H. L. P. Resnik, eds. *Emergency Response to Crisis.* London: Prentiss-Hall International, 1986: 183.

17. Lazarus, R. S. "Why we should think of stress as a subset of emotion." In: L. Goldberger, and S. Breznitz, eds. *Handbook of Stress: Theoretical and Clinical Aspects*. New York: Free Press, 1993: 21–39.

18. Lazarus, R. S., and S. Folkman. *Stress, Appraisal, and Coping*. New York: Springer Verlag, 1984.

19. Keinan, G. "Confidence expectancy as a predictor of military performance under stress." In: N. A. Milgram, ed. *Stress and Coping in Time of War: Generalizations from the Israeli Experience*. New York: Brunner/Mazel, 1986: 183.

20. Lindy, J. D., and M. Grace. "The recovery environment: Continuing stressor versus a healing psychosocial space." In: B. J. Sowder, and M. Lystad, eds. *Disasters and Mental Health: Contemporary Perspectives and Innovations in Services to Disaster Victims*. Washington, D.C.: American Psychiatric Press, 1986: 147–48.

21. Flach, F. "The resilience hypothesis and posttraumatic stress disorder." In: M. Wolf and A. Mosnaim, eds. *Posttraumatic Stress Disorder: Etiology, Phenomenology, and Treatment*. Washington, D.C.: American Psychiatric Press, 1990.

22. Apfel, R. J., and B. Simon. "Psychosocial interventions for children of war: The value of a model of resiliency." *Medicine and Global Survival* 1996; 3: A2. Internet address: http://www.healthnet.org/MGS.

23. Jones, D. R. "Secondary disaster victims: The emotional effects of recovering and identifying human remains." *American Journal of Psychiatry* 1985; 142: 303–307.

24. Hodgkinson, P. E., and M. Stewart. *Coping with Catastrophe: A Handbook of Disaster Management*. London: Routledge, 1991: 175.

25. Jacobs, G. Personal communication. June 6, 1997.

26. Sparrow, J. "World disasters report. Under the volcanoes: Special focus on the Rwanda refugee crisis." International Federation of Red Cross Red Crescent Societies. IFRC WebPage, May 1995.

27. Kahill, S. "Interventions for burnout in the helping professions: A review of the empirical evidence." *Canadian Journal of Counseling Review* 1988; 22: 310–342.

28. Raphael, B., and J. P. Wilson. "When disaster strikes: Managing emotional reactions in rescue workers." In: J. P. Wilson and J. D. Lindy, eds. *Countertransference in the Treatment of PTSD*. New York: Guilford, 1994.

29. Butcher, J. N., and L. A. Dunn. "Human responses and treatment needs in airline disasters." In: R. Gist and B. Lubin, 1989: 106.

30. Quarentelli, E. L. "What is disaster? The need for clarification in definition and conceptualization in research." In: B. J. Sowder and M. Lystad, 1986: 73.

31. Barron, R. A. "The role of the ARC mental health team in St. Croix Operation; DR#013: Report to Disaster Health Services." Unpublished report. Washington, D.C.: American Red Cross, 1990.

32. Bolin, R. "Disaster characteristics and psychosocial impacts." In: B. J. Sowder and M. Lystad, 1986: 15.

33. Cohen, R. E. "Postdisaster mobilization of a crisis intervention team: The Managua experience." In H. J. Parad, H. L. P. Resnik, and L. G. Parad, eds. *Emergency and Disaster Management: A Mental Health Sourcebook.* Bowie, Md.: Charles Press Publishers, 1976: 382.

34. Hartsough, D. M. "Organizational stressors." In: D. M. Hartsough and D. G. Meyers. *Disaster Work and Mental Health: Prevention and Control of Stress among Workers.* Washington, D.C.: National Institute of Mental Health, 1985: 22.

35. Lorch, D. "U.N. in Rwanda says it is powerless to halt the violence." *New York Times,* April 15, 1994.

36. Myers, D. G. "Mental health and disaster: Preventive approaches to intervention." In: R. Gist and B. Lubin, 1989: 196.

37. Raphael, B. *When Disaster Strikes: How Individuals and Communities Cope with Catastrophe.* New York: Basic Books, 1986: 233.

38. Wilkinson, C. B., and E. Vera. "Clinical responses to disaster: Assessment, management, and treatment." In: R. Gist and B. Lubin, 1989: 252.

39. Perlez, J. "Amid Rwanda's misery, charity battles despair." *New York Times,* August 18, 1994.

40. Burkle, F. M. "Coping with stress under conditions of disaster and refugee care." *Military Medicine* 1983; 148: 800–803.

41. Mitchell, J. Lecture given at Metro-Boston C.I.S.D. course, Braintree, Mass., August 19, 1989.

42. Freud, A. *The Ego and the Mechanisms of Defence.* London: Hogarth Press, 1982.

43. Smith, B., et al. "Health activities across traumatized populations: Emotional responses of international humanitarian aid workers." In: Y. Danieli, N. S. Rodley, and L. Weisaeth, eds. *International Responses to Traumatic Stress.* Amityville, N.Y.: Baywood Publishing, 1996: 412–413.

44. Smith, B., et al., 1996: 414–415.

45. Smith, B., et al., 1996: 415.

46. Agger, I. "A longing for Sarajevo: Understanding the trauma of humanitarian aid workers." From a lecture given at the seminar "Psychotherapeutic Interventions with Victims of Organized Violence." Refugee Studies Program, Oxford University, and Psychosocial Center for Refugees, University of Oslo. August 9–14, 1993. Reference courtesy of Ann Bourgeot.

47. Bolin, R. "Disaster characteristics and psychosocial impacts." In B. J. Sowder and M. Lystad, 1986: 11–35.

48. Green, B. L. "Conceptual and methodological issues in assessing the psychological impact of disaster." In: B. J. Sowder and M. Lystad, 1986: 196.

49. McDaniel, E. G. "Psychological response to disaster." In: P. Baskett and R. Weller, eds. *Medicine for Disasters*. London: John Wright, 1988: 237–238.

50. American Red Cross. *Disaster Services Regulations and Procedures*. ARC 3050M. Washington, D.C.: American Red Cross, 1991.

51. Kenardy, J. A., et al. "Stress debriefing and patterns of recovery following a natural disaster." *Journal of Traumatic Stress* 1996; 9: 37–49.

52. Deahl, M. P., et al. "Psychological sequelae following the Gulf War: Factors associated with subsequent morbidity and the effectiveness of psychological debriefing." *British Journal of Psychiatry* 1994; 165: 60–65.

53. Le Fanu, J. "The nightmare of recurrent dreams." *London Sunday Telegraph*, July 16, 1995.

54. McCall, M., and P. Salama. "Selection, training and support of relief workers: An occupational health issue." *BMJ* 1999; 318: 113–116.

55. Smith, B., et al., 1996: 421.

56. International Committee of the Red Cross. *Humanitarian Action in Conflict Zones: Coping with Stress*. Geneva: ICRC, 1996.

57. Smith, B., et al., 1996: 398.

58. Solomon, S. D. "Enhancing social support for disaster victims." In: B. J. Sowder and M. Lystad, 1986:123–124.

59. Krug, E. Remarks delivered at workshop entitled "Complex Needs of the Disaster Worker." The First Harvard Symposium on Complex Disasters. Harvard Medical School. Boston, April 11, 1995.

60. Wright, K., et al. "Individual and community responses to an aircraft disaster." In: M. Wolf and A. Mosnaim, *Posttraumatic Stress Disorder: Etiology, Phenomenology and Treatment*. Washington, D.C.: Psychiatric Press, 1990.

61. Noy, S., Z. Solomon, and R. Benbenishti. "The forward treatment of combat stress reactions: A test case in the 1982 conflict in Lebanon." In: N. A. Milgrim, 1986: 110–116.

62. Lindy, J. D., and M. Grace. In: B. J. Sowder and M. Lystad 1986: 157.

63. Smith, B., et al., 1986: 402–403.

64. Hendin, H., et al. "Meanings of combat and the development of posttraumatic stress disorder." *American Journal of Psychiatry* 1981; 138: 11.

65. Meichenbaum, D., and D. Fitzpatrick. "A constructivist narrative perspective on stress and coping: Stress inoculation applications." In: Goldberger, L., and S.

Breznitz, eds. *Handbook of Stress: Theoretical and Clinical Aspects.* New York: Free Press, 1993: 707–723.

8 THE NEW ETHICAL BOUNDARIES

1. Toole, M. J., and R. J. Waldman. "Refugees and displaced persons: War, hunger, and public health," *JAMA* 1993; 270: 600–605.
2. Loescher, G. "The United Nations, the UN High Commissioner for Refugees, and the global refugee problem." In: R. Coate, ed. *U.S. Policy and the Future of the United Nations.* New York: Twentieth Century Fund, 1994: 143.
3. Longworth, R. G. "UN buckling under new role." *Chicago Tribune,* September 12, 1993: 1
4. Task Force on Ethical and Legal Issues in Humanitarian Assistance. *The Mohonk Criteria for Humanitarian Assistance in Complex Emergencies.* New York: World Conference on Religion and Peace, 1994: 14.
5. Ryan, R. "As slaughter prevails, aid groups assess role." *Boston Globe,* May 14, 1994: 1.
6. Helm, S. "Third world blocks Major's relief plan." *The Independent,* July 23, 1991: 8.
7. Hume, D. *An Enquiry Concerning the Principles of Morals.* Indianapolis: Hackett, 1983: III, 1: 20–23.
8. Shklar, J. N. *The Faces of Injustice.* New Haven: Yale University Press, 1990: 2.
9. Dickens, C. *The Life and Adventures of Martin Chuzzlewit.* Oxford: Oxford University Press, 1971.
10. Schweitzer, A. *On the Edge of the Primeval Forest.* London: A & C Black, 1922.
11. International Committee of the Red Cross. *Fundamental Rule of International Humanitarian Law Applicable in Armed Conflicts.* Geneva: ICRC, 1979.
12. Franck, T. M., and N. S. Rodley. "After Bangladesh: The law of humanitarian intervention by military force." *American Journal of International Law* 1973; 67: 275–305.
13. Scheffer, D. J. "Toward a modern doctrine of humanitarian intervention." *University of Toledo Law Review* 1992; 23: 293.
14. Walzer, M. *Just and Unjust Wars.* New York: Basic Books, 1977.
15. Bok, S. *Secrets: On the Ethics of Concealment and Revelation.* New York: Pantheon Books, 1982: 102–115.
16. Sidgwick, H. "Some fundamental ethical controversies." *Mind* 1889; 14: 473–487.
17. Sidgwick, H. *Practical Ethics.* London: Swan Sonnenschein & Co., 1898: 68.

18. Sidgwick, H. *The Methods of Ethics* (1907). New York: Dover Publications, 1966: 246.

19. Hierocles. Cited in: Long, A. A., and D. N. Sedley. *The Hellenistic Philosophers,* vol. 1. Cambridge: Cambridge University Press, 1987.

20. Nussbaum, M. "Patriotism or cosmopolitanism?" *Boston Review,* October/November 1994: 3–6.

21. Singer, P. *The Expanding Circle.* New York: Farrar, Straus & Giroux, 1981.

22. Schweitzer, A. *Out of My Life and Thought* (tr. A. B. Lemke). New York: Henry Holt and Company, 1990.

9 HUMAN RIGHTS CHALLENGES

1. United Nations. *United Nations Charter.* New York: United Nations, 1945.

2. United Nations. *Universal Declaration of Human Rights.* New York: United Nations, 1948.

3. De Lupis, I. D. *The Law of War.* Cambridge: Cambridge University Press, 1987.

4. Keegan, J. *A History of Warfare.* London: Random House, 1993: 382–383.

5. Contamine, P. *War in the Middle Ages.* Oxford: Basil Blackwell, 1984: 260–302.

6. Brauman, R. "The Médecins sans Frontières experience." In: K. Cahill, ed. *A Framework for Survival: Health, Human Rights, and Humanitarian Assistance in Conflicts and Disasters.* New York: Basic Books, 1993: 202–220.

7. Médecins sans Frontières–Holland. Conference on the cooperation between humanitarian organizations and human rights organizations. Final report of the conference held in Amsterdam, the Netherlands. Amsterdam: MSF-Holland, February 9, 1996.

8. Hansch, S., et al. *Lives Lost, Lives Saved: Excess Mortality and the Impact of Health Interventions in the Somalia Emergency.* Washington, D.C.: Refugee Policy Group, November 1994: 3–9.

9. Prendergast, J. "The gun talks louder than the voice: Somalia's continuing cycle of violence." Washington, D.C.: Center of Concern, July 1994: 3–7.

10. Perlez, J. "Chaotic Somalia starves as strongmen battle." *New York Times,* October 4, 1992: A1.

11. Africa Watch. "Somalia: A fight to the death? Leaving civilians at the mercy of terror and starvation." New York: Africa Watch, February 13, 1992.

12. United Nations. Security Council Resolution 794. New York: United Nations, December 3, 1992.

13. Omaar, R., and A. de Waal. "Humanitarianism unbound? Current dilemmas facing multi-mandate relief operations in political emergencies." Discussion Paper no. 5. London: African Rights, November 1994.

14. Russbach, R., and D. Fink. "Humanitarian action in current armed conflicts: Opportunities and obstacles." *Medicine and Global Survival* 1994; 1: 188–199.

15. Natsios, A. S. "Humanitarian relief interventions in Somalia: The economics of chaos." Paper presented at Conference on Somalia, Princeton University, March 1995.

16. Michaels, M. "Lemon aid: How Somalian relief went wrong." *New Republic,* April 19, 1993.

17. Schemo, D. J. "Donors find much Somali aid stolen." *New York Times,* February 9, 1993: A10.

18. Office of U.S. Foreign Disaster Assistance (OFDA). "Somalia—civil strife." Situation Report no. 7. Washington, D.C.: OFDA, Agency for International Development, January 30, 1992.

19. International Commission on the Balkans. *Unfinished Peace.* New York: Aspen Institute/Carnegie Endowment for International Peace, 1996.

20. Bernstein, R. "UN flight from Bosnia's reality." *New York Times,* July 25, 1993: A8.

21. Scroggins, D. "Aid to Muslims diverts UN from ending war, envoy says." *Atlanta Journal/Atlanta Constitution,* April 13, 1993: A4.

22. van Heuven, M. "Understanding the Balkan breakup." *Foreign Policy* 1996; 103: 175–188.

23. Pavlowitch, S. K. "Who is 'Balkanizing' whom? The misunderstandings between the debris of Yugoslavia and an unprepared West." *Daedalus* 1994; 123: 203–223.

24. Freedman, L. "Why the West failed." *Foreign Policy* 1994–95; 97: 53–69.

25. Destexhe, A. "Foreword." In: F. Jean, ed. *Populations in Danger 1995.* London: Médecins sans Frontières, 1995: 14–15.

26. Priest, B. "Coalition calls for action in Bosnia." *Washington Post,* August 1, 1995: 1.

27. Stover, E. "In the shadow of Nuremberg: Pursuing war criminals in the former Yugoslavia and Rwanda." *Medicine and Global Survival* 1995; 2: 140–147.

28. Destexhe, A. "The third genocide." *Foreign Policy,* Winter 1994–95; 97: 3–17.

29. Prunier, G. *The Rwanda Crisis: History of a Genocide.* New York: Columbia University Press, 1995.

30. Dillner, L. "Human rights group condemns UN in Rwanda." *British Medical Journal* 1994; 309: 895.

31. Kinzer, S. "European leaders reluctant to send troops to Rwanda." *New York Times,* May 25, 1994: A1, 12.

32. Des Forges, A. "Human rights in Burundi and Rwanda and U.S. policy." Testimony. U.S. Senate Committee on Foreign Relations. Congressional Record. Washington, D.C.: U.S. Government Printing Office, July 27, 1994.

33. U.S. Committee for Refugees. *World Refugee Survey 1996.* Washington, D.C.: USCR, 1996: 73–76.

34. Gourevitch, P. "Zaire's killer camps." New York Times, October 28, 1996: A19.

35. Joint Evaluation of Emergency Assistance to Rwanda. *The International Response to Conflict and Genocide: Lessons from the Rwanda Experience. Study 2: Early Warning and Conflict.* Copenhagen: Steering Committee of the JEEAR, 1996: 58–65.

36. Reuters News Service. "Aid workers fear violence by Rwandans." *New York Times,* August 26, 1994: A3.

37. Rosenblatt, R. "The killer in the next tent." *New York Times Magazine,* June 5, 1994: 39–47.

38. Faber, V. "Rwanda two years after: An ongoing humanitarian crisis." In: Médecins sans Frontières. *World in Crisis: The Politics of Survival at the End of the 20th Century.* New York: MSF, Routledge, 1997: 161–180.

39. Rieff, D. "Charity on the rampage." *Foreign Affairs,* January/February 1997: 132–138.

40. International Committee of the Red Cross. *ICRC International Review,* November–December 1996; 315:588.

41. Jean, F. "The problems of medical relief in the Chechen war zone." *Central Asian Survey* 1996; 15: 255–258.

10 COMPLEX EMERGENCIES AND NGOs

1. Rietveld, A. Presentation slide packet. Harvard Center for Population and Development Studies, Complex Emergencies Course. Spring semester. Cambridge, Mass., 1995.

2. Bok, S. *Common Values.* Columbia, Mo.: University of Missouri Press, 1995.

3. International Committee of the Red Cross. "Six ICRC delegates assassinated in Chechnya." Geneva: ICRC, December 17, 1996.

4. *New York Times,* February 6, 1997: 13.

5. CARE. Annual Report. Atlanta: CARE, 1996.

6. Merrin, M. *The Road to Hell: The Ravaging Effects of Foreign International Charity.* New York: Free Press, 1997.

7. F. Jean, ed. *Life, Death and Aid.* London and New York: Médecins sans Frontières, 1993;

8. Prendergast, J. "Helping or hurting? Humanitarian intervention and the crisis response in the Horn." Discussion Paper no. 6. Washington, D.C.: Center of Concern, January 1995.

9. Perrin, P. "The impact of war on disaster response: The experience of the International Committee of the Red Cross." First Harvard Symposium on Complex Humanitarian Disasters. Cambridge, Mass. April 9–10, 1995.

10. Anderson, M. "Do no harm: Supporting local capacities for peace through aid." Cambridge, Mass.: Local Capacities for Peace Project, 1996.

11. Anderson, M. "International assistance and conflict: An exploration of negative impacts." Local Capacities for Peace Project, Issues Series no. 1. Cambridge, Mass.: Local Capacities for Peace Project, July 1994.

12. Anderson, M., and P. Woodrow. *Rising from the Ashes: Development Strategies in Times of Disaster.* Boulder: Lynne Rienner, 1998.

13. International Relief/Development Project. "Disaster and development workshops: A manual for training in capacities and vulnerabilities analysis." Cambridge, Mass.: Graduate School of Education, Harvard University, December 1990.

14. Diamond, L., and J. McDonald. *Multi-track Diplomacy: A Systems Approach to Peace.* Washington, D.C.: Institute for Multi-Track Diplomacy, 1993.

15. Prendergast, J., and C. Scott. "Aid with integrity: Avoiding the potential of humanitarian aid to sustain conflict." Occasional Paper no. 2. Washington, D.C.: Office of U.S. Foreign Disaster Assistance, Bureau of Humanitarian Assistance, U.S. Agency for International Development, March 1996.

16. Minear, L. "The international relief system: A critical review. Parallel national intelligence estimate on global humanitarian emergencies." Washington, D.C.: Meridian International Center, September 22, 1994.

17. Prunier, G. *The Rwanda Crisis: History of a Genocide.* New York: Columbia University Press, 1995: 264.

18. Joint Evaluation of Emergency Assistance to Rwanda. *The International Response to Conflict and Genocide: Lessons from the Rwanda Experience.* Copenhagen: Steering Committee of the JEEAR, 1996.

19. African Rights. *Rwanda: Death, Despair, and Defiance.* London: African Rights, 1995.

20. Author interviews with CARE Rwanda staff. January 13–23, 1997.

21. United Nations. "CARE International's Perspective on the Great Lakes Region. Security Council Briefing." New York: United Nations, February 12, 1997. (Written testimony by David Bryer, executive director of Oxfam UK, Peter Krug, New York representative of ICRC, Jacques de Miliano, president of Médecins sans Frontières, and Marc Lindenberg, senior vice president for program, CARE USA.)

22. French, H. "Mobutu and rebels said to agree to talks." *New York Times,* April 18, 1997: 6.

23. Erlanger, S. "UN refugee chief warns Zaire crisis a nightmare." *New York Times,* May 4, 1997: 1.

11 COORDINATION OF HEALTH RELIEF

1. Carter, W. *Procedures and Guidelines for Disaster Preparedness and Response.* Honolulu: Pacific Disaster Preparedness Project, 1984.
2. Simmonds, S., P. Vaughan, and S. W. Gunn. *Refugee Community Health Care.* Oxford: Oxford University Press, 1983.
3. Pan American Health Organization. *Emergency Health Management after Natural Disaster.* Scientific Publication no. 407. Washington, D.C.: PAHO, 1981.
4. Centers for Disease Control and Prevention. "The public health consequences of disasters" (monograph). Atlanta: CDC, 1989.
5. American Red Cross. "Planning for disaster response, ARC 3010." Washington, D.C.: American Red Cross, 1996.
6. American Red Cross. "Foundations of the disaster services program, ARC 3000." Washington, D.C.: American Red Cross, 1994.

12 MILITARY SUPPORT OF RELIEF

1. Gaydos, J. C., and G. A. Luz. "Military participation in emergency humanitarian assistance." *Disasters* 1994; 18(1): 48–57.
2. Luz, G. A., et al. "The role of military medicine in military civic action." *Military Medicine* 1993; 158: 362–366.
3. Cuny, F. C. "Dilemmas of military involvement in humanitarian relief." In: L. Gordeneker and T. G. Weiss, eds. *Soldiers, Peacekeepers, and Disasters.* New York: Macmillan, 1992: 52–81.
4. Sharp, T. W., R. Yip, and J. D. Malone. "U.S. military forces and emergency international humanitarian assistance: Observations and recommendations from three recent missions." *JAMA* 1994; 272: 386–390.
5. Sharp, T. W., J. D. Malone, and J. Bouchard. "Humanitarian assistance from the sea." Proceedings of the U.S. Naval Institute 1995; 121: 70–75.
6. Greenhut, J. "Medical civic action in low-intensity conflict: The Vietnam experience." In: J. W. Depauw and G. A. Luz, eds. *Winning the Peace—The Strategic Implications of Military Civic Action.* New York: Prager, 1992: 135–161.
7. Foster, G. M. *The Demands of Humanity: Army Medical Disaster Relief.* Washington DC: Center of Military History, U.S. Army, 1983: 3–47.
8. Toole, M. J. "Military role in humanitarian relief in Somalia." *Lancet* 1993; 342: 190–191.

9. VanRooyen, M. J., and J. B. VanRooyen. "Somalia: Medicine and the military." *JAMA* 1994; 271: 904–905.

10. Walker, P. "Foreign military resources for disaster relief: An NGO perspective." *Disasters* 1992; 16.

11. Burkle, F. M. "Complex, humanitarian emergencies: I. concepts and participants." *Prehospital and Disaster Medicine* 1995; 10(1): 36–42.

12. Turner, T. B., and I. V. Hiscock. "Problems of civilian health under war conditions—general concepts and origins." In: J. Lada, ed. *Preventive Medicine in World War II*, vol. 8: *Civil Affairs/Military Government Public Health Activities.* Washington, D.C.: Office of the Surgeon General, Department of the Army, 1976; 3–25.

13. "First complex disasters symposium features dramatically timely topics." *JAMA* 1995; 274(1): 11–12.

14. Baudon, D, A. Spiegel, and G. Sperber. Rôle de la Bioforce militaire lors l'épidémie de méningite cérébro-spinale au Chaud en 1988." ("Role of the military Bioforce during an epidemic of cerebro-spinal meningitis in the Republic of Chad in 1988.") *International Review of Armed Forces Medical Services* 1989; 62: 127–131.

15. Dunant, J. H., and M. Rosetti. "Mass casualty and disaster medicine teaching in Switzerland." *International Review of Armed Forces Medical Services* 1989; 62: 228–231.

16. Fitzsimmons, D. W., and A. W. Whiteside. *Conflict, War, and Public Health.* Conflict Study no. 276. London: Research Institute for the Study of Conflict and Terrorism, 1994.

17. Van Crevald, M. *The Transformation of War.* New York: Macmillan, 1991.

18. Stix, G. "Fighting future wars." *Scientific American,* December 1995: 92–98.

19. United States Mission to the United Nations. *Global Humanitarian Emergencies, 1996.* New York: ECOSOC Section of the United States Mission to the United Nations, 1996.

20. Hunter, H. L. "Ethnic conflict and operations other than war." *Military Review,* November 1993: 18–24.

21. Centers for Disease Control and Prevention. "Public health consequences of acute displacement of Iraqi citizens—March–May 1991." *Morbidity and Mortality Weekly Report* 1991; 40: 43–446.

22. Yip, R., and T. W. Sharp. "Acute malnutrition and diarrhea: Lessons learned from the Kurdish relief effort." *JAMA* 1993; 270: 587–590.

23. Shears, P. "Health effects of the 1991 Bangladesh cyclone, a comment." *Disasters* 1993; 171: 66–168.

24. Smith, C. R. *Angels from the Sea: Relief Operations in Bangladesh, 1991.* Wash-

ington DC: History and Museums Division, Headquarters, U.S. Marine Corps, 1995.

25. "Disaster management." Editorial. *Lancet* 1976; 2 (8000): 1394–1395.

26. "Disaster epidemiology." Editorial. *Lancet* 1990; 336 (8719): 845–846.

27. Hooper, R. R. "United States hospital ships." *JAMA* 1993; 270: 621–623.

28. Bina, W. F. "US hospital ships: more public health, less high tech." *JAMA* 1993; 270: 2927–2928.

29. Sharp, T. W., et al. "Illness in journalists and relief workers during international relief efforts in Somalia, 1992–93." *Journal of Travel Medicine* 1995; 2: 70–76.

30. Sharp, T. W., et al. "Diarrheal disease among U.S. troops in Somalia, 1992–93." *American Journal of Tropical Medicine and Hygiene* 1995; 52(2): 188–193.

31. Hyams, K. C., et al. "The Navy forward laboratory during Operations Desert Shield/Storm." *Military Medicine* 1993; 158: 729–732.

32. Burans, J. P., et al. "The threat of hepatitis E virus in Somalia during Operation Restore Hope." *Clinical Infectious Diseases* 1994; 18: 80–83.

33. "Military supports civil authorities during California wildfire fight." *Hazard Technology,* Fall 1994: 23–25.

34. Gambel, J. M., and R. G. Hibbs. "U.S. military overseas medical research laboratories." *Military Medicine* 1996; 161: 638–645.

35. Crutcher, J. M., M. A. Laxer, and J. B. Beecham. "Short-term medical field missions in developing countries: A practical approach." *Military Medicine* 1995; 160(7): 339–343.

36. *National Military Strategy of the United States of America.* Washington, D.C.: Chairman of the Joint Chiefs of Staff, 1995.

37. Centers for Disease Control and Prevention. "Famine-affected, refugee, and displaced populations: Recommendations for public health issues." *Morbidity and Mortality Weekly Report* 1992; 41 (no. RR-13): 1–76.

38. Toole, M. J., and R. J. Waldman. "Prevention of excess mortality in refugee and displaced populations in developing countries." *JAMA* 1990; 263: 3296–3302.

39. Anderson, M. B., and P. J. Woodrow. *Rising from the Ashes—Development Strategies in Times of Disasters.* Boulder: Lynne Rienner, 1998.

40. Chowdhury, M., Y. Choudhury, and A. Bhuiya. "Cyclone aftermath: research and directions for the future." In: H. Hossain, C. P. Dodge, and F. H. Abed, eds. *From Crisis to Development: Coping with Disasters in Bangladesh.* Dhaka, Bangladesh: University Press, 1992: 101–133.

41. United Nations High Commissioner for Refugees. *A UNHCR Handbook for the Military on Humanitarian Operations.* Geneva: United Nations High Commissioner for Refugees, 1994.

42. Cobey, J. "Donation of unused surgical supplies: Help or hindrance." *JAMA* 1993; 269: 986.

43. de Ville de Goyet, C. "Post-disaster relief: The supply management challenge." *Disasters* 1993; 17: 169–171.

44. Arbelot, A., ed. *Nutrition Guidelines.* Paris: Médecins sans Frontières, 1995.

45. Natsios, A. "The international humanitarian response system." *Parameters* 1995; 3: 68–81.

46. Zinni, A. C. "Psychological operations in support of Operation Restore Hope." In: *Report of Unified Task Force, Somalia, 9 December 1992—4 May 1993.* Camp Pendelton, Calif.: I Marine Expeditionary Force, 1993.

47. Seiple, C. *The U.S. Military Relationship and the Civil Military Operations Center in Times of Humanitarian Intervention.* Carlisle, Pa.: Peacekeeping Institute, U.S. Army War College, 1996.

48. Cobey, J. C., A. Flanigin, and W. H. Foege. "Effective humanitarian aid: Our only hope for intervention in civil war." *JAMA* 1993; 270: 632–634.

49. Shawcross, W. *The Quality of Mercy.* New York: Simon and Schuster, 1984.

50. Anderson, M. B. "Humanitarian NGOs in conflict intervention." In: C. A. Crocker, F. O. Hampson, and P. Aall, eds. *Managing Global Chaos.* Washington, D.C.: United States Institute of Peace, 1996.

51. Weinberg, J., and S. Simmonds. "Public health, epidemiology, and war." *Social Sciences and Medicine* 1995; 40: 1663–1669.

52. Toole, M. J., S. Galson, and W. Brady. "Are war and public health compatible?" *Lancet* 1993; 341: 1193–1196.

53. Flanigin, A. "Somalia's death toll underlines challenges in post–cold war world." *JAMA* 1992; 268: 1985–1987.

54. Lamon, K. P. *Training and Education Requirements for Humanitarian Assistance Operations.* Alexandria, Va.: Center for Naval Analysis, 1996.

55. Lillibridge, S. R., F. M. Burkle, and E. K. Noji. "Disaster mitigation and humanitarian assistance training for uniformed service medical personnel." *Military Medicine* 1994; 159: 397–405.

56. Dunlap, C. J. "The origins of the American military coup of 2012." *Parameters* 1992; 2: 20–35.

57. Nunn, S. "Roles, missions under scrutiny." *The Officer* 1993; 69: 20–24.

58. Burkle, F. M., et al. "Strategic disaster preparedness and response: Implications for military medicine under joint command." *Military Medicine* 1996; 161(8): 442–447.

59. Gallagher, D., M. Moussalli, and D. Bosco. "Civilian and military means of providing and supporting humanitarian assistance during conflicts: A comparative analysis." Washington, D.C.: Refugee Policy Group, March 1997.

13 MILITARY SECURITY

1. 2 Timothy 2:4, Revised Standard Version.

2. International Rescue Committee. *Country Brief: Tuzla, Bosnia-Herzegovina.* February 1996.

3. Hansch, S. "How many people die of starvation in humanitarian emergencies?" Working Paper. Washington, D.C.: Refugee Policy Group, June 1995: 11.

4. Medical Division, International Committee of the Red Cross. Unpublished data. ICRC, Geneva, December 1996.

5. Wurmser, D., and N. B. Dyke. "The professionalization of peacekeeping: A study group report." Washington, D.C.: U.S. Institute of Peace, 1993: 34.

6. Cook, F. J., et al. "The Defense Department's role in humanitarian and disaster relief." Policy Analysis Paper no. 93-02: 6–7. Cambridge, Mass.: National Security Program, John F. Kennedy School of Government, Harvard University, 1993.

7. Dennehy, E. J., et al. "A blue helmet combat force." Policy Analysis Paper no. 93-01: 22–26. Cambridge, Mass.: National Security Program, John F. Kennedy School of Government, Harvard University, 1993.

8. Blechman, B. M., and J. M. Vaccaro. "Training for peacekeeping: The United Nation's role." Report no. 12. Henry L. Stimson Center, July 1994: 1–36.

9. International Federation of Red Cross and Red Crescent Societies. *World Disasters Report 1996.* "Statistical analysis: Good data for effective response." Geneva: IFRC, 1996: 136–138.

10. United Nations Department of Public Information. Charter of the UN and Statute of the International Court of Justice. DPI/511. New York: United Nations, 1945.

11. Weiss, T. G. "A research note about military-civilian humanitarianism: More questions than answers." *Disasters* 1997; 21: 95–117.

12. Minear, L., T. G. Weiss, and K. M. Campbell. "Humanitarianism and war: Learning the lessons from recent armed conflicts." Occ. Paper no. 8. Providence: T. J. Watson Jr., Institute for International Studies, Brown University, 1991.

13. Humanitarian Assistance Coordination Center. J-5 Briefing Report. Central Command, Florida, January 1992.

14. "The UN crawls to the rescue: Living with a recalcitrant U.S." *The Economist.* Cited in *World Press Review,* September 1994, 41 (9): 6.

15. Pan American Health Organization. "Humanitarian assistance and the forgotten majority. Disaster: Preparedness and mitigation in the Americas." Washington, D.C.: PAHO, July 1993; 55: 7.

16. Picard, A. "World accused by its own silence." *Toronto Globe & Mail,* July 25, 1994: A1.

17. McGrecl, C. "Balladur pleads with UN to speed up plan for Rwanda." *The Guardian,* July 12, 1994.

18. Summers, H. "Clinton administration revamps foreign policy." *Fayetteville Observor-Times,* August 4, 1994: 4E.

19. Daniel, D. C. F. "U.S. perspectives on peacekeeping: Putting PDD 25 in context." Occ. paper of the Center for Naval Warfare Studies Strategic Research Department. Research Memorandum 3-94. Newport, R.I.: U.S. Naval War College, 1994.

20. International Federation of Red Cross and Red Crescent Societies. *World Disasters Report 1995.* "Humanitarians in uniform?" Geneva: IFRC, 1995: 60.

21. Rieff, D. "The peacekeepers who couldn't." *Guardian Weekly,* December 25, 1994: 15.

22. United Nations Security Council. UNPROFOR Mission Statement. New York: United Nations, 1994.

23. Natsios, A. S. "The international humanitarian response system." *Parameters,* Spring 1995: 70–72.

24. Slim, H. "The continuing metamorphosis of the humanitarian practitioner: Some new colours for an endangered chameleon." *Disasters,* June 1995; 19(2): 110–126.

25. Zelden, T. *An Intimate History of Humanity.* New York: Harper Collins, 1994: 458–459.

26. United Nations Department of Humanitarian Affairs. *MCDA Field Manual.* New York: United Nations, May 1995: 4.29–30.

27. Air Land Sea Application Center. "Multiservice procedures for humanitarian operations: FM100-23-1." Norfolk, Va., October 1994: 4.0–4.21.

28. Burkle, F. M., et al. "Complex humanitarian emergencies: III. Measures of effectiveness." *Prehospital and Disaster Medicine* 1995; 10(1): 48–56.

29. "House votes against UN peacekeeping fund." Editorial. *Washington Times,* September 14, 1992: 4.

30. Marks, E. "Peace operations: Involving regional organizations." Strategic Forum. Washington, D.C.: Institute for National Strategic Studies, National Defense University, April 1995; 25: 1–4.

31. Chopra, J., and T. C. Weiss. "Sovereignty is no longer sacrosanct: Codifying humanitarian intervention." *Ethics and International Affairs,* 1992; 6: 95–117.

32. de Cuéllar, J. P. "Anarchy or order. Reports of the Secretary-General on the work of the organization, 1982–1991." New York: United Nations, 1991.

14 THE RISKS OF MILITARY PARTICIPATION

1. United Nations. *United Nations Charter, Article 42.* New York: United Nations, 1945.

2. Russbach, R., and D. Fink. "Humanitarian action in current armed conflicts: Opportunities and obstacles." *Medicine and Global Survival* 1994; 1: 188–199.

3. Cranna, M., and N. Bhinda, eds. *The True Cost of Conflict/Seven Recent Wars and Their Effects on Society.* London: Earthscan Publications, 1994.

4. International Committee of the Red Cross. "The mission of the International Committee of the Red Cross (ICRC)." Geneva: ICRC, 17 June 1996 (rev.).

5. International Federation of Red Cross and Red Crescent Societies. *World Disasters Report 1997.* Oxford: Oxford University Press, 1997: 29.

6. International Committee of the Red Cross. *Geneva Conventions of August 12, 1949.* Geneva: ICRC, 1949.

7. International Committee of the Red Cross. *Protocols Additional to the Geneva Conventions of 12 August, 1949.* Geneva: ICRC, 1977.

8. Coupland, R. M., and A. Korver. "Injuries from antipersonnel mines: The experience of the International Committee of the Red Cross." *British Medical Journal* 1991; 303: 1509–1512.

9. *Convention on Prohibitions or Restrictions on the Use of Certain Conventional Weapons Which May Be Deemed to Be Excessively Injurious or to Have Indiscriminate Effects; Protocol on Blinding Laser Weapons (Protocol IV).* Geneva: ICRC, October 13, 1995.

CONCLUSION

1. Mawlawi, F. "New conflicts, new challenges: The evolving role for non-governmental actors." *Journal of International Affairs* 1993; 46: 391–413.

2. International Federation of Red Cross and Red Crescent Societies. *World Disasters Report 1997.* Geneva: IFRC, 1997: 9–22.

3. Minear, L., and T. G. Weiss. *Humanitarian Action in Times of War.* Boulder: Lynne Reinner Publishers, 1993.

4. Toole, M. J. "Identifying applied research priorities to improve responses to complex humanitarian emergencies." Background document prepared for WHO consultation. Geneva: World Health Organization, October 1997.

5. Anderson, M. *Do No Harm: Supporting Local Capacities for Peace through Aid.* Cambridge, Mass.: Collaborative for Development Action, 1996.

6. Moore, J. "The UN and complex emergencies." Geneva: UN Research Institute for Social Development, 1996.

7. Macrae, J., and A. Zwi. "Famine, complex emergencies, and international policy

in Africa: An overview." In: J. Macrae and A. Zwi, eds. *War and Hunger: Rethinking International Responses to Complex Emergencies.* London: Zed Books, 1994.

8. Girardet, E. R., ed. *Somalia, Rwanda, and Beyond: The Role of International Media in Wars and Humanitarian Crises.* Dublin: Crosslines Global Report, 1995.

9. Prunier, G. *The Rwanda Crisis: History of a Genocide.* New York: Columbia University Press, 1995.

10. Lyerly, W. Seminar presentation in Conference on Conflict and Security. U.S. Agency for International Development, Washington, D.C., July 1996.

11. Macrae, J. "Conflict, the continuum, and chronic emergencies: A critical analysis of the scope for linking relief, rehabilitation, and development planning in Sudan." *Disasters* 1997; 21: 223–243.

12. World Bank. *A Framework for World Bank Involvement in Post-Conflict Reconstruction.* Washington, D.C.: World Bank, 1997.

13. "Post-conflict justice: The role of the international community." Vantage Conference. Wye River Conference Centers, Queenstown, Md., April 1997.

14. Anderson, M. B. "International assistance and conflict: An exploration of negative impacts." Cambridge, Mass.: Collaborative for Development Action, July 1994.

15. Yahmed, S. B., and P. Koob. "Health sector approach to vulnerability reduction and emergency preparedness." In: *World Health Statistics Quarterly.* Geneva: World Health Organization, 1996; 49: 172–178.

16. Nafziger, E. W., and J. Auvinen. "War, hunger, and displacement: An econometric investigation into the forces of humanitarian emergencies." Working Paper no. 142. Helsinki: World Institute for Development Economics Research, United Nations University, September 1997.

17. Cahill, K. M. *Preventive Diplomacy: Preventing Wars before They Start.* New York: Basic Books, 1996.

18. Carnegie Commission on Preventing Deadly Conflict. *Preventing Deadly Conflict: Final Report.* New York: Carnegie Corporation, 1997.

19. Rotberg, R. I. *Vigilance and Vengeance: NGOs Preventing Ethnic Conflict in Divided Societies.* Cambridge, Mass.: World Peace Foundation, 1996.

ACKNOWLEDGMENTS

The editors wish to acknowledge first and foremost the enormous contribution that John Loretz has made to the development and production of this book. In support of the lead editor, he worked closely with the authors and publisher throughout all phases of manuscript preparation. His methodical attention to detail, his gracious and thoughtful communications skills, and his discerning editorial capacities were tremendously helpful and are deeply appreciated.

We are very grateful to Michael Fisher, Executive Editor for Science and Medicine at Harvard University Press, whose enthusiasm, support, and patience have made this book possible, and whose advice provided superb focus and guidance. We extend as well our warmest thanks to our manuscript editor, Elizabeth Gilbert, for her engaged, constructive, and unfailingly deft editorial suggestions and comments.

We also wish to thank the Harvard Center for Population and Development Studies and the Common Security Forum, which together provided an intellectual home for two of us (Leaning and Chen) for much of the time this book was under discussion and development.

We would like to thank Carole Lyons, R.N., Janice Chernicki, and Frederick Gallaher for their assistance with the early phases of this project.

Reproduction rights for the photographs from the archives of the International Committee of the Red Cross were donated by the ICRC. We thank them, particularly photo librarian Anouk Bellaoud, for their generosity and support.

The author of Chapter 4 would like to acknowledge Robin Coupland, M.D., and John Navein, M.D., for their most helpful comments on an early draft of this chapter.

Chapter 8 was originally published, in slightly different form, in the December 1994 issue of *Medicine & Global Survival;* and it provided the basis for chapter 5, "Complex Humanitarian Emergencies," in the author's book *Common Values* (Columbia, Mo., 1996, © copyright Sissela Bok).

The authors of Chapter 12 thank Dr. John Whidden and Dr. Kim Kenney for their contributions in the preparation of this chapter, and wish to state that the views and opinions expressed in their chapter are those of the authors and do not necessarily represent the views of the Department of Defense, the Department of the Army, or the Department of the Navy.

CREDITS

Introduction   (Kurdish refugees in northern Iraq, March 1991.) Courtesy of Michael J. Toole, M.D.

Chapter 1   (Cyangugu refugee camp, Rwanda, July 1994.) ©International Committee of the Red Cross. Photo Patrick Fuller. All rights reserved. Reprinted by permission.

Chapter 2   (Immunization of Kurdish refugees in Iraq, March 1991.) Courtesy of Michael J. Toole, M.D.

Chapter 3   (Field surgery in Kabul, Afghanistan, October 1990.) ©International Committee of the Red Cross. Photo Didier Bregnard. All rights reserved. Reprinted by permission.

Chapter 4   (Digfer Hospital, Mogadishu, February, 1992.) ©1992, Peter Menzel. All rights reserved. Reprinted by permission.

Chapter 5   (Kurdish refugee woman and child, 1991.) ©International Committee of the Red Cross. Photo Jean Mohr. All rights reserved. Reprinted by permission.

Chapter 6   (Cambodian boy with skulls from of mass killings during Pol Pot era, Phnom Penh, June 1997.) Photo Marcus Haleri. Courtesy of Richard F. Mollica, M.D., Harvard Refugee Trauma Center.

Chapter 7   (ICRC delegate in displaced persons camp, Rwanda, August 1993.) ©International Committee of the Red Cross. Photo Luc Chessex. All rights reserved. Reprinted by permission.

Chapter 8   (Orphan in Wajid, Somalia, September 1992.) Newsweek–Peter Turnley ©1992, Newsweek, Inc. All rights reserved. Reprinted by permission.

Chapter 9   (Severed hand from mass grave in Kibuye, Rwanda, January 1996.) ©Physicians for Human Rights, file photo. Reprinted by permission.

Chapter 10   (Water distribution in Sarajevo, October 1992.) ©1992, Reuters–Corinne Dufka–Archive Photos. All rights reserved. Reprinted by permission.

Chapter 11   (Convoy of ICRC relief trucks, Sierra Leone near border with Guinea, April 1996.) ©International Committee of the Red Cross. Photo Jon Spaull. All rights reserved. Reprinted by permission.

Chapter 12 (U.S. soldier with injured children in clinic.) Courtesy of Frederick M. Burkle, Jr., M.D.

Chapter 13 (Somali man killed in Mogadishu when Pakistani peacekeepers opened fire, June 13, 1993.) ©1993, Agence France-Press. Photo Alexander Joe. All rights reserved. Reprinted by permission.

Chapter 14 (ICRC hospital, Mogadishu, February 1992.) ©1992, Peter Menzel. All rights reserved. Reprinted by permission.

Conclusion (U.S. soldier with Somali woman in Baidoa, Somalia, December 1992.) ©Detroit Free Press–David Turnley. All rights reserved. Reprinted by permission.

INDEX

active humanitarianism, 230, 236
acute stress disorder, 149
Afghanistan, 4, 16, 52, 212
age-specific mortality rates, 25
Aidid, Mohammed Farah, 200
American Red Cross (ARC), 121, 152, 247;
  Disaster Mental Health Service
  (DMHS), 164; 3000 Series, 249, 266;
  Disaster Operations Center, 249, 259;
  Disaster Services, 249, 252–255; Disaster
  Services Human Resources (DSHR) Sys-
  tem, 250
American Refugee Committee, 5
Amin, Idi, 186
Angola, 4, 16, 212
Annan, Kofi, 245
arc of crisis, 4
armed conflict, 212
Armenia, 21, 181
Armero volcano, 70, 266
austere environment, 70
Azerbaijan, 16

Baidoa, 27, 225
Bangladesh, 16, 60, 278, 289
Barre, Siad, 199, 296
barter shops, 229
beriberi, 49
biological weapons, 75
Bosnia and Herzegovina, 4, 16, 52, 201,
  294, 299, 302
Breuer, Josef, 144
Buffalo Creek flood, 100, 102, 106
Burkle, F. M., 158

burnout, 153
Burundi, 18, 230

Cambodia, 4, 16, 30, 126, 203; refugee
  crisis, 61
CARE International, 5, 221–223,
  245
casualty collection sites, 76
Catholic Relief Service, 5, 218
Chechnya, 4, 16, 206, 216
chemical weapons, 75
child soldiers, 214
Chinese famine, 186
chlorination, 48
cholera, 30, 35, 47, 205
Civil-Military Operations Center
  (CMOC), 302
civilian disaster response, 69
Clinton, William Jefferson, 206
coalition military forces, 295
Cocoanut Grove fire, 145
cold chain, 34, 259
collective trauma, 106
command, control, and communications,
  301
confidentiality, 113
conflict prevention, 320
Congo/Zaire, 4, 91, 245
convenience sample surveys, 23
Convention on Genocide, 197, 209
Convention on the Elimination of All
  Forms of Discrimination against
  Women, 196
Convention on Torture, 196

375

housing rehabilitation programs, 240–242
human circle, 191
human rights, 7, 195–211, 313
humanitarian corridors, 222
humanitarianism, 188
Hume, David, 182
Hurricane Andrew, 257, 261
Hurricane Hugo, 156, 256, 262–264
Hurricane Marilyn, 265
Hutus, 7, 46, 204, 230

IFOR (Intervention Force), 299, 302
immunization, 57, 282
impartiality, 289, 309, 314, 318
Impuzamugambi, 231
indefinite quantity contracts, 224
Indonesia, 203
infant mortality, 18
Interahamwe, 231
internally displaced populations, 17, 42, 326
International Committee of the Red Cross (ICRC), 2, 197, 207, 211, 220, 247, 266, 294, 298, 307, 312
International Council of Voluntary Agencies (ICVA), 226
International Court of Justice, 313
International Covenant on Civil and Political Rights, 196
International Federation of Red Cross and Red Crescent Societies (IFRC), 5, 121, 152, 248, 266
international human rights law, 196
international humanitarian law (IHL), 2, 83, 197, 313, 315, 326
International Rescue Committee (IRC), 173, 224
International War Crimes Tribunal for the Former Yugoslavia, 202
Internet, 121
Iraq, 17, 29, 266, 276, 295

Jacovich, Victor, 202
Janet, Pierre, 144
Joint NGO committees, 225
Jones, D. R., 151
Jonestown, 151

Kabila, Laurent, 7
Kabul, 85–86, 314
Karadžić, Radovan, 202
Kenya, 44
Khmer Rouge, 42, 126, 128, 203
Kigali, 204, 233
King, Martin Luther, Jr., 189
Korean War, 274
Kouchner, Bernard, 301
Kurdish refugee crisis, 29, 44, 58, 296
Kuwait, 266

Lake Kivu, 47
land mines, 6, 16, 212, 316
Laos, 42
Liberia, 16
Lifton, Robert J., 146
Lindemann, Eric, 146
local market economies, 49
Loma Prieta earthquake, 260

malaria, 17, 30, 35, 42
Malawi, 18
malnutrition, 17, 30–33, 42
mass casualty incidents (MCIs), 70
mass violence, 125
meals, ready to eat (MREs), 287
measles, 17, 34, 48, 53, 57
measures of effectiveness, 62, 303
Médecins sans Frontières (MSF), 59, 89, 205, 218, 245, 266, 298
Mengistu, 204
meningitis, 30
mental health, 126; post-disaster symptomatology, 104, 106–110
mid-upper arm circumference (MUAC), 31
military capabilities, 276–282
military civil affairs, 281
military medicine, 280, 285
Mine Ban Treaty, 316
Mitchell, Jeffrey, 160, 164
Mladić, Ratko, 202
Mogadishu, 6, 278
moral aspects, 186
Mozambique, 4, 16, 44, 311
Myanmar, 16

trauma story, 116, 128–133
traumatic injury, 89
triage, 73–77, 87–88; field medical, 73–74
Turkey, 44
Tutsis, 7, 46, 204, 230
Tuzla, 52

Uganda, 16, 186, 204, 230
unaccompanied children, 33
United Nations, 180, 313; High Commissioner for Refugees (UNHCR), 5, 34, 121, 205, 213, 266, 286, 318; UNICEF, 5, 121; Security Council, 202, 206, 245, 295, 298; Department of Humanitarian Affairs (DHA), 302
United Nations Charter, 195, 294, 309
UNOSOM II, 297
UNPROFOR, 201, 299, 304
U.S. Agency for International Development (USAID), 4, 224, 266
U.S. Army Institute for Chemical Defense, 281
U.S. Army Medical Research Institute for Infectious Diseases, 282
U.S. Army Special Forces (USASF), 280
U.S. Center for Mental Health Services, 121
U.S. Centers for Disease Control and Prevention (CDC), 260
U.S. Public Health Service, 101, 266

Universal Declaration of Human Rights, 195

vaccination, 33
ValuJet crash, 256
vector control, 56
victimization, 101
Vietnam War, 99, 144, 275
vitamin deficiencies, 57

war causes, 310; definition, 310; humanitarian consequences, 311; victims, 311
waste disposal, 55
water, 34, 44
water systems, 52, 242
water-borne diseases, 46
weight-for-height (WFH), 31
World Food Program (WFP), 224
World Health Organization (WHO), 52, 57, 59, 259
World Trade Center, 72
World War I, 16, 144
World War II, 1, 16, 144, 203, 274

Yeltsin, Boris, 206
Yemen, 44

Zaire, 17–18, 230, 280
Zenica, 52
Z-score, 31